Energized!

Energized!

ontributions
rom more than
65 health professionals
nd inspirational writers

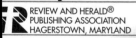
REVIEW AND HERALD®
PUBLISHING ASSOCIATION
HAGERSTOWN, MARYLAND

Compiled by
Jan W. Kuzma, Ph. D., president, Sentinel Research Services
Kay Kuzma, Ed.D., president, Family Matters
DeWitt S. Williams, Ed.D., director, Department of Health Ministries,
North American Division of Seventh-day Adventists.
Forewords by Ted Hamilton, M.D., vice president, Florida Hospital and
Elmar P. Sakala, M.D., M.P.H., School of Medicine, Loma Linda University.

The authors assume full responsibility for the accuracy of all facts and quotations as cited in this book.

Texts credited to Amplified are from *The Amplified Bible.* Copyright © 1965 by Zondervan Publishing House. Used by permission.

Scriptures credited to EB are from *The Everyday Bible, New Century Version,* copyright © 1987, 1988 by Word Publishing, Dallas, Texas 75039. Used by permission.

Bible texts credited to Jerusalem are from *The Jerusalem Bible,* copyright © 1966 by Darton, Longman & Todd, Ltd., and Doubleday & Company, Inc. Used by permission of the publisher.

Texts credited to Message are from *The Message.* Copyright © 1993. Used by permission of NavPress Publishing Group.

Scripture quotations marked NASB are from the *New American Standard Bible,* © The Lockman Foundation 1960, 1962, 1963, 1968, 1971, 1972, 1973, 1975, 1977.

Texts credited to NEB are from *The New English Bible.* © The Delegates of the Oxford University Press and the Syndics of the Cambridge University Press 1961, 1970. Reprinted by permission.

Texts credited to NIV are from the *Holy Bible, New International Version.* Copyright © 1973, 1978, 1984, International Bible Society. Used by permission of Zondervan Bible Publishers.

Texts credited to NKJV are from The New King James Version. Copyright © 1979, 1980, 1982, Thomas Nelson, Inc., Publishers.

Bible texts credited to NRSV are from the New Revised Standard Version of the Bible, copyright © 1989 by the Division of Christian Education of the National Council of the Churches of Christ in the U.S.A. Used by permission.

Texts credited to REB are from *The Revised English Bible.* Copyright © Oxford University Press and Cambridge University Press, 1989. Reprinted by permission.

Bible texts credited to RSV are from the Revised Standard Version of the Bible, copyright © 1946, 1952, 1971, by the Division of Christian Education of the National Council of the Churches of Christ in the U.S.A. Used by permission.

Bible texts credited to TEV are from the *Good News Bible*—Old Testament: Copyright © American Bible Society 1976; New Testament: Copyright © American Bible Society 1966, 1971, 1976.

Verses marked TLB are taken from *The Living Bible,* copyright © 1971 by Tyndale House Publishers, Wheaton, Ill. Used by permission.

This book was
Edited by Gerald Wheeler
Designed by Patricia S. Wegh
Illustrations by Matthew Pierce
Typeset: 9/10.5 Sabon

PRINTED IN U.S.A.

01 00 99 98 97   5 4 3 2 1

R&H Cataloging Service
Energized! Contributions from more than
    165 health professionals and inspirational
    writers. Compiled by Jan W. Kuzma, Kay
    Kuzma, and DeWitt S. Williams.

    1. Devotional calendars. 2. Health. I. Kuzma, Jan
W., comp. II. Kuzma, Kay Judeen Humpel, 1941-   , comp.
III. Williams, DeWitt S., comp.

242.2

ISBN 0-8280-1141-9

THE
COMPILERS

Jan W. Kuzma

Kay Kuzma

DeWitt S. Williams

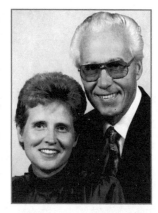

Jan W. Kuzma directs Sentinel Research Services, a nonprofit organization that produces the syndicated radio spot "Got a Minute for Your Health?" For 27 years he taught at Loma Linda University's School of Public Health, serving as chair of the Biostatistics Department and director of research.

Kay Kuzma is president of Family Matters. The author of numerous books for families, she hosts the daily radio spot "Got a Minute for Your Family?" and cohosts the 3ABN television series "Family Matters."

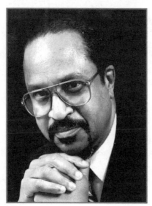

DeWitt S. Williams is director of the Department of Health Ministries for the North American Division of Seventh-day Adventists. A lecturer on healthy living and a crusader against drug addiction, he has also served as a missionary leader in Africa and in the Communication Department of the General Conference. He authored *She Fulfilled the Impossible Dream* and edited the publications *Tell* and *Adventist Health Ministry*.

WORDS OF INTRODUCTION

DeWitt S. Williams

I will praise thee; for I am fearfully and wonderfully made" is how David expressed his awe of God's human creation (Ps. 139:14). The more I learn about how our bodies function, the more I sing this psalm with David. The science of salvation and the science of creation are studies that will certainly keep us enthralled for millennia in heaven.

Since 1848, when Ellen G. White, God's special messenger, received her first temperance vision, and 1863, when she had a larger vision on health, the Seventh-day Adventist Church has been promoting respect for God's wonderful creation. And the results have been impressive.

Consider what research has shown us, for example. Medical science has conducted numerous studies on the Adventist population, the largest being the longitudinal Adventist Health Study at Loma Linda University, in process since the 1960s. Researchers have published more than 225 articles worldwide on the Adventist population, and international studies have been conducted in the Netherlands, Norway, and Poland, that all substantiate the general finding that *those who follow most closely the "health message" are the healthiest and live the longest.* One study conducted by Jan W. Kuzma even suggested that following good health principles adds about nine years to your life!

But on a more personal level, here's just one of thousands of personal testimonies I could share with you of what this lifestyle can do.

Denise weighed 207 pounds, her business was barely surviving, and she was undergoing various trials. On May 14, 1994, she had her house dedicated to the Lord as she was beginning a home-based business. That same day her life took a drastic change for good. First she started a fast, then began eating a more simple plant-based diet and started walking 10 miles a day. In addition, she chose to spend a couple hours a day studying the Bible and praying. She said that "after about six weeks the muscles in my legs were firm, my abdomen took on a stronger appearance, my arms weren't flabby, and I began to look like a 'temple' God could use in His work." Ten months later she was down from a size 16/18 dress to size 6/8. She continues: "My neighbors, clients, friends, and suppliers have seen the change and ask, 'What are you doing? You look great!'"

But what is even more impressive is the witnessing opportunities it opened for Denise. "Four households of my six neighbors have begun a walking and/or exercise program. My vegetarian lifestyle is the talk of the neighborhood barbecues. Two of my clients have visited the Emmanuel-Brinklow Seventh-day Adventist Church. Another 20 or more in this short time have inquired as to what faith I belong to, and one client has become a member of the Seventh-day Adventist Church."

I rejoice with Denise and others who have chosen to live a healthier lifestyle and are reaping the benefits. But as I look around, I have at times been surprised with the zealous dedication to a healthy lifestyle that many nonbelievers profess, while those who have grown up with this information have become lukewarm and at times rebellious in their health practices.

How important it is to turn our minds daily to these wonderful bodies that God has given us, and to choose to live in such a way that God's natural blessing of a more vibrant life will be ours—physically, mentally, and spiritually.

When we first took on the challenge of doing a devotional book, it was an overwhelming job for our little office staff. We believe God directed us to Jan W. and Kay Kuzma, who were willing to put their time, energy, and talent into making this volume a reality. I appreciate the help and support of Alice Hsu, Lenny Pearson, Barbara Choo, and Dorothy Keith. I also want to thank those who helped gather stories from various institutions and colleagues. A special thanks to Dr. Elmar Sakala for rallying the troops at Loma Linda University, the primary medical training center for the Seventh-day Adventist Church for nearly 100 years.

At the time of this writing the Seventh-day Adventist Church operates worldwide 154 hospitals and sanitariums and 336 dispensaries, clinics, health launches, and medical planes, plus 17 medical or paramedical educational centers. Then there are a score of health education and lifestyle centers worldwide. These are administered by Seventh-day Adventists but funded privately, and include the Lifestyle Center of America (Oklahoma), Weimar Institute (California), Wildwood Institute (Georgia), and Uchee Pines Institute (Alabama) in North America. All offer health education, cooking schools, and natural remedy therapy and have live-in facilities for health restoration. In many of the major cities, such as New York, San

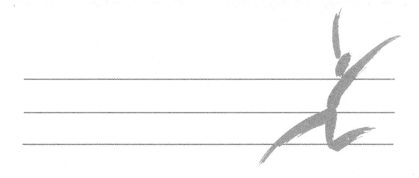

Francisco, Boston, and Los Angeles, health van ministries offer health screening and information.

Perhaps you first became acquainted with Seventh-day Adventists by attending one of the thousands of preventive health seminars, such as the stop-smoking plan currently called *Breathe Free*™, or a stress seminar or cooking school. Or maybe you read one of the many books that Ellen G. White wrote on health, such as *The Ministry of Healing, Temperance, Counsels on Health, Counsels on Diet and Foods*, or *Medical Ministry*. Perhaps you picked up the bimonthly health magazine, *Vibrant Life*, or one of the temperance magazines, *Listen* or *Winner*. Or maybe you have frequented one of the many Country Living health food restaurants located in the major cities of the world. Yes, Seventh-day Adventists believe health is important!

But none of these programs and none of this information will do much good unless people like you catch the message, live the message, reap the benefits from the message, and share the message with others.

This is a new year. It is a time to rally the rank and file of God's people once again to follow the practices God initiated at Creation with His original diet, and which He reiterated to the Jewish population as He led them out of slavery and promised that if they would follow God's prescription for health, "none of these diseases" would come upon them (Ex. 15:26). Then God gave the instruction once again to His people during the past century. We need to be reminded that there is an inexplicable tie between our physical, mental, and spiritual health. Our bodies are the temples of the Holy Spirit (1 Cor. 6:19), but some of our bodies need a little cleaning up and refurbishing before they are fit dwellings for the Deity.

And so let me challenge you as you read this book written from the perspective of more than 165 health professionals and inspirational writers. It is my prayer that you will catch the message and run with it! And may God's Holy Spirit fill you as you read these daily devotional messages.

WORDS OF INTRODUCTION

Jan W. and Kay Kuzma

> Dear friend, I pray that you may enjoy good health and that all may go well
> with you, even as your soul is getting along well. 3 John 2, NIV.

This is God's desire for your life: a healthy body, mind, and soul. But the path to what we call "wholly" health is not always an easy one. It requires choices and decisions. Sometimes we need to make changes in long-term lifestyle and thinking habits, getting rid of those not conducive to the vibrant life. As you face the challenge of living your life according to God's instructions, make this your motto: "I can do all things through Christ who strengthens me" (Phil. 4:13, NKJV).

Now is the time to change to a more healthy lifestyle—spiritually, physically, socially, emotionally, and mentally. No one is perfect. All of our lives have room for improvement. And so we bring you this book so that every day it can remind you of what God's ideal is for your health.

May this year bring you renewed strength, energy, and happiness as you follow God's guidelines on how to live a more vibrant life.

To your health—and a more energized life!

WORDS OF APPRECIATION

To our colleagues, friends, family, and others who so generously shared their inspirational stories, expertise, and words of wisdom. We thank you!

To Elmar Sakala, who personally contacted his colleagues at Loma Linda University, and to those who responded with devotional messages that bring a depth of knowledge and experience to the pages of this book. And an additional thanks for professionally reviewing this manuscript.

To those who wrote but for some reason we were unable to include your stories. We thank you.

To Ted Hamilton, who reviewed this manuscript through the eyes of a physician and the heart of a good friend.

To those of you who read these selections and find yourself challenged to change, frustrated with your wilted willpower, touched by the self-disclosure of others, and angered when your toes are stepped on. We encourage you!

And to our Creator, who designed our bodies—shaped them out of clay and then kissed that first human creation with the breath of life. We praise You!

—Jan and Kay Kuzma

FOREWORD

Ted Hamilton, M.D.

Vice President,
Florida Hospital

Much of Jesus' teaching consisted of telling stories and asking questions. This book does both with skill and grace. The postscript notes at the end of each passage are delightfully pertinent and provocative.

One finds repetition of themes, which one would expect in a book of this nature, but it does not become tedious or boring because of the freshness of viewpoint provided by the various authors. The expressions of personal challenge, struggle, faith and despair, defeat and victory are powerfully compelling.

This book has been a blessing to me, and I'm convinced that its potential for blessing to others is deep and far-reaching.

FOREWORD

Elmar P. Sakala, M.D., M.P.H.

School of Medicine,
Loma Linda University

The idea of a devotional book on health is entirely consistent with Christ's declaration "I am come that they might have life, and that they might have it more abundantly" (John 10:10). The abundant life is truly one of optimum physical as well as spiritual health. To work with Jan and Kay Kuzma to put together a multiauthored volume such as this has been an awesome experience. The eagerness to participate that I received from the wide range of health professionals in many disciplines at Loma Linda University was truly inspiring. I sincerely thank each one who contributed.

Now as I read the final copy through the eyes of an academic physician, I find the product deserving of your time. This is not a medical textbook, yet there are many references to solid scientific facts. The spectrum of viewpoints reflects a diversity of the life experiences of the many authors. At times this can tend toward more subjectivity than science, yet it brings a richness and authenticity to the whole.

One of the rewards of my specialty field of obstetrics is that for the most part I work with healthy women and deliver healthy babies. I spend much of my time encouraging and counseling my patients on how to prevent problems—both physically and psychologically. In addition, as speaker for the *Got a Minute for Your Health?* radio program, I am daily presenting health information to encourage listeners to live a healthier lifestyle.

The motto of Loma Linda University is "To Make Man Whole." This seeks wholeness not just physically, but also emotionally, mentally, and spiritually. I believe this health devotional is an idea whose time has come—a book that will help men and women of all ages to become "whole" and experience the blessings of health God intended all of us to enjoy.

BIOGRAPHICAL SKETCHES

To thank those who contributed to this book.

We want to thank each of the following individuals for contributing to this book. We hope you will enjoy learning more about these special people.

Ouila Abraham is the treasurer, Community Services leader, and school representative at the Maranatha SDA Church in Etobicoke, Ontario. She is married to Theo Abraham, an educator. **Aug. 4.**

Dianne Affolter, wife of Gary, who is vice principal of Georgia-Cumberland Academy, is the mother of three grown children. Dianne is a teacher specializing in English, art, and music. A former missionary in Nigeria and Singapore, she is known for her bell choirs and creative design. **Apr. 1, Nov. 1.**

Wilber Alexander, Ph.D. With many years dedicated to teaching theology and working with chaplains, Wilber is now special assistant to the president of Loma Linda University for spiritual life and wholeness. **May 21.**

Therese L. Allen, paralyzed since 1972 from an automobile accident, now writes from her home in Los Angeles, where she passionately enjoys watching her favorite teams play hockey at the Forum. **Mar. 17, Apr. 27, Aug. 19, Oct. 14, Dec. 22.**

Demetra Andreasen has her degree in social sciences and has worked as a medical social worker at Madison, St. Helena, Parkview Community, and Royal Newcastle hospitals. Presently in community relations at Andrews University, she is the wife of Niels-Erik. They have one grown son, Michael. **Sept. 13, Nov. 8.**

Niels-Erik Andreasen, Ph.D., president of Andrews University, has been president of Walla Walla College, religion professor at Loma Linda University, Pacific Union College, and Avondale College in Australia, and author of three books, including *The Christian Use of Time* and *The Old Testament Sabbath*. **July 3, Sept. 13, Nov. 8.**

William C. "Conn" Arnold has been a dean of boys, teacher, principal, pastor, administrator of various conference departments, and executive secretary-treasurer of ASI (Adventist-Laymen's Services and Industries). He and his wife, Dot, have two children, and his message is still "Straight Ahead." **Sept. 14.**

Linda B. lives in the country in the great Northwest. Married with two children, she loves hiking, music, gardening, people, and church. Her greatest joy, next to God and family, is to share her experience, strength, and hope with other food addicts. **Aug. 7.**

Leonard L. Bailey, M.D., is professor of surgery at Loma Linda University Medical Center. Known for his pioneering efforts in infant heart transplants, he has performed heart surgery in Greece, Brazil, Korea, China, Saudi Arabia, and Nepal. He and his wife, Nancy, a critical-care nurse, have two sons. **July 6, Oct. 11.**

Delbert W. Baker, Ph.D., is president of Oakwood College. Formerly, he was an administrator at Loma Linda University and before that he was editor of *Message* magazine. He is the author/editor of four books. **July 11, Oct. 3.**

Bernell E. Baldwin, Ph.D., is a neurophysiologist and science editor of *The Journal of Health & Healing* at Wildwood Lifestyle Center and Hospital, Wildwood, Georgia. He was formerly on the faculty of the Schools of Medicine and Health, Loma Linda University. **Jan. 16, Feb. 15.**

Marjorie V. Baldwin, M.D., is editor of *The Journal of Health & Healing* and a physician at Wildwood Lifestyle Center and Hospital, Wildwood, Georgia. She was formerly on the faculty of the Schools of Medicine and Health at Loma Linda University. **Jan. 7, Mar. 1.**

Linda Barton is a dedicated mother of four and wife of Vernon, a family practice physician in Payette, Idaho. She is active in her local church and church school, and is enjoying the next generation. **May 16.**

David B. Beardsley is president of Heritage Healthcare Management, headquartered in Cleveland, Tennessee. He and his wife, Donnalene, and their two children, Doug and Stacey, enjoy traveling and taking trips with Maranatha Volunteers International. **June 27, Dec. 19.**

Linda Bell, R.N., M.S.N., C.C.R.N., has been a nurse in critical care and education for 24 years. She is currently working in an advanced practice role at Loma Linda University Medical Center. Her secondary interest is in clinical ethics. **Dec. 26.**

Wallace "Buddy" Blair, C.P.A., lost his fight for life on April 20, 1996. He was a certified public accountant for more than 30 years. He and Elsie have two grown children, Lisa and Kenneth. Buddy was known by all for his kind, gracious, optimistic, and generous spirit. Thousands prayed for Buddy during these five challenging years. **May 20.**

Dennis Blum, Dr.P.H., M.P.H., president of Lifestyle Center of America in Oklahoma, was former director of public health and preventative medicine at the University of Montemorelos in Mexico, and taught at Columbia Union College, Weimar College, and Hartland College. **Feb. 22, June 13, July 19.**

Olive Blumenshein, R.N., was a missionary nurse at Malamulo Hospital in Malawi and Mwami Hospital in Zambia. Her husband, Arthur, died in 1985, and she now lives in Springer, Oklahoma, where she and her sister, Anna May Vaughan, enjoy studying the Bible and holding small group meetings in their home. **Feb. 17.**

Gerri Bradley is a real estate agent and was number one in her office for 1995. She enjoys family and country living in Ellijay, Georgia, where Gerri loves to garden, can foods, ski, and participate in all types of water sports. **Mar. 8.**

Debby Bullock is working with the Patient Education Department at the Royal University Hospital with the Fibromyalgia Association. She and her husband, John

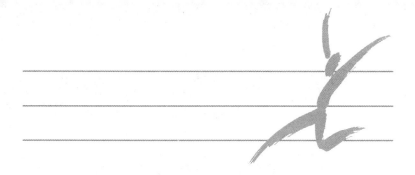

(treasurer of the Manitoba/Saskatchewan Conference), have three boys. She has assisted in stop-smoking programs, cooking schools, and summer camp work. **Jan. 6.**

Kenneth I. Burke, Ph.D., R.D., is a professor in the Department of Nutrition and Dietetics in the School of Allied Health Professions at Loma Linda University. **May 13, July 9, Oct. 4.**

Paul Cannon, former pastor, is executive director, and **Carol Cannon** is clinical director at The Bridge, a treatment center for dependency disorders in Bowling Green, Kentucky. The Bridge specializes in treating workaholism, perfectionism, and other "clean" addictions as well as chemical dependency and codependence. **Feb. 19, Dec. 7.**

Elden M. Chalmers, Ph.D., is a licensed psychologist and has served as director of counseling in the Georgia-Cumberland Conference. He has been a pastor, evangelist, and professor at Columbia and Pacific Union colleges and Andrews University. He and his wife, Esther, live in Yountville, California. **Feb. 13, June 1.**

Barbara Choo writes from Silver Spring, Maryland. A graduate of Kettering College of Medical Arts, she converted from Buddhism into the Seventh-day Adventist faith. Her interest in the health and wellness of the underprivileged has inspired her to concentrate her medical service on hospice patients. **Mar. 25.**

Kay Collins, R.N., graduated from Madison College and has worked with her husband in evangelism since 1973 as a gospel ministry team. Currently in the Michigan Conference, she is a former Bible instructor for Amazing Facts, and is now a credentialed commissioned minister. **Mar. 3, Apr. 12, May 11, June 30, Dec. 9.**

Norma J. Collins is associate director at the Ellen G. White Estate, in which she serves as office manager, answering correspondence from around the world. She has two children and two grandchildren. In addition, she has a private pilot's license and enjoys reading and shopping. **May 4.**

Bert Connell, Ph.D., R.D., teaches in the Department of Nutrition and Dietetics in the School of Allied Health Professions, Loma Linda University. **June 24.**

Kathy Corwin codirects with her husband, Harvey, the Family Life Department of the Oregon Conference of Seventh-day Adventists. They are popular speakers and present a variety of seminars on various family health issues. One of their most popular is "Love Takes Time." **May 8.**

Jim Cox pastors in Cohutta, Georgia, and is also the chaplain of the Dalton Police Department, the Georgia state representative for the International Conference of Police Chaplains, and a member of the Whitfield County Juvenile Court. His wife, Carol, is a psychiatric and mental health-care nurse. **Apr. 7, May. 7, June 6.**

Andrea Creed is a mission reporter for Springs of Life Foundation in Poland. An American with a missionary heart, Andrea has dedicated her writing skills to promoting the health message in the heart of Poland. **Nov. 2.**

Tim Crosby is editor at large of the Review and Herald Publishing Association, author of a number of books, and a concert keyboard artist. He is married to Carol, an R.N., and they are enjoying their first foster child. **Oct. 22**

Faith Crumbly is editor of *Sabbath School Leadership* magazine. She and her husband, Edward, have five healthy grown children and have worked hard to keep them in good health. The Crumblys conduct tasting events for the Vegetarian Supper Club of Hagerstown, Maryland. **Feb. 9.**

Dona Daniel is a certified nurse's aide who works with her husband, Terry, in home health care with hospice. She teaches health and nutrition classes at her church. They have six children and five grandchildren. Dona loves nature and gardening at their home in Colton, Oregon. **Sept. 9.**

Richard M. Davidson, Ph.D., is chair of the Old Testament Department at the SDA Theological Seminary. He and Jo Ann and their two children lived in Israel for a year, where they observed firsthand the Jewish celebration of Shabbat. He has authored *A Love Song for the Sabbath* and *In the Footsteps of Joshua.* **June 2.**

M. Jerry Davis, M.A., Rel.D., is chair of the Department of Chaplains, Loma Linda University Medical Center, and regional director of the Pacific Region Association for Clinical Pastoral Education. He and his wife, Sylvia, have two grown boys. **July 10.**

Nicceta Davis, M.S., P.T., also known as "Nikki," is originally from Camden, New Jersey. She is an alumna of Pine Forge Academy, Oakwood College, Loma Linda University, and Temple University. A licensed physical therapist, she has served on the faculty of Loma Linda University. **Aug. 11.**

Dan Day, M.Div., is senior vice president of Coppinger and Affiliates, a company specializing in photoprocessing. He's the author of dozens of books, the most recent *Hanging On by Your Fingernails* and *Kids, Teens and Wives.* He has five children and loves writing. **Aug. 22, Nov. 19.**

David J. DeRose, M.D., M.P.H., is on the medical staff of Lifestyle Center of America in Oklahoma. His wife, Sonja, is also a physician. David writes health education material and radio scripts, publishes the *HealthWise Newsletter* on the Internet, and serves as assistant editor of *The Journal of Health & Healing.* **Feb. 23, Mar. 4, Apr. 6, Nov. 18.**

Samuel L. DeShay, M.D., D.Min., and his wife, Bernice, served in Nigeria for 12 years and now live in Takoma Park, Maryland, with their two daughters. He is in private practice, is the director of medical services for Hadley Memorial Hospital, and has coauthored with Bernice the health book *Plus Fifteen.* **Apr. 28, July 26.**

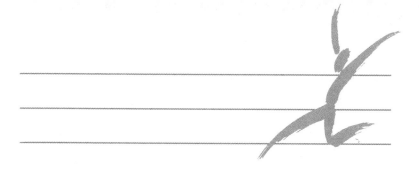

Bernice A. DeShay, R.N., received her degree from Loma Linda University and has done graduate work in midwifery and pediatrics. She was program coordinator and office manager for Plus Fifteen, a health products company she and her husband founded, and now teaches nursing at Columbia Union College. **Apr. 28.**

John DeVincenzo, D.D.S., is a practicing orthodontist in San Luis Obispo, California. His avocation is plant research. He and his wife, Bobbie, enjoy developing their "Gopher Glen" apple farm as well as visiting their three grown children and grandchildren. **June 11, Aug. 13.**

Hans Diehl, Dr.P.H, M.P.H., president of Lifestyle Medicine Institute in Loma Linda, California, is an outstanding motivational speaker and writer on health behavior change. He conducts CHIP (Coronary Health Improvement Project) seminars and is married to Lily, a professional musician. **Jan. 11, Dec. 30.**

Dick Duerksen is vice president for communication, marketing, and creative ministries of the Columbia Union Conference, and has been a college administrator, high school teacher and principal, campus minister, and youth leader. He and Brenda have three children, Jeremy, Julene, and Joy. **May 24, Oct. 8, Dec. 17.**

Connie M. Dunn, M.A., is a doctoral candidate in clinical psychology, with a master's degree in theology. She enjoys spending her leisure time with her husband and her dogs, Mugsy and Molly. After completion of her degree she hopes to work as a neuropsychologist and counselor. **Nov. 17.**

Winona Eichner, R.N., is a nurse manager for the Pediatric and Adult Rehabilitation Unit at Loma Linda University Medical Center. She and her husband, Ron, who is a general contractor, have two sons, Michael and Christopher. They enjoy camping and all outdoor activities. **Nov. 21.**

Rose Shafer Fuller is an academy English and physical education teacher, pastor's wife, and mother of three active teenagers. Any spare time left in her hectic schedule gets filled with camping, sports, a walking/exercise program, baking, or reading. **July 5.**

Judith T. Getchell teaches and is registrar at Ouachita Hills Academy in Arkansas. She and her husband, a civil engineer for the Forest Service, have three children, April, Paul, and Adam. Her greatest love is studying the Scriptures and walking with her neighbors, which she considers her most effective witnessing tool. **Oct. 23.**

Carla Gober, R.N., M.P.H., M.S., is coordinator of the spiritual care program in the Nursing Division at the Loma Linda University Medical Center and assistant professor of relational studies, faculty of religion. A popular seminar speaker and a columnist for *Women of Spirit*, she loves adventure. **Dec. 15.**

Rosemary D. Graham, a 1974 graduate of Oakwood College, was diagnosed with lupus erythematosus in 1984. Although disabled, Rosemary currently serves on several national and local health committees. She also does presentations and conducts workshops on health. **Feb. 2.**

David Grellmann, M.D., M.P.H., is a family practitioner in Michigan who has been practicing acute care and public health in the U.S. and in developing countries, including five years of mission service in West Africa. **Carrie Grellman,** P.T., is a physical therapist. David and Carrie have two girls, Kelsey and Shelly, and a son, Jason. **Sept. 11, Oct. 28.**

Dane J. Griffin is director of Sure Word Productions in North Carolina, where he produces health education videos, slides, booklets, recipes, and other health resources. He and his wife, Vicky, are the parents of two children, Gina and Anthony. **Jan. 14, Feb. 6, Mar. 15, Oct. 1, Dec. 16.**

Nancy Hadaway works as an administrative secretary in Children's Hospital Nursing Administration at Loma Linda University. **Sept. 10.**

Steven L. Haley, M.Div., is a former police officer who, after studying righteousness by faith, became a pastor to share the good news of salvation with others. He grew up in Maryland and married Malinda, a registered nurse. They have two children, Brenden and Carissa. He currently pastors the Bowman Hills church in Cleveland, Tennessee. **May 10, Aug. 9, Sept. 27, Nov. 5.**

Madlyn Hamblin has authored one book and coauthored three books with Cari Haus. Madlyn is the public relations director of the Hamblin Company, a family-owned business founded by her husband in 1974. They are parents of two grown children and reside in Adrian, Michigan. **Feb. 3.**

Jean Hametz, R.N., is a nurse and health educator who serves as the health and temperance leader at the Warrenton Seventh-day Adventist Church in Virginia, and in the Health Ministries Department of Hartland College. **Jan. 12.**

Ted Hamilton, M.D., is family physician and medical director of Florida Hospital Central Care in Orlando, Florida. Previously he was the executive director for Loma Linda University Faculty Medical Group and medical director for an HMO in Georgia. Ted and his wife, Jackie, have two grown daughters, Jennifer and Jessica. **Apr. 22, July 27, Sept. 2.**

Fred Hardinge, Dr.P.H, R.D., C.H.E.S., is president of Total Life Creations, which produces health enhancement videos and seminars—such as *Fatigue Busters*. He is particularly interested in the relationship of physical health to spiritual life. Fred enjoys hiking, climbing, and skiing with his wife and two children. **June 7, Dec. 21.**

Mervyn G. Hardinge, M.D., Ph.D., Dr.P.H., founded the School of Public Health at Loma Linda University and became its first dean. He received his medical degree from

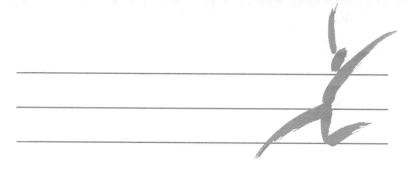

Loma Linda University, a doctorate in pharmacology from Stanford, and a doctorate in public health from Harvard, and is a former editor of *Vibrant Life*. **Jan. 8.**

Cliff and **Freddie Harris** are codirectors of Drug Alternative Program (DAP). They operate a men's drug recovery home and outpatient drug support groups from their headquarters in Grand Terrace, California. **June 29, Sept. 18.**

Cari Haus, C.P.A., a certified public accountant/freelance writer, supplies the contents for tax and accounting newsletters, has coauthored four books, and is founding editor of the newsletter *Creative Parenting* and editor of *Prime Time for Parents*. Cari and David have two sons, Michael and Matthew. **Feb. 3.**

Harvey Heidinger, M.D., M.P.H., is an associate professor in the School of Public Health at Loma Linda University, teaching in the areas of maternal and child health since 1976, and practicing in the area of university health services at the University of California at Riverside. He and Elizabeth have three adult children. **Oct. 10.**

Georgia E. Hodgkin, Ed.D., R.D., is an associate professor at Loma Linda University's Schools of Allied Health Professions and Public Health. She chaired the Lay Advisory Council for Southeastern California Conference, is a member of the Pacific Union Conference executive committee, and head elder of the Loma Linda University church. **May 23.**

Betty M. Hoehn, M.A., M.P.H., a former medical technologist who worked in the United States, Canada, and Jamaica, now lives in Cleveland, Tennessee, and coordinates health programs for Family Matters retreats. She has two daughters and two grandsons. **Aug. 5, Nov. 27, Dec. 5, Dec. 6.**

Joyce W. Hopp, Ph.D., M.P.H., is dean of the School of Allied Health Professions and professor of health promotion and education, School of Public Health, Loma Linda University. She has contributed to the science-health textbooks of the North American Division for 25 years. **June 23, Aug. 3.**

Todd Hoyt is assistant director of Family Matters. A communication major from Union College, he has been a student missionary in Australia and Guam, where he worked for Adventist World Radio. **Mar. 22.**

Auldwin T. Humphrey was a pastor and at one time served as the director of health and temperance in the Lake Union Conference. Currently the director of adult ministries for the North American Division of Seventh-day Adventists, he baptized Larry in his 1981 evangelistic seminar. **Apr. 20.**

Silvia Jacobson and her husband, Tim, have a publishing ministry, Jacobson Publications, and are lay pastoring in the Florida Keys with their two boys, Eric and Ken. **Apr. 23.**

Jennifer Jas and her husband, Raul, live in Chattanooga, Tennessee, where she

21

works in corporate communications at McKee Foods and Raul is a personal fitness trainer. They have one child. In addition, they take care of foster children on weekends as well as overnight emergency situations for children with intense behavior problems. **July 23.**

Janene Jenkins, R.N.C., M.S., is an obstetrical nurse educator who works with the Perinatal Outreach Program at Loma Linda University. She has been honored as Teacher of the Year in the School of Nursing. **Aug. 8.**

Linda Willman Johnson, R.N., Ph.D., is executive director of nursing for Loma Linda University Children's Hospital and Total Care Birth Center. She has dedicated the majority of her nursing career to the care of children. Her doctoral studies focused on self-esteem and identity development in adolescents with cancer. **Nov. 6.**

Patricia K. Johnston, Dr.P.H. M.S., R.D., is the associate dean of the School of Public Health, Loma Linda University. **May 29, June 16, Nov. 20.**

Jill Kennedy is a speaker and seminar presenter for Family Matters. She and her husband, Allan, an administrator and pilot, have been presenters for Marriage Encounter for many years. Jill has home-schooled Jeremy and Jonathan and has worked in Sabbath school, Vacation Bible School, and women's ministries. **Dec. 14.**

Dianne Kosarin is a professional violinist who won the Rome Festival Orchestra Solo Competition and was the youngest member ever of the Charleston Symphony Orchestra. She met Oscar (a conductor and arranger) at the University of Cincinnati College Conservatory of Music, and they have two children. **Nov. 7.**

Edwin H. Krick, M.D., M.P.H., is associate professor of medicine at Loma Linda University and has charge of the Rheumatology Fellowship Training Program. He spent eight years in Japan as a missionary and was dean of the School of Public Health at Loma Linda. He and his wife, Beverly, enjoy traveling. **Apr. 19, Aug. 1, Sept. 28, Dec. 8.**

Robert Kuczek is the president of Springs of Life Foundation, established to promote lay ministry and outreach in Poland. It operates a printing press, a publishing house, a farm, and three health food stores, and is affiliated with Outpost Centers Incorporated. **Oct. 27.**

George Kuzma, M.D., is a family practice physician in Albion, Michigan. He enjoys gardening, skiing, camping, and ocean beaches. His motto is: "He changed my life." **Nov. 11.**

Kathy Kuzma, R.N., is a homemaker with five children—Macaiah, Samuel, Mary Elizabeth, Joseph, and Daniel—who keep her busy day and night. She sews, cooks, reads, and enjoys time with her physician husband, George. **June 17.**

Jan W. Kuzma, Ph.D., formerly the chair of the Department of Biostatistics and di-

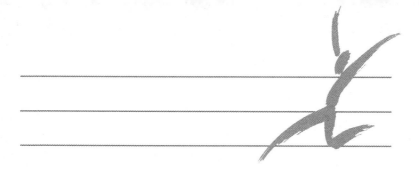

rector of research at the School of Public Health, Loma Linda University, is currently president of Sentinel Research Services, a nonprofit organization that provides statistical consultation in medical areas, and produces the *Got a Minute for Your Health?* daily radio program. **Jan. 20, Jan. 25, Feb. 4, Feb. 16, Feb. 26, Mar. 27, Apr. 24, May 6, May 26, June 20, July 13, July 24, Aug. 21, Sept. 26, Oct. 20, Oct. 24, Dec. 20.**

Kay Kuzma, Ed.D. is speaker, author, and founder of Family Matters, an organization that provides information and services for families through a daily radio program called *Got a Minute for Your Family,* through television, through a quarterly newspaper called *Family Times,* through newspaper columns, and through the Welcome Baby outreach program for families. **Feb. 6, Feb. 10, Feb. 14, Feb. 21, Mar. 5, Apr. 17, May 31, June 5, June 21, June 28, July 4, Aug. 12, Aug. 31, Sept. 6, Sept. 12, Sept. 21, Sept. 30, Oct. 13, Oct. 16, Nov. 3, Nov. 14, Nov. 22, Nov. 24, Nov. 29, Dec. 24, Dec. 25, Dec. 27.** Coauthored with **Jan W. Kuzma: Jan. 2, Jan. 9, Jan. 15, Jan. 18, Feb. 7, Mar. 9, Mar. 19, Apr. 3, Apr. 29, May 15, Aug. 6, Oct. 9, Nov. 9.**

Kevin Kuzma writes from southern California, where he attends La Sierra University and surfs. He spent a year in Majuro teaching third grade, and because of that experience is planning a career in elementary teaching. **Apr. 9.**

Betty M. Larson, R.N., C.C.B.E., is a certified child birth educator who has taught at San Bernardino County Medical Center, San Gorgonio Pass Memorial Hospital, and Chino Institution for Women. Also a home health nurse doing postpartum visits, she enjoys her three children. **Mar. 18.**

Benjamin Lau, M.D., Ph.D., is professor of microbiology and immunology at the School of Medicine, Loma Linda University. **Mar. 12, May 14, Sept. 4.**

Caris H. Lauda is former president of the Carolina, Minnesota, and Potomac conferences and executive secretary of Adventist-Laymen's Services and Industries (ASI). He and his wife, Mary, were popular camp meeting speakers. He always said: "As long as the Lord gives me breath, I'll sing, teach, preach, and live the love of Jesus." **Aug. 30, Sept. 20.**

Mary Paulson Lauda has worked in administrative health care since 1947 and served on various church and community committees. Her first husband died in 1977, and she married Caris Lauda in 1989. She is listed as one of the 1995 Notable Adventist Women, and has three daughters, six grandchildren, and two great-granddaughters. **Aug. 10.**

George M. Lessard, Ph.D., professor of biochemistry, has taught in the Schools of Medicine and Dentistry at Loma Linda University since 1972. His interests include educational philosophy and curriculum. He instructs in the areas of biochemistry, nutrition, and oral health. **May 12, June 8, July 25.**

Kenneth H. Livesay is a retired pastor. In addition he was personal ministries director and Adventist-Laymen's Services and Industries (ASI) director of Southeastern California Conference, and former secretary/treasurer of ASI. Ken and Ruth live in Paradise, California, and have two children, Don and Karen. **June 4.**

Aileen Ludington, M.D., is a board-certified physician whose major interest is lifestyle change. She has a staff appointment with Weimar Institute, coauthors materials with Hans Diehl, and is a popular seminar speaker. She and her physician husband are practicing in a lifestyle center in Thailand. **Feb. 25, Mar. 26, July 31, Sept. 16.**

Dale Marcotte, M.D., has enjoyed his career in opthalmology and is now doing cattle ranching. He truly loves people and is involved in his church. With his wife, Phyllis, he lives in Boulder, Colorado. **June 25.**

Edwin Martin is a retired hospital and nursing home administrator who enjoys golfing with friends and traveling around the world with his wife, Mary Belle. They have the best of both worlds, living in Cleveland, Tennessee, during the summer and enjoying Florida sunshine in the winter. **Mar. 2.**

Henry C. Martin, vice president of communications and development at Weimar Institute, is responsible for promoting off-campus seminars and working with students doing health screening. Henry and his wife, Robin, have two grown children, and their hobby is bringing people to God. **Jan. 13, Apr. 8, Oct. 12.**

Dan Matthews, M.A., is the executive director of Faith for Today television and host of the weekly television program *Lifestyle Magazine*. Previously Dan was a pastor, church administrator, and public relations director. He and his wife, Betsy, have three grown boys and are currently enjoying grandparenting. **Jan. 3, July 16, Aug. 15, Sept. 29, Nov. 26, Dec. 13.**

Alberta Mazat, M.S.W., R.N., who is a licensed marriage, family, and child counselor, chaired the Department of Marriage, Family, and Child Counseling at Loma Linda University and has authored books and articles on sexuality. She and her physician husband, Alfred, have four children. **June 9, July 29, Sept. 1.**

Mary McDonald, Ph.D., is a Stanford graduate and researcher in developmental psychology who is now writing children's books. The 1995 winner of a prestigious award in her field of writing, she and her physician husband, Craig, have four children: Dane, Dawn, Shay, and Luke. **Aug. 16.**

Norma McKellip is a junior accountant in the General Conference Transportation and International Personnel Services, where she works with interdivision employees. She was raised in Minnesota, attended Union College, enjoys her children, and is in-

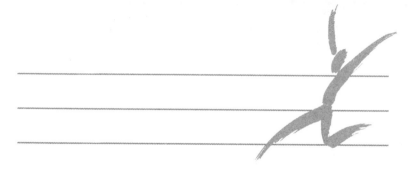

terested in reading, flowers, and handiwork. **Jan. 21.**

Lonnie Melashenko, M.Div., is director-speaker for the Voice of Prophecy, the oldest continuous religious broadcast in North America. Formerly he was a pastor and associate director-speaker for the *It Is Written* telecast. He and his wife, Jeannie, have conducted large evangelistic campaigns in Brazil, Russia, and the Philippines. **Feb. 8.**

Mark Messina, Ph.D., is a leading authority in the field of soy foods and cancer prevention. He and his wife, **Virginia Messina,** R.D., M.P.H., have coauthored the book *The Simple Soybean and Your Health.* Virginia was director of nutrition services for the George Washington University Ambulatory Medical Center. **Jan. 5, Sept. 23.**

Raymond Moore, Ph.D., and **Dorothy Moore,** M.S., are pioneers of the home school movement and have cofounded the Moore Foundation, which offers consulting and seminars in home schooling. They travel extensively and are well-known presenters and authors of numerous books, including *Home Made Health.* **Nov. 10.**

Jerry Muncy, D.D.S., has a private dental practice in Safford, Arizona. Active in his local church and involved with prison ministries, he enjoys flying and volunteering with various mission projects. He and his wife, Patti, have three grown children and are now enjoying grandchildren. **Jan. 17.**

Patti Muncy has her own interior decorating business, teaches a Revelation study group, and is chair of an interdenominational Christian women's club in southeastern Arizona. Formerly a dental assistant and office manager of her husband's practice, she has taught flying as a certified flight instructor. **Jan. 31.**

Cecil Murphey is a freelance author who has written more than 100 books, one of which is on health and was coauthored by Jan W. Kuzma. Some of his best-sellers are *Gifted Hands* and *Think Big,* coauthored with Dr. Ben Carson. **Jan 25, Feb. 4, Feb. 26, Mar. 27.**

Patricia B. Mutch, Ph.D., R.D., is dean of the College of Arts and Sciences at Andrews University. Formerly director of the Institute for Prevention of Addiction, she was also director of nutrition and dietetics and assistant director of the General Conference Health and Temperance Department. **July 7, Aug. 24, Aug. 25, Aug. 26, Aug. 27, Oct. 21, Nov. 4, Nov. 23, Dec. 11.**

Richard Neil, M.D., M.P.H., is director of Relinco Associates, a health consulting and human resource management organization in Grand Terrace, California. Formerly associated with Loma Linda University's School of Public Health, he is an author and a dynamic speaker. He and his wife, Verlene, have three children. **Apr. 16.**

Christine Neish, Ph.D., M.P.H., C.H.E.S., is chair of health promotion and education in the School of Public Health, Loma Linda University. She and her husband,

Ron, live near beautiful Oak Glen, California. **June 26.**

Velda Nelson is a retired English teacher and mother of four married daughters and grandmother of eight. She enjoys reading, crossword puzzles, quilting, and raising roses. She teaches a Sabbath school class, chairs her church flower and library committees, and edits two newsletters. **Apr. 11.**

Nancy Newball works at Home Study International as a graphic designer and writer for the Office of Institutional Advancement. She enjoys freelance writing as well as corresponding with her friends all over the world. **Jan. 19, Feb. 5, Mar. 23, Sept. 3.**

Don L. Nicolay, M.D., is a general surgeon in Boulder, Colorado, who on the side enjoys peach farming, hiking, and skiing. He and his wife, Lynn, have three children and one grandchild. **June 25.**

Lynn Nicolay, R.N., has recently chosen to shift her focus from her nursing career to spend more time in youth projects, Community Services, and with her family. **May 17, June 25.**

Pat Nordman writes from Deland, Florida, where she works at Stetson University and is a freelance writer of articles and books. She and her husband, Charles, have four living children. Her philosophy is "not to ask for more before saying thank you for what you have already received." **Jan. 24, Apr. 18, Aug. 20, Oct. 6, Dec. 28.**

Jacalyn Nosek, M.P.H., is director of Lancaster Educational Associates, a private practice offering academic therapy, study skills, organizational skills, and tutoring in math and science. Currently she is also a volunteer teacher in mathematics at the Browning Memorial Elementary School and South Lancaster Academy. **Jan. 30, Apr. 14, Dec. 4.**

Connie W. Nowlan is a wife and mother of two grown children—one of whom has had special needs from birth. Also she is a former girls' dean, an English teacher, a preschool director, and a writer who loves God's outdoors. **Mar. 29, July 17.**

C. A. "Bill" Oliphant, Ph.D., has been a book editor for Southern Publishing Association, a public relations director, a magazine editor, and a professor of journalism at Memphis State University, Marshall University, Andrews University, Southern Adventist University, and La Sierra University. He's written five books. **Apr. 30.**

Karis Osadchuck, M.S., P.T., a physical therapist, writes from San Francisco, where her husband, Vasiliy, is in graduate school. They plan to return to Russia, where Vasiliy will be teaching at Zaokski Theological Seminary. They are the parents of a boy. **Mar. 30.**

Carlos Pardeiro is founder and president of Creation Enterprises, Inc., a ministry to supply inspirational and health-oriented books and materials to others. He and his

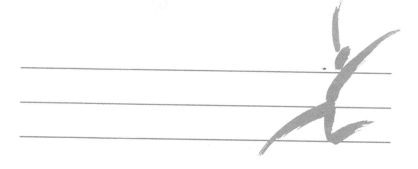

wife, Nancy, live in Gentry, Arkansas, where he is helping to develop a television satellite network. **Dec. 23.**

Lois (Rittenhouse) Pecce works in a medical office. Her special interests lie in family, writing, corresponding with inmates, nursing home visitation, chapel services, and assisting with cradle roll at church—along with gardening, sewing, knitting, and traveling with husband Ed. **Feb. 27, July 14, Nov. 13, Nov. 30**

Joan Pierce, active leader in the Beaumont, California, Seventh-day Adventist Church, is the mother of two grown children and wife of Dick, a social worker in Banning, California. Her special interests are flower arranging and decorating for weddings. **May 30.**

Betty Pierson is the recording secretary of the North American Division. She and her husband, Don, who is an associate treasurer of the North American Division, have three grown daughters and have served in Nigeria, Ghana, Ivory Coast, and England. **Oct. 13.**

Stoy Proctor, M.P.H., is associate director of the Health and Temperance Department of the General Conference of Seventh-day Adventists. His wife, Leilani, works with a health resource service, the Health Connection. **Jan. 28.**

Rob Purvis heads Purvis Construction Welding in Riverside, California. He is currently the associate head deacon at the Azure Hills Seventh-day Adventist Church, where he and **Debbie** are actively involved in Sabbath school, and where **Matthew** is enjoying his little sister, Traci. **July 12.**

Kathryn Ann Raethel, R.N., M.P.H., M.H.A., is the administrative director for nursing quality management at Loma Linda University Medical Center. She and her husband, Hilton, are the parents of one daughter, Ashley Elizabeth. **Oct. 19.**

Rise Rafferty writes from Washington, where she and her husband are part of the Light Bearers Ministry and are enjoying their young son. **Aug. 17, Sept. 19.**

Vivian Raitz is a certified vegetarian cuisine instructor, through the General Conference of Seventh-day Adventists. The wife of a Georgia physician, she has been active in nutrition, stress-control, weight-management, and smoking-cessation seminars for more than 15 years. **July 22, Aug. 14, Sept. 7, Oct. 29.**

E. John Reinhold, who writes from Florida, is the executive director of the Christian Care Ministry, an organization in which sharing Christians meet medical needs. He and his wife, Dona, enjoy family (four children and two grandchildren) and traveling. **Mar. 11.**

Marilyn Renk, M.S., M.P.H., is assistant director of the Health Department and Community Services at the Oregon Conference. She has taught home economics at the college level and has been a health educator in the Adventist Health System.

Marilyn is married to Wes and lives on a five-acre "farm." **Apr. 2.**

Jimmy Rhodes is director of music services for Life Care Centers of America. His keyboard artistry has inspired thousands as he has traveled for Faith for Today, Mission Spotlight, and evangelistic crusades, taught music at various academies, and produced 15 albums. His wife, Pam, is an accomplished vocalist. **Apr. 5.**

Larry Richardson, Ph.D., is president of Richardson Health Services. He taught communications and drama at Pacific Union College and La Sierra University. Both he and his wife, Becky, have earned their black belts in karate, and they have two teenagers, Damon and Lauren. **Jan. 29, Feb. 18, Mar. 16, Apr. 4, May 3, June 3, July 1, Aug. 2, Sept. 8, Oct. 15, Dec. 31.**

Nancy Rockey, Ph.D. and her husband, Ron, are currently a part of the Faith for Today family health ministry. They have master's degrees in family therapy and doctorates in counseling psychology. **Feb. 12, July 8, Oct. 26.**

Antonio M. Rosario was born in the Dominican Republic, where he became acquainted with the Adventist message in 1970. After graduating from Antillian Adventist University, he pastored in Puerto Rico. He now pastors in New York. His wife, Wanda, is an R.N., and they have three children. **Apr. 21, Dec. 3.**

John H. Ryan is a retired administrator for the New York City Housing Authority. He enjoys gardening, singing, playing the piano, and serving as a local elder at the Honesdale, Pennsylvania, Seventh-day Adventist Church. **Aug. 29.**

Elmar P. Sakala, M.D., M.P.H., is director of medical student education in the Gynecology and Obstetrics Department at Loma Linda University. Elmar has delivered thousands of babies, and is the host of the daily syndicated radio program *Got a Minute for Your Health.* He and his wife, Darilee, have two grown children. **Jan. 4, Mar. 13, June 19, Aug. 23, Sept. 24, Oct. 11, Oct. 25.**

Dawna Sawatzky, R.N., M.P.H., has spent much of her time during the past few years in international health evangelism in Russia. Her book *Handy Guide for Teaching Kids About Health* has been published in Russia along with a series of health lessons. She and her dentist husband, Hans, live in Willits, California. **Jan. 26, May 9, June 22, July 28, Aug. 6, Oct. 31, Nov. 25.**

Jackson A. Saxon, M.D., is a board-certified anesthesiologist still practicing medicine. He has written many lay medical articles, two health booklets, and currently publishes a monthly health newsletter. In addition, he has conducted more than 250 stop-smoking programs, helping several thousand people to "kick the habit." **Apr. 13.**

L. J. Saxon is an automotive technologist and industrial electrician. Married, with two children, Lawrence became ill while working in the copper mines in Arizona. **Mar. 7.**

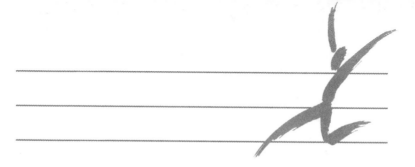

Richard A. Schaefer is director of community relations at Loma Linda University Medical Center. He is the author of *Legacy*, which tells the incredible story of past and ongoing miracles that make up the heritage of Loma Linda University and are the basis of the Seventh-day Adventist health message. **June 15, Sept. 5.**

John Scharffenberg, M.D., M.P.H., physician and nutritionist, is an elder, personal ministries leader, and health leader for his local church, plus consultant to the General Conference Health and Temperance Department and adjunct professor of nutrition at Loma Linda University. He and Carmyn Joyce live in North Fork, California. **Mar. 10.**

Blondel E. Senior, Ph.D., and his wife, Gloria, are cofounders and directors of Advent Home Youth Services, a licensed residential treatment program for boys in Calhoun, Tennessee. Blondel is a licensed professional counselor and a certified instructor in nonviolent crisis intervention. **Feb. 20, May 2, Oct. 5.**

Harold Shryock, M.D., is a retired physician who spent his entire professional career teaching medical students at Loma Linda University, which included 10 years as associate dean of the School of Medicine. Harold has written books and articles on all aspects of health. **Jan. 22, Mar. 20, Apr. 10, May 5, July 15.**

Jane Sines, R.N., M.P.H., designed and coordinated the health booth at the 1982 World's Fair in Knoxville, Tennessee, and is the director of Healthfest, held each year in Chattanooga. In addition, she manages her husband and son's dental practice and has four grown children and 13 grandchildren. **Dec. 2.**

Jerre St. Clair and her husband, Glenn, have dedicated their lives to mission service. She is an administrative secretary, and her husband is the administrator of the Masanga Leprosy Hospital and ADRA director for Sierra Leone and West Africa. **Mar. 31.**

Kari St. Clair, M.S., P.T., is a physical therapist who works in home health care. She and her husband, Jeff, live in La Follette, Tennessee, where he is in construction. Kari loves horses, cooking and canning, and people—but most of all, she loves the Lord. **Nov. 15.**

Roxy St. Clair and her husband, Fred, have been active lay leaders in Alabama where they lived for many years. They are continuing to minister in Costa Rica. **June 10.**

Connie Coble Starkey works at the Georgia-Cumberland Conference office as an administrative secretary and enjoys people, reading, and travel. She and her husband live in Calhoun, Georgia, where they enjoy time with extended family and friends. Connie's dad passed away on May 11, 1995. **Oct. 2.**

Lincoln Steed is editor of *Listen*, a drug education magazine for teens, and associate director of the International Commission for the Prevention of Alcoholism and Drug

Dependency. In addition, he has been book editor at Pacific Press and assistant editor of *Good Health* in Australia. He and his wife, Rosa Delia, live in West Virginia. **Oct. 17.**

Elizabeth Sterndale is former director of women's ministries for the North American Division and former associate in the Health and Temperance Department. Holding degrees in psychiatric nursing and administration, she enjoys traveling and volunteer mission service, and is a real friend to women in all cultures. **May 1.**

Nicole Sydenham is the wife of a pastor, Ron. They and their four children live in Winnipeg, Manitoba, where she serves as women's ministries director and works as an administrative assistant at the French School Division. She loves traveling and is a speaker for Family Matters. Nicole's accident happened in 1995. **July 20.**

Arlene Taylor, Ph.D., M.P.H., R.N., is founder and president of Realizations Inc., an educational, consulting, and brain profiling service. She is also director of risk management and infection control at St. Helena Hospital. Her latest self-help books are *Back to Basics* and with Lorna Lawrence, *Thresholds to Thriving.* **Dec. 29.**

Walter C. Thompson, M.D., is a surgeon and author of a book on how to make lifestyle changes dealing with stress, weight management, alcohol, tobacco, and sex through the power of God's love. He is married to Avonne, and they have four grandchildren. Walt helps various ministries and works with stained glass and cameras, and plays the guitar. **Feb. 24, May 27, June 14, July 18, Sept. 17, Oct. 7, Nov. 16.**

Agatha Thrash, M.D., is cofounder with her physician husband, Calvin, of Uchee Pines Institute in Seale, Alabama. She is a well-known authority on natural remedies and lifestyle medicine. She has lectured widely and written many books, including one on pets and the prevention of disease. **Apr. 25.**

Max C. Torkelsen II, M.P.H., is the health and communication director of the Upper Columbia Conference in Spokane, Washington. He and his wife, Linnea, have two daughters, Annalisa and Kirsten. Previously the family lived for eight years in Hawaii, "the healthiest state in the union." **Mar. 21, Dec. 10.**

Homer Trecartin, former pastor and teacher, is now the director of development at Georgia-Cumberland Academy. He and his wife, Barbara, have three children and enjoy outdoor activities and traveling. **Jan. 27.**

Therese Valin, Mar. 24.

J. Rita Vital, M.P.H., has been a teacher for kindergarten through college, a colporteur, Bible instructor, and health educator. She started Junior Adventurers in 1966 in Connecticut, established a church, and now is directing the Boston Van Ministry. She has three grown children. **Dec. 12.**

Pam Vredevelt, M.S., is a licensed counselor and works with Behavior Health Care

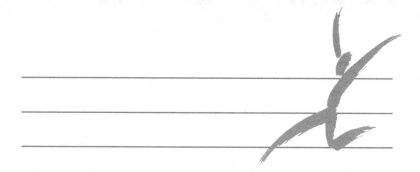

Northwest in Portland, Oregon. She's a pastor's wife with three children. Her youngest, Nathan, is a special needs child. Her story comes from her book *Empty Arms*, published by Questar Publishers and used with permission. **Jan. 10.**

Caroline Watkins is a human resource developer and member of the North American Division AIDS ad hoc committee. She serves on community advisory boards in the metro Atlanta area. Her love and dedication to the Lord inspire her to spread the health message to others. **Aug. 18, Sept. 25.**

Izak Wessels, M.Med., F.R.C.S.E., F.R.C.Ophth., F.A.C.S., lives in Chattanooga, Tennessee, with his wife, Elaine, and their three children. Born and raised in South Africa, Izak was an associate professor of opthalmology at Loma Linda University. Elaine works with women's ministries. **May 18, July 2, Oct. 18, Nov. 12, Dec. 18.**

Raymond O. West, M.D., former professor of epidemiology in the School of Public Health, Loma Linda University, is enjoying his retirement in Belfair, Washington, with his wife, Julie. **Feb. 28, May 25, Nov. 28.**

Ellen G. White, spiritual leader, inspirational author, and cofounder of the Seventh-day Adventist Church, was born November 26, 1827, and died July 16, 1915, at the age of 87. Through her lectures and thousands of written pages, Ellen White inspired many to live a more healthy lifestyle. **July 21.**

Crystal Whitten, M.S., R.D., teaches at the School of Allied Health Professions, Loma Linda University. **May 22, Sept. 22.**

DeWitt S. Williams, Ed.D., M.P.H., is director of the Department of Health and Temperance of the North American Division and previously served as president of the Central African Union. He and his wife, Margaret, who is an English teacher, have two grown daughters, Deitrice and Darnella. **Jan. 1, Mar. 6, Apr. 26, Oct. 30.**

Jeffrey K. Wilson is director of planned giving at Andrews University, and has been in development work at Faith for Today and in the Ohio Conference. He and Sharon, a nurse, have three children, Kimberly, Kevin, and Kari. His hobby is researching Abraham Lincoln's life and the events surrounding it. **Feb. 1, Apr. 15, Sept. 15, Dec. 1.**

Neal C. Wilson served as the world leader of the Seventh-day Adventist Church for 12 years. He and Elinor, his wife, have two children, Ted, who is president of the Review and Herald Publishing Association, and Shirley, who chairs the Department of Nursing at Columbia Union College. **Mar. 28.**

Richard Winn, M.A., M.Div., former president of Weimar Institute and associate professor of religion at Pacific Union College, is currently doing marketing consulting with Faith for Today. **May 28.**

Gregory R. Wise, M.D., M.P.H., is associate professor of medicine and head of the

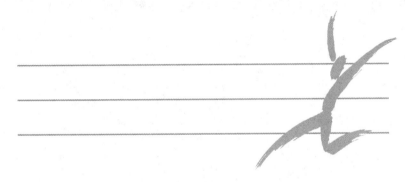

Division of General Internal Medicine and Geriatric Medicine at Loma Linda University. Before returning to Loma Linda, he spent six years in mission service at Bella Vista Hospital in Mayaguez, Puerto Rico. **May 19.**

Mary Wong, Ph.D., has served as an English teacher and chair of the English Department in several Adventist schools and colleges in Asia for many years. Her first love is teaching. Reading, music, and traveling are some of the hobbies she enjoys. **June 18, July 30.**

Roger D. Woodruff, M.D., is a family practice physician in Spokane, Washington. He and his wife, Krista, have two children. They are active in their local church and enjoy planting and harvesting produce from their land. **June 12.**

Ron Wylie, J.D., is a partner in the Washington/Baltimore law firm of Harriman, Jansak, Levy, and Wylie and has served as assistant to the administrator of the federal Medicare and Medicaid programs and as a member of the Health and Human Services Secretary's Task Force on Minority Health. Feb. 11.

THE HABIT
OF HAPPINESS

January 1

DeWitt S. Williams

A cheerful heart is good medicine, but a crushed spirit dries up the bones. Prov. 17:22, NIV.

Happiness is an illusive butterfly. If pursued directly, it flits away beyond our reach. But if we sit down contented with what we have, it's likely to perch on our shoulder. Perhaps that's why only 10 to 15 percent of Americans consider themselves truly happy.

As John Powell (author of *Happiness Is an Inside Job*) puts it, happiness "is not like putting so many coins into a happiness-dispensing machine. Then suddenly out comes the candy bar of happiness!" Happiness, he says, is an inside job. To the extent we think our happiness will come from outside things or other persons, our dreams are destined to die.

The sad fact is that almost half of all first marriages end in divorce, as do 65 percent of all second marriages! Disillusion always seems to follow when we expect someone (like a spouse or friend) or something (such as fame or fortune) to make us happy.

Yet we are all capable of acquiring the habit of happiness, regardless of the depressing world in which we live. When we watch television and see what's happening around us—child and spousal abuse, chemical dependency, teenage pregnancy, gangs, bulging prisons, wars, AIDS—it is not surprising that the World Health Organization has singled out depression as the world's most widespread disease. One third of all Americans wake up depressed every day. *But you don't have to be one of them!*

Are you happy with your work? This may be the most important question one can ask that relates to life expectancy. If you are not happy with your work, you should either get happy with it or change your job.

Are you happy at home? Invite Christ in. "With Jesus in the family, happy, happy home."

Are you happy with yourself? You can become the person you and God want you to become. But regardless, Jesus still loves you. Why shouldn't you like yourself if God already does?

So as we begin our journey together to a more vibrant life, I wish you a *happy* new year. Not just today or during the month of January, but all through the year and until Jesus comes again. Choose happiness and live!

Choose happiness. Resolve to replace every negative thought with thoughts of God's blessings. You can have a happy new year!

E-2

33

Jan W. and Kay Kuzma

Do you not know that in a race all the runners run, but only one gets the prize? Run in such a way as to get the prize. 1 Cor. 9:24, NIV.

I f you have no vision of your potential, you have no hope of victory. Circumstances will control your life, and you'll find yourself sitting on the sidelines. You need to climb the mountains in your life and give it your best.

Peter Nelson, a 45-year-old dentist from San Luis Obispo, California, was asked to join an expedition climbing 29,028-foot Mount Everest. It was very unusual for a man his age who was not a professional climber to be asked to join the 10-member team. But because he lived a healthy vegetarian Adventist lifestyle, he was one of the most fit.

During the final stages of the climb the group, wanting someone to set a good pace, put Peter in the lead. Hoping to get to camp 4 by nightfall and finish the climb of 2,000 feet to the top the next day, he pushed to climb 5,000 feet that day.

As he approached camp 4 his lungs began to fill with fluid from altitude sickness (pulmonary edema), which sometimes kills in 20 to 40 minutes. He spent the night sitting up, breathing oxygen, fighting for each breath, and praying.

In the morning he began his trip down the mountain, while his team went on to the top without him.

When someone asked Peter how he felt having failed to reach the top, he replied, "Victory is in running the race. I had an opportunity to climb Mount Everest. Reaching the top would have been wonderful, but what's really important is that you climb all the mountains in your life with courage and joy."

What "mountains" are you facing today? Why not ask God to give you His courage and joy for the climb?

SPIRITUAL
FREEDOM

January 3

Dan Matthews

Now the Lord is the Spirit, and where the Spirit of the Lord is, there is freedom. 2 Cor. 3:17, RSV.

When you ask people to name the most spiritual person they know, you get an amazing array of answers. Some think of people in the Middle Ages who walked on cold floors with bare feet and made sure their stomachs were always growling. Those who admire this kind of individual have a dark suspicion that submitting to harsh circumstances and even cruel superiors must be very spiritual. Perhaps it's because they think of God as harsh and cruel.

Others will suggest people who are quiet and gentle—pious individuals who never make quick moves or loud sounds and who certainly never do anything spontaneous or fun. Perhaps again their admirers worship a very uptight God.

But it's clear this is not what Paul had in mind when he looked for the signs of a truly spiritual person. He knew that when the Lord's Spirit touches the core of someone's life, they discover freedom. Paul thought of people whose faces are brighter, whose steps are lighter, and who know a wonderful creativity and boldness as they face life.

We're not talking about a reckless freedom, an irresponsible license to indulge hurtful desires. Rather we're discussing freedom from the fear of rejection, freedom from the need to ask other people's permission to forgive oneself. This is freedom to grasp life at a new level and grow in directions of one's own choosing. It is freedom from the fears of failure that have haunted us since childhood and kept us from launching into life as a daring adventure. Such freedom taps our most creative juices and allows us to become the unique, one-of-a-kind persons God intends for us to be.

Jesus spent a lot of His ministry setting people free from the false notions about His Father taught by the religious establishment of the day. His fresh understanding of spirituality still lurks today on the edges of our souls, waiting to break us free! We must believe His words: "So if the Son makes you free, you will be free indeed" (John 8:36, RSV). That's good news!

How is your spiritual health? What can you do to experience the freedom Jesus offers you?

35

PRAYER IS
THE BREATH
OF THE SOUL

January 4

Elmar P. Sakala

> But I call to God, and the Lord saves me. Evening, morning and noon
> I cry out in distress, and he hears my voice. Ps. 55:16, 17, NIV.

While the baby is still in the uterus, it is obviously unable to breathe air into its lungs. Yet as soon as it is born it must be ready to start breathing within seconds. For the baby to go from living comfortably in a bath of warm water for nine months to suddenly surviving in cold, dry air takes a lot of preparation. How can this happen? Does the Creator leave it to chance? No! In His usual ingenious manner God has designed that the baby will perform special exercises to get ready for this vital event.

Before birth the baby regularly exercises the chest muscles used to breathe air after birth. Such breathing exercises start early in pregnancy and are a normal part of what the baby does when it is awake. The closer the baby gets to the time to be born, the more it does its special exercises. When the baby is asleep it lies still, allowing the breathing muscles to rest.

Even though the baby cannot take air into its lungs when it moves its chest, the exercises are very important. As well as keeping the breathing muscles strong, the breathing movements help the millions of tiny air sacs in the lungs to develop normally. The baby will need to fill the air sacs with air when he or she takes his or her first breath after birth.

Babies unable to perform breathing movements in the uterus not only have weak breathing muscles and get tired quickly, but their lung air sacs may not develop properly.

Prayer is the breath of the soul. Like a baby exercising its breathing movements before it needs it, we must be exercising our spiritual "breathing movements" regularly, or our spiritual muscles will be weak, our spiritual growth will be limited, and we won't have the spiritual health we need to make it through tough times.

Am I getting the spiritual exercise I need to
grow spiritually strong and healthy?

THE MIRACLE BEAN

Mark and Virginia Messina

Every good endowment and every perfect gift is from above, coming down from the Father of lights with whom there is no variation or shadow due to change. James 1:17, RSV.

Webster defines a miracle as "an extraordinary event manifesting divine intervention in human affairs." Usually we think of miracles as events that are beyond our limited human understanding of the natural world. They inspire awe and bring us to our knees in the humbling presence of God's power and mercy, such as during a spontaneous healing of a life-threatening disease.

But most of us recognize that even some easily explained, everyday occurrences so reflect God's goodness and magnificence that they contain a touch of the miraculous. No matter that science explains their occurrence. They still take our breath away and fill us with awe just the same, whether it be the cry of a newborn baby or a perfect rainbow.

But some miracles seem to escape our notice because we don't look hard enough or we forget that God's gifts to us are not always earth-shattering.

Nutritionists who study plant-based diets have found such a "miracle." Soybeans are rich in the highest quality protein. Inexpensive and easy to grow, they produce 20 times more protein an acre than an acre devoted to raising beef. So versatile is the soybean that in one form or another it appears in nearly every kind of dish imaginable. Packaged in this little bean is a host of natural substances that have impressive health protective effects, earning soy the nickname "miracle bean." Scientists have found in soybeans substances called isoflavones, which appear in no other commonly consumed food. Isoflavones have been linked to a reduced risk for cancer, heart disease, and osteoporosis.

A miracle? Webster might not agree that soybeans meet the strictest definition of that word. But God's people know that the true miracle is His never-ending desire to bless us with gifts for our welfare and happiness. Each of these gifts is a miraculous sign of His great love for us. They come in big and small packages, and often escape our notice. But our lives are enriched when we recognize and are grateful for each gift—whether it be healing, a baby, a rainbow, or a little brown bean.

Lord, teach me to see the many gifts with which You bless my life, and to be always thankful for all the good things You provide.

SUBSTITUTING
PRAISE
FOR PAIN

January 6

Debby Bullock

I will praise you, Lord, with all my heart. I will tell all the miracles you have done. I will be happy because of you. God Most High, I will sing praises to your name. Ps. 9:1, 2, EB.

Sometimes it seems as if the whole world comes crashing in on you at once. My husband's back problem threatened to leave him a helpless cripple. My father-in-law died. Benji, our firstborn, hemorrhaged and was facing surgery. Then it happened . . .

A blowout forced me to the side of the road. I remember bending down to fit the jack, and the next thing I knew, I was picking myself up from down the embankment. Someone had sideswiped my car.

Not until a couple hours later did the pain hit—excruciating, nauseating pain shot down from my shoulder through my body, leaving my head throbbing. "Probably just a pulled muscle," the doctor said.

A couple weeks later I became incapacitated with pain spasms so severe that I'd lose consciousness. I was hospitalized for a month, then bedridden at home for six months with pain so intense that I almost existed on morphine. Later a doctor in Edmonton said he'd never seen such a severe reverse whiplash and exclaimed, "You should have been killed instantly!" I owe my life to being in peak physical condition. My body simply bent instead of breaking! But as a result of the stress on my system I had come down with Fibromyalgia, a disease that now forces me to live in constant pain.

At first I fought it, became depressed, and felt a burden to my family. My negative attitude put a chasm between me and God. But as I began to read and pray, I came to realize that I was responsible for my own health and happiness. I needed to accept my condition and live life within my limits. My worth was not tied to my works.

I believe God is in the process of healing me. I may never be free of pain. The miracle is that He is giving me an attitude of praise that supersedes the pain. When I begin to count my blessings—when I focus on praising Him—I don't notice the pain.

*What are you thankful for today? How can you
live in an attitude of praise all day?*

LOOK BEFORE YOU SWALLOW

January 7

Marjorie V. Baldwin

Test everything. Hold on to the good. 1 Thess. 5:21, NIV.

Swallowing is such an easy thing to do. It is one of the things we do best. We pop in the food, give it a crunch or two, swallow—and it's gone.

But hold on a minute. That swallow, so simple, constant, and automatic, is a very complicated physiological action. It requires the carefully orchestrated and cooperative efforts of more than 30 muscles or groups of muscles! And once the symphony is begun, you can't stop it at will. The act of swallowing moves on to the completed act—that of digesting and absorbing the food that eventually becomes you.

The process begins in your brain. You see a beautiful apple with a mouthwatering aroma. Grasping it, you bite into it. If as you begin to chew you note half a worm in the uneaten portion, you can easily eject what is in your mouth. No problem. But once you have swallowed apple and worm, only much more violent and unpleasant measures can prevent digestion and the worm becoming part of you.

So it is with truth and error. You perceive an inviting concept and ingest it into your mental and spiritual "mouth." If on closer examination and comparison with the criteria of truth it remains acceptable, you may swallow and integrate it into your character. If, however, it hides error, hopefully you reject it before you swallow.

Being indifferent to what you think about, or neglecting to evaluate things critically, will permit the accepted error to become part of your mental and spiritual self—your character. Only by violent, painful effort can you heave it out.

Joseph fled pressured temptation, even at the sake of losing his coat, his reputation, and his freedom, in order to preserve his integrity and loyalty. Job said, "I made a covenant with my eyes not to look lustfully at a girl" (Job 31:1, NIV). Jesus taught us to pray, "Lead us not into temptation" (Matt. 6:13).

Don't swallow sin. Saying no to temptation has its reward—a seat with Jesus on His throne, access to the tree of life, eternal wisdom, health, and vibrant happiness.

Lord, help me to know the difference between truth and error, and to accept and love only truth.

130-YEAR-OLD HEALTH INFORMA- TION CONFIRMED

I desire to do your will, O my God; your law is within my heart. Ps. 40:8, NIV.

In 1863 the Seventh-day Adventist Church officially organized. That same year Ellen G. White received her first vision on the principles underlying health reform. These and subsequent instructions, confirmed by modern science in recent years, shaped the health practices of the church's members. And all this began at a time when bloodletting and the almost indiscriminate use of powerful drugs were the tools of medicine, while the sciences of physiology, biochemistry, microbiology, and nutrition were in their infancy or had yet to emerge. The recommendations she made include:

• Reduce fat, especially animal fat. Now known to increase cholesterol, atherosclerosis, heart disease, and stroke.

• Use whole-grain wheat flour in breadmaking rather than the superfine white flour then considered the best.

• Avoid overeating and being overweight, today recognized as public health problems.

• Use salt sparingly and avoid baking soda and powder in making bread. This given long before research showed their role in high blood pressure and chronic kidney failure.

• Breast-feed babies. This at a time when bottle feeding was becoming popular. Now science recognizes mother's milk as the ideal nutrition for an infant.

• Use grains, fruits, nuts, and vegetables to make the most healthful diet. Ellen White recommended this at a time when many ridiculed a vegetarian diet. Recent research has shown that vegetarian diets provide desirable levels of unsaturated fat, generous amounts of complex carbohydrates, and an abundance of vitamins, minerals, dietary fiber, and other biologically active components. Such a diet protects against coronary heart disease, stroke, hypertension, diabetes, kidney disease, and a variety of cancers. In 1993 the American Dietetic Association officially recognized in a position paper the adequacy and benefits of a vegetarian diet.

And what did Ellen White say of that first health reform vision in 1863? "I saw that it was a sacred duty to attend to our health." Medical science confirms the strong connection between physical well-being and psychological well-being.

What adjustments should you make in your lifestyle to live up to how you know you should be living?

ELLEN WHITE'S STRUGGLE WITH MEAT-EATING

Jan W. and Kay Kuzma

Because the Sovereign Lord helps me, I will not be disgraced. Therefore have I set my face like flint, and I know I will not be put to shame. Isa. 50:7, NIV.

One of the most admired individuals in the 150-year history of the Seventh-day Adventist Church is its cofounder Ellen G. White, who wrote 26 books in current circulation, 4,600 articles, and more than 200 tracts and pamphlets, many of which had to do with some facet of health, and all of which she wrote in longhand.

What's incredible is that Ellen White had such poor health herself that few expected her to survive childhood. She was a cheerful, buoyant, active child until 9 years of age, when a rock thrown by another child hit her in the head. It broke her nose and she remained unconscious for three weeks. The experience left her disfigured, ill, and debilitated. For two years she was unable to breathe through her nose. She was nervous and unable to hold her hand sufficiently steady to write, and the effort to read made her dizzy. Despite poor health she tried repeatedly to attend school, but the effort was too much, and finally she gave up when she was 12.

With this background, how was she able to live to 87 years of age and accomplish so much? It was partially as a result of her willingness to change her lifestyle as new principles of healthful living became plain to her. But it was not without a struggle. For example, she loved meat. But after her 1863 vision in which she learned the dangers of eating flesh foods, she told the cook, "No more meat from now on!"

When the family came for breakfast and there wasn't any meat on the table, Ellen took one look and disgustedly left the room. When she returned at noontime, again there was no meat, and she refused to eat. The next day she felt so hungry that the simple food looked more appetizing to her, so she could finally eat.

If you're struggling to make healthful changes, take courage. Set your face "like flint," and the Lord will help you. Others have struggled before you and have been victorious. You can too.

In what area of health do you need to set your face "like flint" and do what you know you should?

LETTING GO

Pam Vredevelt

And we know that in all things God works for the good of those who love him,
who have been called according to his purpose. Rom. 8:28, NIV.

After our first baby died, there came times when I said to myself, "Pam, you've got to let go and move on with life." It was easier said than done. To break away from someone we have been bonded to tears apart our emotions. The greater the bond, the greater the pain.

Usually when our awareness of our loss increases, so does our pain. A cartoon showed a woman with her head and arms squeezing through the wringer of an old washing machine. Her face was full of anguish. The caption read: "The truth will set you free, but first it will make you miserable." It's very painful to face the full impact of our losses.

Letting go demands that we allow ourselves to feel our pain and ride out the grief. Some of my favorite sayings are "Feeling is healing" and "Birds fly, fish swim, people feel." Numbing our feelings with addictive behavior prolongs and intensifies our grief and blocks us from successfully letting go.

During the painful times of life when I am having to let go of something or someone dear to me, I've found that God is the one to run to.

God has the power to heal the pain. But He will never force us to let go of something to which we cling. Instead, He will wait compassionately for us to release our grip, open our hands, and invite Him to participate in our lives. Once we have invited Him into our lives, we have an eternal guarantee that He will be with us no matter what circumstances bring our way. And He promises to help us let go of our pain a little at a time.

One day we will be able to look back and see how God's hand has been on our lives. But not until history has run its course will we fully understand how "all things work together for good." So for now we must choose a life of faith, which means believing in advance what will make sense only in hindsight.

How do you feel about the phrase "Feeling is healing"?
Why is it so hard to let go?

1 CORINTHIANS 13
FOR HEALTH
PROFESSIONALS

January 11

Hans Diehl

And now these three remain: faith, hope and love.
But the greatest of these is love. 1 Cor. 13:13, NIV.

I may be a famous scientist or practicing physician and display in my office many diplomas and degrees. I may be considered an excellent teacher and a convincing speaker. But if I have no love, my words are worth no more than a noisy gong or a clanging bell.

I may have the gifts of an outstanding clinician, making difficult diagnoses, and understanding all the mysteries of the human body. And I may communicate well to my patients to enable them to make better lifestyle choices. But if I have no love, I am nobody.

I may invest all my money to build the best facilities and purchase the best equipment. I may provide the best staff to treat my patients. I may devote all my time to their care, even to the point of neglecting my family or myself. But if I have not love, it profits me nothing.

Love is nature's medicine. It is natural and does not depress the immune system, but enhances it.

Love can be combined with many remedies; it is an outstanding catalyst. Love relieves pain and maintains life at its best.

Love is tolerated by anyone, never causing allergic reactions or intolerance.

New medicines come and go. What was considered good yesterday may be useless today. What is considered good today may be worthless tomorrow. But love has passed the test of time; it will be effective always.

We now understand things only partially, and new therapies are often only experimental, for our gifts of knowledge and inspired discoveries are only partial.

When all things will be understood, only then we will recognize the true value of love.

Love is the finest agent to create rapport between patients, relatives, and friends. It will help us to act not as children, but as mature adults.

Today many truths appear as blurred images to health professionals. We still don't understand how the things of the Spirit work to maintain life. But one day we shall see all things very clearly.

Still there remains three basic remedies: faith, hope, and love. The greatest of these is love.

Lord, help me not to be so busy doing good that I don't
have time to experience God's love and give it away.

BY THE BLOOD OF THE LAMB

Jean Marie Hametz

They overcame him by the blood of the Lamb and by the word of their testimony; they did not love their lives so much as to shrink from death. Rev. 12:11, NIV.

The way our blood fights the body's enemies offers a wonderful object lesson in how Christ's blood enables us to overcome sin. Every day we encounter hundreds of germs that could make us sick or even kill us. Yet usually we are unaware of them.

What happens inside the body when it is invaded by these tiny enemies? As soon as the body detects an invading object, or pathogen, the body makes what is known as antibodies. They are protein molecules in the blood that fight the pathogen. The next time the same pathogen invades the body, special types of cells known as memory cells detect the infectious agent and quickly act to help the body form the exact antibodies needed to fight the enemy.

At birth a baby receives antibodies from its mother through the placenta and her milk. For the first few months of life the baby actually has resistance to or immunity from the diseases its mother has had even though the child hasn't had the diseases itself. The baby is safe from every pathogen the mother has successfully battled.

In the same way, when we are born again by faith in Jesus Christ we receive power to overcome all sin. Jesus was exposed to all sin for us, so we may overcome through faith in Him. The Bible tells us: "For we do not have a high priest who is unable to sympathize with our weaknesses, but we have one who has been tempted in every way, just as we are—yet was without sin" (Heb. 4:15, NIV).

Jesus took on every sin for us. Imagine if a mother could allow herself to be exposed to every physical disease in the world in order to pass on immunity to her children! Even the most loving mother has never done that. Yet Jesus risked it all so that we could overcome!

Help me to trust You, Lord Jesus, and the power of Your blood to forgive my past sins and give me the ability to overcome current temptations.

CAUGHT WITH HIGH BLOOD PRESSURE

Henry C. Martin

> The thief comes only to steal and kill and destroy; I have come that they may have life, and have it to the full. John 10:10, NIV.

Your blood pressure is markedly elevated. Have you seen your doctor?" That was the first warning that I had hypertension. Attending a national convention in San Francisco, I found myself attracted to a routine health screening booth in the Moscone Convention Center exhibit hall. Since then I have learned that sometimes the first symptom of heart disease is sudden death. Anxiously I went to the telephone to call a physician friend.

My father had died from heart disease just 10 days after my mother succumbed to diabetes and depression. Of course, I had inherited genes from my parents. The husbands of both of my younger sisters had strokes. Now I discovered myself suffering from high blood pressure, and I didn't want to have it!

Having heard of the natural lifestyle medicine taught at Weimar Institute, I contacted Dr. Vernon Foster, who urged me to enter the NEW-START lifestyle program that had just begun. While there I learned the eight natural remedies that put me on the road to better health: nutrition, exercise, water, sunlight, temperance (self-control), air, rest, and trust.

Eighty percent of men are able to discontinue blood pressure medication in less than three weeks. After adopting a whole plant food diet and regular exercise, I observed a steady drop in my weight, blood pressure, and cholesterol. Now more than 10 years later I continue to be blessed with improved health. I have just returned from a 41-mile family backpack trip in the Rogue River Wilderness. Ten years ago I'm not sure I would have made it!

The good news is that you don't have to be what you are. You and I can take charge of our lives right now. You can use your power of choice to select healthy, natural foods and choose a stronger immune system. Even the testimony of a healthy Christian is more effective. Jesus came so that we "might have life, and . . . have it more abundantly" (John 10:10).

Are you following God's health principles so you can enjoy the abundant life Jesus wants us to have?

GROWING
OLD HEALTHY

Moses was a hundred and twenty years old when he died, yet his eyes were not weak nor his strength gone. Deut. 34:7, NIV.

The seasoned leader sat alone, saddened by the reality of impending death. His life's dream lay below him in awesome splendor and inspiring beauty. His disease-free heart thrilled within him as he considered entering the Promised Land, but his crystal-clear mind reminded him that he would not set foot in Canaan.

Moses sat upon Mount Nebo in good health, waiting to die! His eyesight, perfect in his advanced age, took in the rapture of the scene before him. He did not have to squint or adjust his glasses. Though he had just climbed the mountain, he felt no fatigue, nor was his heart pounding from the strain of the climb. "His eyes were not weak nor his strength gone."

At 120 years of age Moses was in good health, a living testimony of the result of following the Lord's lifestyle plan. There was no physical reason for Moses to die, only spiritual. God had told him he would not enter Canaan because he had struck the rock twice. As his life had been an example of the result of obedience to God's natural law, now his death would be an example of disobedience to God's spiritual commands.

Today when someone is diagnosed with colon polyps, the reaction typically is "Oh, well, everyone gets these by the time they're 60; it's just part of growing old." When a doctor informs a retired man that he has cataracts and needs expensive surgery, what's the response? "Well, I should have known this would happen. Cataracts are a part of growing old."

But is it? Here are some interesting statements to consider: "Obedience to God's law in every respect would save men from . . . disease of every type" *(Temperance,* p. 228). "Every practice which destroys the physical, mental, or spiritual energies is sin" *(The Ministry of Healing,* p. 113). "The burden of sin, with its unrest and unsatisfied desires, lies at the very foundation of a large share of the maladies the sinner suffers" *(Testimonies,* vol. 4, p. 579).

Maybe old age isn't to blame! It's something to think about, isn't it?

Sickness and disease don't need to be an expected part of growing older if you maintain your body with God's lifestyle plan.

Let the morning bring me word of your unfailing love, for I have put my trust in you. Show me the way I should go, for to you I lift up my soul. Ps. 143:8, NIV.

There's no great accomplishment just in living many years," said an active 91-year-old. "Nursing homes are filled with medicated survivors—as if that has to be the fate of those who reach old age. But to live to those ages and still be independent, physically active, and mentally alert, *that* is an accomplishment."

And that's exactly what Charlotte Hamlin has been doing as she sets walking and cycling records across the country. "The closer we live by the laws of nature," she says, "the better we will feel and the longer we will live." And what are the laws of nature? According to Charlotte, the secret's in the acronym FRESH START: Fresh air, Rest, Exercise, Sunshine, Happiness, Simple diet, The use of water, Abstemiousness, Restoration, and Trust in divine power.

Charlotte, nearing her eightieth birthday, cycles from 50 to 80 miles a day and has proved to millions that we can stay productive and healthy at any age. From 1973 until she retired in 1986 she organized and directed a summer health-screening program, and founded the three C's, a risk evaluation program that tested for potential risk for coronaries, cancer, and CVA (stroke).

In 1986 Charlotte retired as assistant professor of nursing at Andrews University and established FRESH START, a health-conditioning live-in program. When she was 68 she and her son, Gene, formed a nonprofit organization, Global Trek International.

The same year she walked and cycled from coast to coast, leaving southern California in March 1987 and arriving 67 days later at Charleston, South Carolina. She made a 32-day trek across Europe that fall. The following year her 9,000 miles of pedaling took her through portions of Israel, Pakistan, India, Thailand, China, Japan, Guam, and Hawaii, and she finished at her birthplace in Canada on her seventieth birthday.

An article about Charlotte carried the title "Too Fit to Quit." Not a bad slogan as she pedals around the world, reminding us that God has a work for us to do, regardless of our age.

What could you be doing to help you earn
the slogan "Too Fit to Quit"?

USE IT
OR
LOSE IT!

January 16
Bernell E. Baldwin

Wisdom is supreme; therefore get wisdom. Though it cost all you have, get understanding. Esteem her, and she will exalt you; embrace her, and she will honor you. Prov. 4:7, 8, NIV.

At the University of California in Berkeley scientists put rats into four different environments to test the effect on their brains.

Group 1 experienced *solitary confinement*. The rats were given food and water only.

Group 2 experienced *social enrichment*. Three animals occupied each cage.

Group 3 experienced *environmental enrichment*. In addition to three in a cage, a new toy or device was added every day for 30 days.

Group 4 experienced a *natural environment*. Instead of a cage, the rats were put in a large area with a buried fence, with stars and sky for ceiling and earth for floor. For challenges they had hawks by day and owls by night looking to make them fresh meals! Immediately the rats were motivated into action. They dug holes and tunnels to obtain food, water, and friends.

In group 3, in which the rats had environmental enrichment, their average brain weight increased 7 or 8 percent. They had more and better dendrites, which are the long fingers of nerve cells—the input connectors in the brain. Their brains had increased amounts of the chemical choline acetylase (ah-SEAT-ul-ase), which is important in intelligence. (Note: this is the chemical that decreases in Alzheimer's disease.) Hexokinase (hex-o-KIN-ase), the chemical that helps energy get from the blood into the brain, also increased. In addition, the rats were faster and smarter in getting through a maze.

But the most amazing finding was with the group 4 rats in the *natural environment*. Their brain weight went up 12-13 percent, almost twice as much as those in the artificially enriched environment of group 3.

Why did this happen? It is called the *law of atrophy of disuse*. Simply stated, "Use it or lose it."

I'm reminded of Ellen White's words: "Action is a law of our being. Every organ of the body [including the brain] has its appointed work, upon the performance of which its development and strength depend" *(The Ministry of Healing, p. 237)*.

The question is What are you doing for your brain? Are you in group 1: lonely and feeling sorry for yourself? group 2: with friends, but inactive? or in group 3: getting a lot of artificial stimulation? Hopefully, you're a group 4 person, enjoying God's natural environment and motivated activity.

Lord, help me to use it—not lose it!
Increase my wisdom and understanding.

SUGARCOATED
SIN

January 17
Jerry Muncy

> He [Moses] chose to be mistreated along with the people of God rather than
> to enjoy the pleasures of sin for a short time. Heb. 11:25, NIV.

'll never forget the first time we flew into the poverty-stricken village of
Ocoroni, Mexico, to hold a dental clinic. The minute we touched down
on that tiny 1,500-foot dirt landing strip more than 100 children ran to
the plane, hoping for handouts. When they smiled up at us, my heart sank.
Many of them had their front teeth rotted off to the gums because of the
habit of sucking on sugarcane.

The children suffered from ignorance and poverty. Sugarcane made
them feel good. But they had no one to tell them it was a deceptive pleasure that would end up destroying their teeth, causing them incredible pain
and eventual loss.

We could do little with those who flocked to our open shed where we
set up our dental clinic but pull teeth. One woman kept trying to move
ahead in the line. Through an interpreter we learned that because of the
pain she was suffering she had walked 30 miles (50 kilometers) to get to the
clinic, and would have to go back home that day. I pulled 15 of her teeth,
each one so rotted down to the gums that I hardly had anything to get a grip
on. If only these people had realized the hidden dangers of sugarcane!

Then I thought about the children in my country whose front teeth had
begun to rot. Not from sugarcane, but from apple juice, soft drinks, and
soda pop given in a bottle from the time they were tiny babies. Some parents didn't know how dangerous it was to allow a child to suck on juice or
milk and fall asleep with their teeth literally "sugarcoated." Others, not
wanting to put up with a fuss at bedtime if they removed the juice-filled
bottle, allowed their innocent children the pleasure that would later result
in damaged teeth.

It made me think about how much sin is like sugarcane or the sugar-
sweet liquid in a bottle. It tastes good at the time, but without realizing it,
we are being destroyed. The pleasures of sin, even for a short time, can
have long-lasting and painful consequences.

Lord, open my eyes to the hidden dangers of "sugarcoated" sin.

CURE WORRY
WITH A SONG

January 18
Jan W. and Kay Kuzma

Therefore I tell you, do not worry about your life, what you will eat; or about your body, what you will wear. Life is more than food, and the body more than clothes. Luke 12:22, 23, NIV.

J. C. Penney, the genius behind one of the world's largest chains of department stores, had built his business to a multimillion-dollar level when he lost $40 million in the crash of 1929. Three years later, when he was 56 years of age, he had to sell out to satisfy his creditors, leaving him virtually broke. He worried so much that he couldn't sleep. The stress from his chronic fatigue depressed his immune system, and he suffered a relapse of the chicken pox virus that had been dormant in his nerves since he had had the rash as a child. The recurrence of this virus, called shingles, causes severe pain. He was hospitalized at the Battle Creek Sanitarium and given sedatives, but he still tossed and turned all night. Broken physically and mentally, he was overwhelmed with a fear of death and wrote farewell letters to his wife and son, since he didn't expect to live until morning.

Then he awoke to the staff singing in the hospital chapel, "Be not dismayed whate'er betide, God will take care of you . . ." Following the music to its source, he slipped into a back row. Mr. Penney said something happened at that moment that he couldn't explain. "I felt as if I had been instantly lifted out of the darkness of a dungeon into warm, brilliant sunlight. I felt the power of God as I had never felt it before. I realized that I alone was responsible for all my troubles. I knew that God with His love was there to help me. From that day to this, my life has been free from worry. I am 71 years old, and the most dramatic and glorious minutes of my life were those I spent in that chapel that morning."

As a result of the renewing of J. C. Penney's mind through the power of a song, he went on to rebuild his financial empire to well over the billion-dollar mark and celebrated with his family and friends his ninety-fifth birthday.

When you're tempted to worry,
what song could you think of or sing to relieve the stress?

BREAKING AN ADDICTIVE HABIT

I can do all things through Christ who strengthens me. Phil. 4:13, NKJV.

Again and again you've tried to quit. You're tired of the guilt that comes from your dependance on food, coffee, sex, pills, cigarettes, alcohol, drugs, or whatever. How can you obtain freedom from your addiction? The following seven steps may be your answer.

Step 1: *Exercise.* A brisk walk, a swim, or a bike ride will help by physically removing you from the temptation. Exercise produces endorphins that encourage feelings of optimism and happiness. It gives you energy and relieves the stress that drives you to your habit.

Step 2: *Practice positive self-talk.* High self-esteem enables you to see your potential instead of your failures. Remind yourself of your talents and abilities. Stop putting yourself down. When you get up in the morning, look in the mirror and say, "I like myself just the way I am!" (including bulges, hang-ups, and all).

Step 3: *Focus on peace of mind.* Turmoil and unrest cause you to revert to your bad habits. A sense of contentment can silence that inner unrest. When you feel upset, read Psalm 23 and focus your thoughts on that green pasture and still water that God has promised you.

Step 4: *Accept the fact that you're human and that you may blow it occasionally.* All people have setbacks as they try to break an addictive habit. But feelings of failure lead to guilt and discouragement, which in turn may drive you back to your habit for comfort. It's a vicious cycle, so don't get caught in it. Don't expect yourself to be perfect.

Step 5: *Develop an "I can" philosophy.* The ability to break your addictive habit is to a great extent dependent on your attitude. If you truly believe you can do it, you will be more likely to succeed.

Step 6: *Develop your power of choice.* Willpower is the best tool to use when trying to break a habitual behavior. It's the ability to say no to something you want and know you shouldn't have.

Step 7: *Ask for Jesus' power.* Even though you may have the desire to quit, remember, the power to do so comes from outside yourself. Claim the promise "I can do all things through Christ who strengthens me."

God longs to give you the peace and power you need to change your bad habits. Remember, with God all things are possible.

WHAT RESEARCH SAYS ABOUT THE ADVENTIST LIFESTYLE

January 20

Jan W. Kuzma

My son, do not forget my teaching, but keep my commands in your heart, for they will prolong your life many years and bring you prosperity. Prov. 3:1, 2, NIV.

The year 1967 was a landmark year for Adventist health. That year the School of Public Health began at Loma Linda University, and the *Adventist Review* published the article "The Life Expectancy of SDAs" (Dec. 14, 1967), based on research that indicated that SDAs outlived the average American by several years. The results gave the first quantitative figures to substantiate what Adventists have long believed—that by adopting healthy lifestyles individuals could make a difference in how long they lived.

Researchers at Loma Linda believed that the difference in life expectancy resulted primarily from not smoking. However, questions were being raised about the role of a vegetarian lifestyle, exercise, and weight loss.

Using the same life table analyses used in the 1967 article, researchers published in the June 29, 1989, *Adventist Review* an article on the lifestyle and life expectancy of SDAs. The results, based on 26 years of follow-up, revealed the life expectancy of a 35-year-old SDA male to be 8.9 years longer than an average California male, and that of a 35-year-old SDA female to be 7.5 years longer. Researchers found that vegetarian men outlived nonvegetarian men by 3.7 years. Those who exercised outlived others by as much as five years, and there was a two-year difference in men who were trim versus those who were at least 20 percent overweight. Such findings substantiated the effectiveness of the health principles long advocated by the church.

Dr. T. Abelin from Harvard University noted that the increase in life expectancy observed by SDAs exceeded all the gains in life expectancy made in the previous 40 years in this country, including advances in medical skills and knowledge and in the environment.

So why did God entrust us with the knowledge of healthful living? Was it so that we could live longer and better and have fewer diseases? Was it so we could radiate more of the joy of living? Was it so we could be better examples to others so that they can enjoy life more? Or was it so we would be more receptive to what God is trying to communicate to us and what He would like us to do?

What do I need to change in my lifestyle to be more receptive to God's will for me?

IT ISN'T FAIR!

Norma J. McKellip

If you listen carefully to the voice of the Lord your God and do what is right in his eyes, if you pay attention to his commands and keep all his decrees, I will not bring on you any of the diseases I brought on the Egyptians, for I am the Lord who heals you. Ex. 15:26, NIV.

t's just not fair! I thought. *Why doesn't God keep His promise? Is He really who He says He is?* I was upset with God. It seemed as if my faith were trapped in a dark valley.

My mom, a genuine Christian, had experienced relatively good health for 80 years. Because she loved God, she served Him faithfully. She walked in the "good works" Paul spoke of in Ephesians 2:10: "For we are God's workmanship, created in Christ Jesus to do good works, which God prepared in advance for us to do" (NIV).

In her 80s my mom began experiencing nausea and extreme vomiting. The physicians diagnosed her with cirrhosis of the liver. I thought cirrhosis was a disease of alcoholism, and my mother didn't drink—never had! At the most she had probably had one or two tablespoons in medicine when a child.

The doctor read my puzzled look and said, "I know, you're wondering how can this be? We don't know either. When this happens, we suspect the individual had a childhood disease that damaged the liver. Do you know if that could be true of your mother?" I then remembered her telling me she had had jaundice as a child.

Angry with God over my mother's illness, I now questioned His goodness, honesty, and promises. Still, I continued to communicate with Him, sharing my hurt, disappointment, and misgivings. Eventually His Spirit broke through my hurt, and I realized that because my mom had lived as God suggested is best for all of us—refraining from alcoholic beverages—He *had* kept His promise. I had been privileged to have a mother for 30 to 40 years beyond what I would have had had she drunk liquor. Many alcoholics die in their 40s or 50s. He had withheld the disease from her well beyond that! Because of her health practices and God's blessings, she lived a full 85 years, glorifying God. Why should I mistrust Him? Instead, I will say, "To you, O Lord, I lift up my soul; in you I trust, O my God" (Ps. 25:1, 2, NIV).

Sometimes our faith is tested. Today praise God for the blessings He promises and provides.

CHERISH YOUR VITALITY

> Then because so many people were coming and going that they did not even have a chance to eat, he said to them, "Come with me by yourselves to a quiet place and get some rest." So they went away by themselves . . . to a solitary place. Mark 6:30-32, NIV.

Jesus knew His personal ministry on earth wouldn't last long, and one of His main objectives was to train His disciples to carry on when He was gone. Therefore, it was important to use every opportunity for them to gain the instruction and experience they would need. It was an intense course of study.

Even at the end of each day their work was not finished. If they were to take time out, many of the needy people would not receive the help they needed. So it was only natural that they would try to work continuously lest they neglect any opportunity. But even so, the Master arranged for a period of relaxation and rejuvenation. He placed a higher priority on the need for preserving vitality and efficiency than on continuously responding to whatever cried for their attention.

It is clear that working beyond one's capabilities, even in a worthy enterprise, carries the risk of defeat. Take the case of Margery, a 34-year-old schoolteacher and mother of three, who was beginning to suffer from migraine headaches. Typical of most persons who suffer from migraine, she was a highly organized and efficient mother, homemaker, and teacher. She did all this, however, by sheer determination and at the price of not having time to consider the beauties and blessings that surrounded her. Margery felt personally responsible for her pupils' progress and her family's comfort and welfare. But she was not taking time to replenish the energy she was consuming.

What would remedy the headaches? Should she quit? Not necessarily. Margery needed to reconsider her personal limitations and adopt a new lifestyle in which she shared her responsibilities with others. She could petition the school board to provide a volunteer aid for her classroom and could counsel with her husband and children to see how she could be relieved of some routine home duties. Most of all, she needed time to be by herself and think, pray, and relax.

Just as Jesus summoned His disciples apart to replenish their energy, He is calling you. What changes do you need to make in your life so you can do as He urges?

A BREATH
OF FRESH AIR

Let everything that has breath praise the Lord. Praise the Lord. Ps. 150:6, NIV.

Zipping up my jogging suit, I step out into the early-morning light. The dew-freshened air grabs at my cheeks. My face tingles. I head down the path, picking up speed as I go. Morning fresh air—there's something special about it. Breathing in, I feel the cool clean air slipping into my body. One deep breath leads to another until I feel exhilarated. Rejuvenated. It's almost like there's life in the air.

Air. It's so common. Yet it's the most vital element in all my environment. I walk in it. I talk with it. I filter it and remove its oxygen for my cells. It calms my mind and lowers my blood pressure. Air helps decrease my cholesterol and even slows the formation of cataracts in my eyes.

Studies have shown that in spite of the fact that it's only about one fortieth of my body's weight my brain needs five times the oxygen of any other organ in my body.

Those morning deep breaths of quality air improve my thinking ability, my alertness, and my physical being. What a way to begin the day!

Often after spending most of the day indoors it's easy to lose one's alertness. A closed, overheated, and crowded area has less oxygen and often high concentrations of harmful chemicals. The thing to do in such a case is to step out for a quick walk or open a window for some fresh, clean air. After a few minutes you'll find your mind awakened, your energy level up, and your spirits ready for some action.

If you find that at some point during the day you're feeling irritable toward your family; if you feel as if your brain's stuck in neutral; if you're tired of dragging around half coherent; take a fresh-air break. The solution to your problem may be as simple as breathing.

Lord, help me always to remember, as I breathe into my body clean,
fresh air, that You are the breath of life to my soul.

FILL YOUR MOUTH WITH LAUGHTER

He will yet fill your mouth with laughing, and your lips with rejoicing. Job 8:21, NKJV.

aughter may indeed be the best medicine after all. In his *Anatomy of an Illness*, published in 1979, Norman Cousins recounts how 10 minutes of solid belly laughter would give him two hours of pain-free sleep. Laughter stimulates heart and blood circulation and promotes respiration. It produces deep relaxation, thereby breaking up our tension.

Just putting on a happy face can be rewarding. Working in a high-rise for senior citizens for several years, I made what I thought at the time was the profound discovery that if I smiled—*whether I felt like it or not*—I would feel better. I knew I couldn't go in to those old people looking like a grump, so I would paste on a smile, and soon I was actually smiling. In an article published in the Orlando *Sentinel*, Ronald S. Miller states that "if we just assume facial expressions of happiness, we can increase blood flow to the brain and stimulate release of favorable neurotransmitters." So when I smile I am releasing neurotransmitters and giving others—and myself—a better day in the process!

Years ago I had a ministry with parents who had lost children. At the risk of sounding like a heretic, I asked them to keep a good joke book beside the Bible. I explained that there would be days when even the Bible might need to be supplemented with a good laugh that could, at least momentarily, lift the incredible weight of pain and loss. My personal daily shot in the funny bone is Lynn Johnston's *For Better or for Worse*. God bless her for her painkiller insight on family life.

One more bit of advice: don't stick around negative people. These are what one writer calls "energy suckers." Do yourself a huge favor and find someone positive and funny and enjoy life.

God wants us to laugh and enjoy the full range of positive emotions He created. Otherwise, He wouldn't have promised to "fill your mouth with laughter and your lips with rejoicing"!

So let's rattle those funny bones today and praise our heavenly Father for the wonderful gift of laughter.

If 10 minutes of laughter helped Norman Cousins sleep pain-free for two hours, what might it do for your health?

GOD'S GIFT
OF TIME

January 25

Jan W. Kuzma and
Cecil Murphey

Remember the Sabbath day by keeping it holy. Six days you shall labor and do all your work, but the seventh day is a Sabbath to the Lord your God. Ex. 20:8-10, NIV.

In our high-tech, stress-filled, busy world of work we need a weekly, 24 hours of downtime. We need to rest from the overstimulation of our body's adrenal system, the root of many modern stress problems. That's why God gave us the Sabbath. "The Sabbath was made for man, not man for the Sabbath" (Mark 2:27, NIV). People were to work for six days and rest for one—a rhythm that history has shown to fit human life.

People have tried other rhythms. For instance, in 1793 the French adopted a calendar of 12 months of 30 days each. Workers stayed on the job for nine days and rested on the tenth. Soon, though, they discontinued that calendar as unworkable because workers didn't want to work nine days before getting a day of rest.

During World War II the United States and Great Britain speeded up the production of war materials. Many factories went to 74-hour work-weeks. Before long they realized that their employees were averaging only 66 hours of actual work. These same factory workers complained about feeling irritable. Morale dropped. Accidents increased. Spoilage soared.

Factory owners soon decreased the workweek. In the United States some factories added more workers and others introduced three eight-hour shifts instead of increasing the hours of the single shift. What were the results? They had higher production, fewer spoiled items, lower rates of absenteeism, and better morale.

In Great Britain when they reduced the number of working hours to 48 a week (eight-hour days, six days a week), production went up. The British then went so far as to declare a mandatory rest of one day each week and gave their workers two weeks of annual vacation.

The idea of resting one full day out of every seven is as old as the beginning of the human race. It was God's gift to the human race to preserve life and health. Isn't it about time we enjoyed God's gift of time?

How can you reap the health benefits from the Sabbath day as God intended?

BELIEVING
THE LAWS
OF NATURE

January 26

Dawna Sawatzky

> And now my life ebbs away; days of suffering grip me. Night pierces
> my bones; my gnawing pains never rest. Job 30:16, 17, NIV.

Something was wrong—very wrong. Despite a definite diagnosis and appropriate medication, Audrey Watts wasn't feeling better. Instead, joint pain, stiffness, and muscle weakness now involved her hands and arms as well as her legs. The pain was increasingly incapacitating, leaving her wheelchair-bound and unable to do even the simplest household duties.

Her husband pastored at a lifestyle center, so she knew "the health rules," and she followed many of them. Her doctors said they didn't matter. Lifestyle changes probably wouldn't help her condition anyway.

As a last desperate resort after long years of suffering, Audrey checked herself into the Weimar Lifestyle Center's three-week live-in program. There she ate a diet free of refined oils, high-fat foods, and refined sugar. She was served an abundance of fresh and unrefined plant foods. Her daily routine included several hydrotherapy treatments, physical exercise, and spiritual renewal. By the end of three weeks Audrey was feeling better than she had in years. She was able to move with less pain, even exercise some.

At home she put the principles she had learned into practice. Concentrating on actually living all eight of the natural laws of health, she reordered her life to eliminate stressful activities, prepared only natural, unrefined foods, exercised outdoors daily in the fresh air and sunshine, conscientiously drank adequate amounts of water, and continued with hydrotherapy and massage treatments. For her, temperance meant not overdoing it and learning to relax and get adequate rest as well as good quality sleep. Daily she renewed her walk with Jesus and her trust in God.

Day by day she had less stiffness and pain. A year later she was off medication, symptom-free, and holding an undemanding job. Her painful symptoms creep up if she slips back into her old health-destroying habits, but God's natural remedies continually work a miracle in her life.

There's no doubt in Audrey's mind or mine about the truth of this statement: "The laws of nature . . . are divine, and . . . only in obedience to them can health be recovered or preserved" *(The Ministry of Healing,* p. 113).

*Lord, thank You for the incredible restorative power my body
has if I just follow God's laws of nature.*

SCREAMS
IN THE
PILLOW

Homer Trecartin

And he brought the present unto Eglon king of Moab: and Eglon was a very fat man. Judges 3:17.

My brothers and I grew up working hard and eating well. We didn't eat between meals, and only occasionally had desserts, but when we ate, we ate plenty. Because of all the outdoor work and play, the amount of food we consumed was not a problem until just before I started eighth grade.

My left hip began to bother me. The doctors said I had two choices: become crippled, or undergo major surgery and use crutches for a year. I knew that meant no more ball games, skiing, or mountain climbing.

The year dragged by. Summer came, and finally I was free. I didn't tell anyone for a long time that my right leg was beginning to hurt, but by the end of the summer Mom had noticed. That meant more doctor's visits, more X-rays, another surgery, and more months on crutches.

On top of that, I was getting fat—maybe not as fat as King Eglon, but far more than chubby! I had friends, but who wanted to date a fat boy on crutches? Many nights I screamed into my pillow in frustration and hurt. I know how it feels to smile at the fat jokes while your heart is breaking. I know what it is like to hold back the tears until you are alone in your room. I know how hard it is to diet and diet and diet without seeing any change.

Months went by. Spring came again, and I abandoned the crutches for good. My exercise increased, and my diets continued until another year had passed. By then I was tall and thin. Today people can't imagine me as a short fat boy, but I remember! And it still hurts when I hear someone laughing and joking about weight.

During those two terribly difficult years I learned that God still held me close. Even while I beat on His chest and screamed in His ear, He never let me go. Sometimes I accused Him of abandoning me, but through it all He loved a little fat boy that everyone else wanted to avoid.

What support can you offer someone who is suffering from obesity?
And if you are the one who is overweight, have you learned
that God still loves you and will help you
even if others say things that hurt?

THE BLIND
SHALL SEE

January 28

Stoy Proctor

In that day the deaf will hear the words of the scroll, and out of the gloom and darkness the eyes of the blind will see. Isa. 29:18, NIV.

Blindness was a widespread and serious disease in the ancient Near East. Although the physicians of the day tried various remedies, they could do little. Blindness was caused by old age, contagious diseases, venereal diseases, and injuries to the eye. Today we also know that much blindness is a result of a defective genetic code.

The retina specialists think that was my situation. I was diagnosed as having retinal tears. In fact, I experienced a series of tears and finally a complete retina detachment over a period of four months.

Now after six months of virtual blindness in my right eye and a series of seven surgeries, as well as lying on my right side and then my left side for 90 percent of every 24 hours, I am beginning to see a little. I can now be much more empathetic with the blind of Isaiah's day. What a blessing it is to be able to see!

Perhaps a few of my colleagues and friends may be questioning, "What did he do wrong?" "Who sinned, this man or his parents?" (John 9:2, NIV). It is easy to blame poor health habits for disease, but that is not true in every case. I do not know for sure what caused my blindness, but I do know one thing—I am praying and hoping for restored sight as the doctors have given me a glimmer of hope. And I look forward to the time when the blind will receive their sight, the deaf their hearing, and the sick complete healing.

Fortunately, for the thousands who have trouble seeing, we live in the twentieth century; microsurgery, cryosurgery, and lasers offer help for many. But even with these procedures, my sight and your sight ultimately depend on the ability of the body to heal itself through the divine power of our Creator.

As I realize how utterly dependent I am on God for healing, I often think of the miracle of sight and sound that I took for granted for so many years. How true the words: "Ears that hear and eyes that see—the Lord has made them both" (Prov. 20:12, NIV).

Lord, I praise You for the miracle of sight and sound,
and for the promise of healing.

SPIRITUAL
HYGIENE

> The Lord does not look at the things man looks at. Man looks at the outward appearance, but the Lord looks at the heart. 1 Sam. 16:7, NIV.

I've noticed that my devotion to hygiene seems to vary depending on the time and place. For example, in the typical restaurant I can be downright finicky. If I was served a meal with a bug in my potato or seated at a table that wasn't free of crumbs or other debris, I would be outraged. Should my plate have dried-on food from the previous meal, I would be indignant. If I dropped my spoon on the carpeted floor, I would demand a replacement. A greasy saltshaker would raise a protest. And if I knew that the cook's hands were dirty, I might even notify the health department.

However, on a weekend backpacking trip a miraculous transformation occurs. When cooking over the open fire, are the chef's hands dirty? No problem—mine are dirty too. Is my plate a little gritty from the last meal? That's OK; it's just food. We dine on the ground with the dirt as our tablecloth and think nothing of it. If we drop a spoon in the dirt, we simply wipe it off on our dirty pants and continue eating. And of course, if a bug flies into our food, we just shovel out the unwanted pest, flick it away, and without disrupting the rhythm of the meal, we dine on. Quite a double standard, I admit!

Jesus condemned the Pharisees for their double standard in the realm of spiritual hygiene. He declared: "Woe to you, teachers of the law and Pharisees, you hypocrites! You clean the outside of the cup and dish, but inside they are full of greed and self-indulgence" (Matt. 23:25, NIV).

Spiritual hygiene calls for cleansing the inside, not a superficial once-over for human praise. When I analyze my own relationship with God, I remember my illogical and intermittent devotion to personal hygiene, and pray the prayer of Simon Peter: "Lord, not my feet only, but [wash] also my hands and my head" (John 13:9).

Dear Lord, wash my heart and mind with Your Holy Spirit
so that I might be spiritually clean. Amen.

REFLECTING
GOD'S BEAUTY

January 30

Jacalyn Nosek

But the Lord said to me, "Do not say, 'I am only a child.' You must go to everyone I send you to and say whatever I command you. Do not be afraid of them, for I am with you and will rescue you," declares the Lord. Jer. 1:7, NIV.

I was born with a dark-red, cavernous hemangioma (birthmark) covering half the right side of my face. It can't be hidden by clothes, covered by makeup, or erased by lasers. When you look at me, it's the first thing you see, and for some people it's all they see.

As I was growing up I learned how cruel people can be to someone who looks different. But whenever I would cry, my mother would reassure me, saying, "You have this special mark because God has a special work for you."

My greatest blessings have come from what this birthmark seems to signify to others. One summer my best friend and I sold religious magazines door-to-door. We'd try to keep pace with each other, but I would often fall behind because some lonely, hurting person would insist I come in. They didn't need or want the magazine, they just needed someone to listen to their heartache. Many times that summer I held hurting individuals in my arms as they cried. I wondered why so many people would react this way to me. It didn't happen to my friend. Eventually I understood. When these people saw my face they knew instinctively that I could empathize with their pain and loneliness.

This was where I learned that my birthmark could open doors for me to tell people about my loving, compassionate Saviour that would not open for someone else. Today as I work with young people I remind them that God calls each one of us to reflect to a hurting world His true character of love. It doesn't matter how our lives have been scarred. We can represent His scarred hands and His gentle, comforting voice to the people we meet daily.

I love singing the song that tells how we will be the only Jesus some will ever see, the only words of life some will ever have a chance to read.

It is my prayer that when someone sees my face, my birthmark, that they will not see the scars, the hurt, and the trials, but rather a reflection of the hope and love with which my Saviour has blessed my life.

Lord, because I am created in Your image, help me
to see the beauty in myself—and in others.

FLYING WITHOUT FEAR

I sought the Lord, and he answered me; he delivered me from all my fears. Ps. 34:4, NIV.

I was terrified of flying. But the day my husband announced he had signed up for flying lessons, I made a decision to overcome my fear. I figured that if I could learn how to fly, then maybe I wouldn't be so frightened.

As it turned out, I loved flying. I liked it so well that I became a flight instructor and taught for several years.

Then one day I was hired to pick up an aerial photographer, fly him to the White Mountains to photograph some land, and then meet a real-estate agent in Quemado, New Mexico, which had a short dirt landing strip known for crosswinds.

I landed without problems, but when I started to take off, I was not able to get the air speed I had planned. At the end of the runway I added some flaps to hop a fence and tried to stay low because of power lines, but a wing tip caught, and we cartwheeled and crashed upside down. I suffered a concussion, but thankfully my passenger climbed out unhurt.

Not only was I terribly embarrassed about the accident; I was now terrified of flying. The crash had shattered my confidence. But I had students who needed to complete their training, so I couldn't walk away. The worst part was that because of the accident I once again had to go through the licensing procedure of flying a plane with an examiner.

The stress was so great that while waiting for the examiner I had a panic attack. I thought I was going to have a heart attack. My heart raced and my body tensed until I could hardly breathe. My chest felt as if someone was sitting on it. So stressed out that I couldn't function properly, I had to force myself into the plane. But somehow I passed.

Fear makes one vulnerable to distress and disability. But there are many things you can't control in life that you just have to trust the Lord to get you through. I've learned that you have to face the fear, walk through it, and get on the other side of it. God is helping me through this one, and I will fly again—without fear.

Fear can be debilitating. But with God's help
you can walk through your fear and "fly" again.

FINDING
PEACE
OF MIND

February 1

Jeffrey K. Wilson

Jesus looked at him and loved him. "One thing you lack," he said. "Go, sell everything you have and give to the poor, and you will have treasure in heaven. Then come, follow me." Mark 10:21, NIV.

He was a man who had everything—a typical baby boomer, rich, successful, handsome, and well educated. But he lacked one thing: peace of mind—the peace of mind that comes with one's assurance of a saving relationship with God. So when he asked what he needed to do to be saved, and Jesus said to sell everything and give it to the poor, he panicked!

"What! Give up my Porche, my Waverunner, my vacation home, my Caribbean holidays, my . . . Impossible!"

What Jesus required of the young man shocked the disciples. But material possessions are often a source of anxiety rather than a means of escaping from it. I learned that lesson recently on a trip to Atlanta. The rental car company gave me a new bright-red Cadillac for the price of the subcompact I had reserved. All night I tossed and turned in my motel bed worrying that someone might steal it! Had I been driving my old jalopy, I would have slept like a baby!

Gaining or maintaining financial success can be stressful: investing, buying, selling, watching the stock market, meeting deadlines, making business luncheons, playing politics. And when you feel driven to do everything that life on the fast track demands, it doesn't leave much time and energy for the Lord.

But impossibilities for humanity are possibilities with God (Mark 10:27). Rich men and women can enjoy peace of mind in this life *if they make God's kingdom their first priority and follow Him.*

Allow God to manage your financial affairs. Make investments in His kingdom rather than Satan's. With God's help, you can lay down your burdens, go through the "eye of a needle" (see Luke 18:25), and find peace of mind.

*Ask God what burden you need to
put down to have true peace of mind.*

GOD'S CALL TO BE A COMFORTER

Rosemary D. Graham

Praise be to the God and Father of our Lord Jesus Christ, the Father of compassion and the God of all comfort, who comforts us in all our troubles so that we can comfort those in any trouble with the comfort we ourselves have received from God. 2 Cor. 1:3, 4, NIV.

The voice on the other end of the phone was crackly and sniffly. "I called the Lupus Foundation to . . ." she said, then paused to weep. I let her cry, praying I could ease her fears. "Have you been diagnosed with lupus?" I inquired.

"Yes," she replied.

Slowly she poured out her story (a familiar tale for me) of fatigue, pain, and weakness. She asked many questions: "How long do I have to live?" "Will I get worse?"

We talked almost an hour, laughing and crying over similar experiences—frequent visits to doctors with condescending attitudes, and strange, sometimes painful, laboratory tests. The conversation ended on a lighter note, and she thanked me for easing her concerns.

Eleven years ago I began experiencing painful body aches, extreme fatigue, and pain. After frequent doctor visits and extensive lab tests, I was diagnosed on Thanksgiving Eve, 1984, with lupus erythematosus, an autoimmune disease in which the body attacks itself. Even today I remember the emotional devastation I felt—the depression, frustration, and uncertainty. I spent many tearful nights praying into the early hours for God to heal me. God's healing spirit began to soothe my mounting fears. He was preparing me to be a "comforter," to testify for Him.

My first assignment as a volunteer for the Lupus Foundation was as a hot line counselor. Each call from an inquirer reflected the emotions and pain I'd felt myself. Now I could lessen their fears, saying, "Yes, I've been through that, and here are some suggestions how you can cope . . ."

At times we experience trials that have no explanation—sometimes we can't even hear God's voice during them. But in all our difficulties He gives us strength to endure—thus strengthening our testimony.

When you experience difficulties and come through as victor, you will in time encounter someone else going through a similar trial. It is then you can confidently say, "Let me share with you what helped me deal with a similar problem." And in comforting others, you will be comforted yourself.

"Praise be to the God and Father of our Lord Jesus Christ, the Father of compassion and the God of all comfort."

Challenge: Share your testimony and faith with someone who's experiencing similar difficulties.

FATALLY
DELUDED
ABOUT SLEEP

There is a way that seems right to a man, but in the end it leads to death. Prov. 14:12, NIV.

Perhaps you may have what appear to be good reasons for your current way of life. You may even believe that none of the questionable things you do will have lasting effects, or that nothing bad can happen to you. That's the way it is with delusions—those pieces of fiction we choose to believe. Often they are fatal—not only to our life now, but also for eternity.

Ellen G. White once wrote: "We are surrounded with temptations [delusions] so disguised that they allure while they taint and corrupt the soul. Satan varies his enticements to suit different minds; and he takes advantage of every circumstance to make his plans for a soul's destruction successful" *(Review and Herald,* Nov. 9, 1886).

And one of the delusions that we talk about in our book *Toxic Trends* is that *it doesn't matter how much sleep you miss.* But here are the facts:

Even one night of shortened sleep can produce adverse effects. People will briefly rise to meet the demands of an occasion, such as playing tennis or giving a speech, but mental concentration, flexibility, and creativity suffer. Two nights of skimpy sleep will cripple rote functioning. During laboratory tests sleep-deprived subjects have trouble adding columns of figures or doing simple repetitive tasks like hitting buttons in a prescribed pattern.

Stanford researcher William Dement's studies show that if you miss sleep one night, your body keeps a record of the "sleep debt." If the debt isn't paid back soon, you'll start nodding off during the day.

"We don't tend to have a good handle on our amount of sleep debt. So when we finally go bankrupt it happens fast," Dement says. "People can go from feeling wide awake to falling asleep in five seconds. If you are behind the wheel of a car, you're dead."

Are you getting enough sleep?
- Are you chronically drowsy?
- Do you lack energy?
- Do you need an alarm to wake up in the morning?
- Do you fall asleep within five minutes?
- Do you nap at will?

If the answer to any of these questions is yes, then you are probably short on sleep.

Avoid the "toxic trend" of too little sleep. Set limits on your working hours and get seven or eight hours of sleep at a regular time each day.

THE HEALING OF THE SUN

February 4

Jan W. Kuzma and Cecil Murphey

For you who revere my name, the sun of righteousness will rise with healing in its wings. And you will go out and leap like calves released from the stall. Mal. 4:2, NIV.

The ship arrived at Antarctica December 24, 1928. Richard Byrd and his crew of 41 unloaded supplies for Little America—the place they would stay for the next 14 months. When they arrived, the sun shone for 24 hours. As the men worked, they knew time only by checking their watches.

Then the length of days began to decrease, and in April they lost the sun. They lived in buildings connected by underground tunnels for five months. During this time the morale of the men deteriorated significantly. Then on August 20, 1929, the sun returned. Norman Vaughn writes in his autobiography *With Byrd at the Bottom of the World:* "How can I explain the joyousness of the first few days of sunlight? We felt like prisoners who had received commutation of our sentences. A brightness appeared on our faces. We walked faster and moved with an energy we had long forgotten."

Do you take the sun for granted? It has incredible health-giving properties such as killing germs, helping our bodies manufacture vitamin D, and improving the function of our pituitary, hypothalamus, and pineal glands. Plus, it's essential for growing our food. The simple fact is, we can't function without the sun. Nor can we function without the Sun of righteousness.

I can just imagine Admiral Byrd's party coming out of their underground homes, seeing the light of the sun, and kicking up their heels with joy, can't you? This same joy can be yours each morning as you welcome God's new day, and as you invite the Sun of righteousness into your life. Experience the reality of the promise in Malachi: "For you who revere my name, the sun of righteousness will rise with healing in its wings. And you will go out and leap like calves released from the stall."

Light is the starting place of life. Perhaps that's why the biblical account of Creation begins this way: "In the beginning . . . God said, 'Let there be light,' and there was light. God saw that the light was good" (Gen. 1:1-4, NIV).

Spend some time today in the light God created for you to enjoy.

67

GETTING INTO
BIBLICAL SHAPE

Enoch walked with God; then he was no more, because God took him away. Gen. 5:24, NIV.

As we look at some of the well-known characters of the Bible, an interesting picture emerges. See Elijah running in front of the horses of Ahab. Imagine David following the sheep mile after mile, and being so physically fit that he could kill a bear with his hands. Picture Abraham trekking about 1,000 miles from Ur of the Chaldees to Canaan on foot. Can you visualize yourself traveling with Jesus as He treads the dusty roads of Palestine? Or follow Paul around on his three missionary journeys?

Do you think you could keep up with any one of these characters if they were to show up today? If not, maybe it's time you got into "biblical shape."

1. *Schedule exercise into your day.* Don't just wait till you "find time" for it. Chances are, you never will.

2. *Exercise frequently, at least every other day.* Daily would be even better.

3. *Enjoy the exercise you choose.* There's no point in trying to improve your body while torturing your mind. Plus, when you exercise with a negative attitude, your body doesn't get as much benefit out of it.

4. *Exercise for at least 30 minutes at a time.*

Exercise can come in many different types, but most people prefer walking. It does wonders for all ages, without the risks involved in more vigorous exercise programs such as jogging or aerobics. Even God walked in the garden of Eden in the cool of the night with Adam and Eve (Gen. 3:8). And Scripture records that centuries later Enoch walked with God.

People who exercise regularly say that it calms their minds and makes them more alert. Perhaps all the walking the Bible greats did was one of the reasons their minds were so perceptive of God's will. They likely spent many hours walking and talking with their Creator. It's a combination that can keep all of us physically as well as spiritually fit. God is eager to bless us, as He did Enoch, Elijah, David, Abraham, Jesus, and Paul, if we will follow their example of maintaining a walking-and-talking-to-Him lifestyle.

> *What is keeping you from getting out of your chair,
> stepping out the front door, and walking with the Lord
> for 30 minutes? God wants you to be physically fit
> as well as spiritually fit.*

WANT AND WASTING DISEASES

Dane J. Griffin
and Kay Kuzma

In the desert they gave in to their craving; in the wasteland they put God to the test. So he gave them what they asked for, but sent a wasting disease upon them. Ps. 106:14, 15, NIV.

After more than 400 years as slaves in Egypt the Jews finally experienced God's deliverance. He led and sheltered them by a cloud during the day and guarded them with a pillar of fire at night. God gave them manna—the very best food for their journey to Canaan. Yet God's people weren't satisfied—they craved flesh food!

God answered their grumbling by sending a massive flock of quail. All that day and night and all the next day the people went out and gathered quail. No one collected less than 60 bushels. Self-satisfied, they sat down to eat their gluttonous feast. What was the result? Their ravenous eating caused a "wasting disease," and they ended up burying those who had craved meat (Num. 11).

Today God has once again given us the very best for our journey to the heavenly Canaan, yet many are craving a meat diet rather than being satisfied with God's original diet of fruits, nuts, grains, and vegetables.

Will we suffer from "wasting diseases" like the Israelites? Reputable scientific researchers have linked cancer, heart disease, stroke, and diabetes—today's four leading "wasting diseases"—with the high-fat, high-protein intake associated with a flesh-based diet.

"When God led the children of Israel out of Egypt, it was His purpose to establish them in the land of Canaan a pure, happy, healthy people" (Counsels on Diet and Foods, pp. 377, 378). He did this by removing flesh from their diet and giving them manna. "Had they been willing to deny appetite in obedience to His restrictions, feebleness and disease would have been unknown among them. Their descendants would have possessed physical and mental strength. They would have had clear perceptions of truth and duty, keen discrimination, and sound judgment. But they were unwilling to submit to God's requirements, and they failed to reach the standard He had set for them, and to receive the blessings that might have been theirs. They murmured at God's restrictions, and lusted after the fleshpots of Egypt" (ibid., p. 378).

Are you praising God for His modern manna—a flesh-free, cholesterol-free diet? Or are you grumbling after the fleshpots of Egypt? What could be the consequences of your choice?

DUES FOR GOD'S HEALTH INSURANCE

February 7

Jan W. and Kay Kuzma

> Worship the Lord your God, and his blessing will be on your food and water. I will take away sickness from among you, and none will miscarry or be barren in your land. I will give you a full life span. Ex. 23:25, 26, NIV.

I can't think of a better health insurance plan than one that guarantees no illness, miscarriage, or infertility, and a full life span, can you? That's what God gave His people more than 3,000 years ago if they would pay the premiums—worship Him and do as He said.

God's insurance plan is a conditional one. It requires certain "dues" that are prerequisite to the health benefits promised. Here are a few of the most important.

• *"Due" follow a simple vegetarian diet.* "Grains and fruits prepared free from grease, and in as natural a condition as possible, should be the food for the tables of all who claim to be preparing for translation to heaven" *(Counsels on Health, p. 42).*

• *"Due" be temperate in all things.* "Intemperance, in drinking tea and coffee, wine, beer, rum, and brandy, and the use of tobacco, opium, and other narcotics, has resulted in great mental and physical degeneracy, and this degeneracy is constantly increasing" *(ibid., p. 49).*

• *"Due" exercise.* "The blood is not enabled to expel the impurities as it would if active circulation were induced by exercise. . . . A walk, even in winter, would be more beneficial to the health than all the medicine the doctors may prescribe" *(ibid., p. 52).*

• *"Due" enjoy fresh air and sunlight.* "A free and abundant use of the air and sunlight—blessings which Heaven has freely bestowed upon all—would give life and strength" *(ibid., p. 54).*

• *"Due" use pure water for drinking and cleansing.* "In health and in sickness, pure water is one of heaven's choicest blessings. Its proper use promotes health. . . . Drunk freely, it helps to supply the necessities of the system and assists nature to resist disease. The external application of water is one of the easiest and most satisfactory ways of regulating the circulation of the blood" *(The Ministry of Healing, p. 237).*

The lifetime benefits of God's health plan can be yours if you worship Him and pay your "dues."

> *What more could you be doing to reap*
> *the benefits of God's health plan?*

A PARK
IN TIME

February 8
Lonnie Melashenko

He [Jesus] went to Nazareth, where he had been brought up, and on the Sabbath day he went into the synagogue, as was his custom. And he stood up to read. . . . "He has sent me to proclaim freedom for the prisoners and recovery of sight for the blind, to release the oppressed." Luke 4:16-18, NIV.

A *park is a refuge in space.* My friends who live in Manhattan tell me how precious Central Park is to them. They live and work surrounded by towering buildings and pavement. The pace of city life is frantic, unrelenting. But when they step into Central Park, everything changes. Trees offer shade. They find grass for spreading a blanket and sharing a picnic. My friends say that while in the park they feel a thousand miles away from the pressure, the stress, the frantic pace.

The Sabbath is a refuge in time. For 24 hours every week God invites us to put aside the struggle to earn a living, to get A's in school, to keep an immaculate house. During those 24 hours He invites us to act out the rest we have in Jesus. The Sabbath is the gospel in dramatic form. For a whole day we rest in the accomplishments of our Saviour. We shut out all the demands and expectations of the world and luxuriate in the promises of God.

Notice how Jesus kept the Sabbath (Luke 4). During a Sabbath worship service Jesus quoted from Isaiah 61, a passage that predicts the coming of the Messiah in the language of the Jubilee, the time when Israelites should release captives and set free the oppressed (Lev. 25:10, 40, 54).

Luke then follows with two healing episodes. Both of them occurred on Sabbath. The first one happened in Capernaum during a Sabbath service at which Jesus healed a possessed man, freeing him from spiritual slavery to a demon (Luke 4:33-37). The second occurred later the same day in the home of Peter, where Jesus and the disciples had gone to eat after church. There Jesus healed Peter's mother-in-law's high fever (verses 38, 39).

Notice the way Luke tells these stories. First Jesus announces His mission as Messiah by quoting Isaiah about freeing the oppressed. Next He brings *spiritual* healing to a man possessed by a demon. Then He gives *physical* healing to a woman suffering from a fever. I think Jesus was telling us something about the meaning of the Sabbath, don't you?

Why do you spend all your time among towering problems
and dead-end pavement, when God has provided a weekly park
in time for you to enjoy? Why not follow the custom of Jesus?

ON THE MEATLESS WAGON

February 9

Faith Crumbly

With him is only the arm of flesh, but with us is the Lord our God, to help us and to fight our battles. 2 Chron. 32:8, NIV.

Robert set off a roar of joyous approval at the Vegetarian Supper Club cooking school when he began explaining his reasons for taking the course: "These are going to be my 'Meataholics Anonymous' meetings. I really have been overdoing my meat consumption, and I want to learn how to prepare another kind of protein." He detailed the extent of his perceived addiction, including the exact ounces of meat he had been devouring daily. Then he set off another rumble of laughter by concluding, "So I came here to get on the wagon."

Americans have been formally getting on the wagon ever since the phrase became popular during the late 1800s. And as anyone who has been on any kind of "wagon" can tell you, eliminating the loved and the familiar requires commitment and fortitude. The friendship and support of other people trying to make the same change or a similar one helps a lot. Robert can tell you all about that. He stuck with his class for all five training sessions.

At the International Tasting Event finale to the cooking school, Robert's face reflected the peace and joy of an overcomer. Several weeks later he announced that he had prepared every recipe in the course manual, and apparently his friends had tasted them all. "When's the next class?" he asked. "I have a lot of friends who want to come!"

The bottom line of support for everyone making lifestyle changes, whether it's getting enough sleep, getting enough exercise, or getting on a meatless diet, is the Great Enabler. He provides the power to hold on and hold out—to stay on the wagon of wholesome change. However, even when we are leaning on Him, it certainly comforts our humanness to have friends who'll encourage us.

That's why I'd suggest joining a support group of people who are eating vegetarian-style or doing (or stopping) whatever you have chosen as your goal. If you don't know anyone nearby to turn to, ask your omniscient Father to direct you to someone He has ordained to supply the encouragement you need.

Lord, You are the Great Enabler. Help me to get on the "wagon" for You.

Whoever loves discipline loves knowledge, but he who hates correction is stupid. Prov. 12:1, NIV.

A n old man once remarked, "When I was a little boy somebody gave me a cucumber in a bottle. The neck of the bottle was small, the cucumber very large. I wondered how it had gotten in there. Out in the garden one day I came upon a bottle that someone had slipped over a little cucumber. Then I understood. The cucumber had grown large after it had been put in the bottle."

Have you ever looked around at all the good, strong, and sensible people you know and wondered why they hang on to their bad habits when they know better? What about yourself?

People with bad habits are like the cucumber in the bottle. They just grew into them while young and now find it impossible to slip out of them. Changing a bad habit is work. Probably the hardest work in the world!

Much of children's early behavior (or misbehavior) is impulsive. They want a piece of candy, so they take it. They feel a little hungry halfway between breakfast and lunch, and spying the cake on the table, take a piece and eat it. Children may feel sad because no one is paying any attention to them, so they eat too many sweets because it makes them feel better. Little acts at first—little impulsive ones. But what if the next time they want something, they take it, or if when they feel hungry, they eat junk food, or if they feel sad and eat candy?

What if no one is around to help them find a better way of coping with their desires and feelings, to help them control their impulsive behavior? They will probably repeat their previous behavior. And like the cucumber growing in the bottle, the more they repeat those actions, the stronger the behavior grows and the more difficult it is to slip out of it.

Obviously, the best way to stop a bad habit is never to start it, but if you've got a habit that's already the size of a cucumber in the bottle, maybe it's time to start cutting it out—or maybe you just ought to break the bottle!

Lord, I know what I should do, but it's so hard. Show me how to "cut out the cucumber" or "break the bottle." Thank You.

THE RESISTANCE FACTOR

February 11
Ron Wylie

Submit yourselves, then, to God. Resist the devil, and he will flee from you. James 4:7, NIV.

Some years ago Purdue University biologists studied the wolves and their prey, the moose, in the unique natural laboratory of Isle Royale in Lake Superior. Some of their observations seem applicable to our struggle with that great predator, Satan, who is viciously "looking for someone to devour" (1 Peter 5:8, NIV).

Cow moose average about 800 pounds, and when they fight against a wolf pack, they are formidable antagonists. During one confrontation a cow, protecting her calf, defiantly faced the pack. As the wolves approached, she leaped at them, lashing out furiously with her forefeet, holding her ground.

The wolves got the message. They scattered in a panic, then stood around considering. After several minutes, much to the surprise of the biologists, the wolves abruptly left.

In another confrontation the cow moose saw the approaching wolves. She hesitated and then began moving away. That seemed to trigger the wolves' pent-up urge, and immediately they approached the moose, lunging at their huge prey. She momentarily fought back, then ran. Soon the wolves swarmed over her, and a few minutes later she was dead.

The scientists recognized that wolves have a prudent fear of their dangerous quarry. Frequently the animals give up and move on when a moose deliberately stands and defies them. The scientists discovered that the wolf pack "tested" 12 moose for every one they killed.

What made the difference in the individual moose reaction? The most significant factor was the general health and fitness of the moose.

Healthy, vigorous moose were unlikely to be victims. Their predators sought weaker prey. Having autopsied wolf-killed moose to determine their state of health, the biologists reported that, on the limited evidence they had, "it seems highly significant that we have found one or more kinds of disability in 45 percent of the adult wolf-killed moose."

As we live through the stressfulness of these last days of the struggle between good and evil, let us determine to be healthy, vigorous, and fit, both in mind and body, so that in cooperation with divine power we can consistently resist the devil, "standing firm in the faith" (1 Peter 5:9, NIV).

When the devil attacks you, does he find you physically and spiritually healthy, vigorous, and fit enough to resist him?

DON'T LET THE DEMONS RETURN

February 12

Nancy Rockey

Oh, that their hearts would be inclined to fear [adore with tender feeling] me and keep all my commands always, that it might go well with them and their children forever! Deut. 5:29, NIV.

It was 7:30 a.m. when the doorbell rang. Still dressed in pajamas, the pastor ran to answer. The tearstained face was unfamiliar, yet it displayed a sense of panic. "Are you the folks who take love off the rocks? I am two days away from my divorce being final, and I need help. I don't want a divorce. I love my wife, but we can't seem to live together. We've been married 30 years, and we just can't get along. Can you help me? Will you?"

His words spilled as freely as his tears.

The pastor and his wife invited Gary in, and for the next three hours they listened to a history of pain and emotional abuse. They wept with him, recalling their own painful marriage. Together they prayed that God would intervene.

After a few months of counseling, Gary and Lucille's marriage had improved greatly. There were still issues needing attention, but they had the necessary tools for resolution. Each week Gary attended Sabbath services, and occasionally Lucille accompanied him. Before a year had passed they recommitted their lives to each other in a special church dedication service.

Nearly another year passed, and the pastor transferred elsewhere. Immediately Gary felt abandoned. He ceased attending church, and before long had reverted to his old abusive and controlling ways with a vengeance. He began to distance himself from his friends at church, and then from his wife and children. His eyes wandered, and finally he chose to leave the marriage.

Today, as I write this, they are again days away from a divorce. He leaves behind a devastated wife and three very angry children.

What must we learn from such an account?

1. All of the tools for character change, without our submission to God and without following God's plan, will not create permanent recovery.

2. God is our life source, not other Christians, who will often disappoint us.

3. When we turn our back on God after once seeing His salvation, our "demons" will return in greater number.

Faith in Jesus and a teachable, submissive spirit will produce character transformation, and when the character changes, the behavior will follow.

Are you relying on others to keep your behavior in line, or are you holding on to Christ to change your character?

75

WHEN YOU'RE IN THE PITS

He redeemed my soul from going down to the pit, and I will live to enjoy the light. Job 33:28, NIV.

L ife isn't always a bowl of luscious cherries—you can end up in the pits! If you've suffered from depression, you know how terrible it is. You feel all alone, and nobody seems to understand. It's difficult to concentrate. Everything takes extra effort. Feeling washed out and tired, you can't make up your mind about anything. And you have no ambition or interest in what is going on around you.

How can you climb out of the pits?

Try eating "cherries" and other wholesome food at regular times, spaced about five hours apart. Regularity is important in controlling blood-sugar levels and in providing your digestive system with its necessary rest.

Many disturbed and easily depressed children come from homes where mealtimes are unimportant. They develop habits of eating junk food (empty calorie food high in fat, sugar, or salt) at all hours. Refined sweets, if used at all, should be eaten sparingly. Carbohydrates should come from fruits and whole-grain food, such as wheat, corn, oats, and millet. You can usually prevent low hemoglobin by meals rich in iron, vitamin C, and vitamin B_{12}—eat plenty of dried fruits, dark, leafy green vegetables, and whole grains.

The second thing you should do when depressed is make a change in your environment. It will help transform your thoughts. Physically move out of the spot where you are and think about something you can do with your hands. Deliberately bring your mind to a new task—scrubbing, digging, planting. Drink a glass of water. Breathe deeply out in the fresh air. Vigorously wash your face and the back of your neck with cold water. Take a warm shower followed by a cold one.

Any of these mechanical methods will tend to shift the circulation of the blood and the firing patterns of your nervous system and make it easier for you to use your willpower to think of the positive, wholesome, and rewarding experiences of your life.

Finally, remember who ultimately brings victory over depression. "Thanks be to God! He gives us the victory through our Lord Jesus Christ" (1 Cor. 15:57, NIV).

Thank You, Lord, for giving me the victory over depression,
and may I consider my problems pure joy knowing that
You are in the process of maturing me.

KEEPING YOUR LOVE CUP FULL

You anoint my head with oil; my cup overflows. Surely goodness and love will follow me all the days of my life, and I will dwell in the house of the Lord forever. Ps. 23:5, 6, NIV.

Down deep in your heart there's a cup. Not of fine china, silver, or gold, but a cup of feeling and emotion that when filled makes life worth living. I call it the love cup. It measures your level of contentment. In essence, it's your psychological well-being.

The love I am writing about is not a romantic love, but agape love—a principle, not necessarily devoid of emotion, but not dependent on it either. It is love given with no strings attached, just because the other person exists. When we experience it, endorphins—substances chemically similar to morphine—flow into the brain, producing a sense of security, peace, and calm. One feels good because one feels intrinsically valuable.

When your cup is running low, you feel unloved, rejected, worthless, and empty—you have nothing to give. A drained cup turns your world negative. Anger, criticism, sarcasm, guilt, and bitterness rush in to fill the void.

God can enter a life that's filled with hate and selfishness. He can change it. In a sense, that's the meaning of conversion. No one is beyond God's healing power of love. But even though God can do it, that doesn't mean we should leave the filling entirely to Him. The Lord gives us the opportunity to be His entering wedge. People starved for love may first need to experience a little love in action—from fellow human beings. It causes them to realize that their lives are empty. Then we can point them to the Source of complete love.

If you feel empty, ask God to fill you. He will speedily respond. And seek out others who can be cup-fillers, too. Then when your cup is filling, or full, reach out and begin filling the empty love cups of the unlovable. You may not feel loving toward them, but that doesn't matter. God asks no one to *feel loving*. He just says to *be loving*. It's the act of love that is important. Love is something you do. And as you love, both you and the one whose cup you are filling will begin to live life abundantly!

Loving Father, fill my cup with Your love so I can fill others. Amen.

WALKING HELPS THE HEART

Bernell E. Baldwin

I have no greater joy than to hear that my children are walking in the truth. 3 John 4, NIV.

A dozen years ago many considered jogging and vigorous exercise the best way to maintain cardiovascular health. But not anymore. Walking is the better choice to get the heart rate up enough to keep it healthy, but not so high that it gets stressed. Research has now confirmed what Ellen G. White wrote in 1872: "There is no exercise that can take the place of walking" *(Testimonies,* vol. 3, p. 78).

Walking helps the vagus nerve slow the heart rate, which is one of the goals of modern cardiology, and it does so without drugs. Formerly the goal of exercise was to race the heart, but for many it overworked the organ. About 25,000 extra deaths occur each year in the U.S. alone because people exercise too briskly.

The December 1993 issue of the *New England Journal of Medicine* reported a study done on 2,000 people in Boston and Augsburg, Germany. When they exercised to the point of panting, as when jogging, playing raquetball or tennis, or pushing cars out of snow, they had twice the risk of getting a heart attack within one hour—even among those who exercised five times a week.

Walking outdoors in nature can also lower the adrenaline in the blood, which means less stress. The less stress, the slower the heart will beat. Jogging and aerobics spill stress hormones into the blood, inflaming the platelets to initiate clotting and depriving the blood of a clot-dissolving enzyme called plasmin or fibrinolysin (fi-brin-o-LY-sin). Competition adds to the problem.

Walking improves the efficiency of the heart. It can increase your HDL (high-density lipoprotein), which works like little dump trucks that pick up last year's cholesterol from the coronary arteries and take it down to the liver, where a high-fiber vegetarian diet can sweep it out of your body forever.

No other exercise can do as much for you, with so little risk, as walking.

I have a feeling that if James had the evidence we now have about the benefits of walking when he wrote "I have no greater joy than to hear that my children are *walking* in the truth," he would have meant walking spiritually in the truth, yes, but also walking physically in the truth demonstrated by scientific evidence.

Ask a friend to go walking with you today and
tomorrow and the next day.

DOES WINE PROTECT THE HEART?

Do not gaze at wine when it is red, when it sparkles in the cup, when it goes down smoothly! In the end it bites like a snake and poisons like a viper. Your eyes will see strange sights and your mind imagine confusing things. Prov. 23:31-33, NIV.

Have you heard that a little wine is supposedly good for your health? The idea all started with a number of studies that seemed to link the drinking of wine to some health benefits. But was wine really good for the heart, as the studies seemed to indicate? How could it be? After all, wine is one of the biggest culprits in alcoholism.

Well, of course as soon as the alcohol industry got wind of the findings that suggested a health benefit to the drinking of wine, they pumped it up for all it was worth and used it to promote their product.

For a number of years health researchers questioned the finding that wine was good for the heart. Now they know why. It's not the wine, it's the grape juice—or better yet, it's the purple Concord grape that offers heart protection.

According to the *University of California at Berkeley Wellness Letter,* unfermented grape juice is the drink of choice, because from it you get heart protection and none of the unhealthful side effects caused by fermentation, such as liver damage or decreased brain function.

Consequently, you can no longer use the excuse that "it's good for my heart" to condone your drinking habit. If you do, you're asking for trouble. A little wine too easily leads to the use of a little more, and before you know it, you're craving something stronger. And the result? Not only physical health problems, but social and family problems as well.

Then what about the Bible text, 1 Timothy 5:23, that says that a little wine is good for the stomach? It doesn't take much effort to realize that the apostle Paul is not endorsing alcoholic beverages, since just a couple chapters before, in 1 Timothy 3:3, 8, he clearly states that godly persons should not be "given to wine." Most likely he was referring to unfermented grape juice being good for the stomach. And that's exactly what the latest research has confirmed.

So enjoy your grape juice; it's good for your heart—and your stomach, too—but beware of the fermented drink that "bites like a snake and poisons like a viper."

Beware of sin that "bites like a snake and poisons like a viper."

DANIEL'S FAST

But Daniel resolved not to defile himself with the royal food and wine, and he asked the chief official for permission not to defile himself this way. . . . So the guard took away their choice food and the wine they were to drink and gave them vegetables instead. Dan. 1:8-16, NIV.

Barbara was a conscientious mother who was willing to do whatever was necessary to provide a good home for her husband and three boys. But they had problems at home and in school. Restlessness, irritability, short attention spans, and poor grades plagued her sons.

Feeling that the Holy Spirit led her to search for answers in the Bible, she read again the story of Daniel as he was taken to Nebuchadnezzar's court in Babylon. Daniel's report of the wonderful results of the experiment with a vegetarian diet encouraged her. Maybe something similar would help her family.

She told the story of Daniel to her husband and children. They discussed what it would mean if they tried what they called "Daniel's fast." It would include not only a change in what they were feeding their bodies but also a difference in what they were feeding their minds. They agreed to give it a try.

Barbara started by removing from the house all books and videotapes that contained anything aggressive or overstimulating, or that seemed to foster antisocial, unhappy behavior. Next she began reducing the amount of meat and animal products she offered her family.

Soon the boys showed an increased interest in reading and studying, and their grades improved.

Today Barbara is very happy with her "new" family. I got acquainted with her when she begged for advice on how to cook vegetables and borrowed my cookbooks. She is now taking Bible studies, for she wants the best for her family physically, mentally, *and spiritually.*

God is impressing others with the need for a healthier lifestyle. What a privilege to be able to help people who are convicted by the Holy Spirit to make major lifestyle changes.

Are you convicted?

Dear Father, please grant me strength as I resolve not to defile myself with the king's food, wine, and entertainment.

PRAISE GOD FOR THE HOPE OF RENEWED YOUTH

He knows how we are formed, He remembers that we are dust. Ps. 103:14, NIV.

My father, a retired physician, several years ago became intrigued with gathering any medical research available on ways to slow down the aging process. For about a year he was a modern Ponce de León in search of the fabled fountain of youth. He wrote more than 1,000 letters to physicians, medical schools, research laboratories, and pharmaceutical houses all over the world, asking for any information, experimental treatments, or proven methods to restore youth or reverse the effects of old age.

He got back hundreds of replies. Some talked about experiments with growth hormone injections that have produced amazing results. One such treatment supposedly reverses 15 to 20 years of aging. The skin tightens, muscles improve, the lungs and heart strengthen. However, the writer warned that dangerous side effects make the procedure unsafe. Other doctors wrote of drugs to improve oxygen utilization. Some discussed various enzyme treatments that have shown promise. Still others recommended certain vitamins to restore lost vitality.

My father—a frail, white-haired man—turns 80 this week. Despite his search for the fountain of youth, he, like Ponce de León, will one day return to the dust from which we were all created. Even the most advanced discoveries in medicine have not been able to stop the clock of time.

We should all strive to live a healthy life, to enjoy the abundant blessings God intended us to experience here on earth. But our heavenly Father knows that we are frail, formed from dust. So I cling to the promise that God is returning to make all things new, including my father—and me! While I do my push-ups and sit-ups, I know that my heavenly Father will restore my youth when He restores my soul.

Like the psalmist, I praise the Lord "who forgives all your sins and heals all your diseases, who redeems your life from the pit and crowns you with love and compassion, who satisfies your desires with good things so that your youth is renewed like the eagle's" (Ps. 103:3-5, NIV).

What can you praise the Lord for today?

WORKING OURSELVES TO DEATH

February 19
Paul and Carol Cannon

> Once when Jacob was boiling pottage, Esau came in from the field, and he was famished. And Esau said to Jacob, "Let me eat some of that red pottage, for I am famished!" . . . Jacob said, "First sell me your birthright." . . . So he swore to him, and sold his birthright to Jacob. Gen. 25:29-33, RSV.

Incredible as it may seem, Esau bartered away his birthright for a kettle of stew. He traded status and security to gratify physical appetite. Why didn't Esau think before he acted? How could anyone be so hungry that he would throw caution to the wind and cast away his inheritance without a second thought?

Obviously, Esau wasn't in his right mind. Was he drunk or "high"? We've known young people who have sold or traded valuable possessions for a pittance to buy drugs, others who have tossed their personal belongings into a campfire when they were high—just to watch them burn. And we've known adults who walked away from things they had struggled a lifetime to accomplish in order to appease some form of appetite.

Achievement, exercise, shopping, and working are a few mood-altering activities with addictive potential if carried to an extreme. Research has established that innocent shoppers seeking a bargain have the same physiological reaction, in terms of brain chemistry, as a hunter stalking his prey. An entrepreneur who pulls a swift business deal experiences a rush of endorphins similar to that of the cocaine user. When people are hooked on their own adrenaline, they don't have to buy drugs on the street. They manufacture their own.

Esau is an excellent example of someone with a "clean" addiction. Obsessed with the thrill of the hunt, he neglected his basic human needs. He didn't pause long enough to eat, and it placed him at risk. Many workaholics act similarly: they refuse to eat or sleep until they have completed the project at hand.

When we compromise our own well-being or the health and welfare of those we love in order to achieve a goal, we place ourselves at risk. If we are so driven that we cannot stop overachieving, overworking, or overdoing something in spite of the fact that it's hurting us, we're acting addictively. Working ourselves to death, eating ourselves into oblivion—such "clean" addictions are as deadly as alcoholism. As Christians, we cannot afford to deny this reality, or refuse to get the help we need to overcome them.

*Do I have "clean" addictions in my life? If so, what can
I do to find help to deal with them?*

JESUS CAN HEAL ATTITUDE PROBLEMS

Your attitude should be the same as that of Christ Jesus. Phil. 2:5, NIV.

Paul, at 15, was overweight, had a poor self-image, and had a long history of failing special educational programs.

As a last resort his parents brought him to the Advent Home Youth Services, a residential program for hurting teenagers. I met Paul in the parking lot and introduced myself.

"Your name is Paul?" I queried.

"Why do you want to know my name?" he retorted.

"To get to know you," I responded lightheartedly, then continued, "How was the flight from California?"

"I hated it," came his hostile reply.

Over the months we counseled Paul and worked closely with him. We met daily in group therapy and talked about all kinds of subjects. Coaxing Paul into trying harder, we cheered him on for every little bit of success.

For the first six months he seemed at a standstill. The only progress we noted was that he was not getting worse.

As the months went by, we nurtured him. Daily we presented the needs of our boys to heaven and prayed that they might be healed from the severe emotional, academic, and spiritual problems they had.

God heard our prayers. Slowly Paul began to make progress. Our healthful diet was having a positive effect on his desires and impulses. We could see changes in his disposition and attitude.

One day Paul and I were having a counseling session in one of the gazebos on the campus. Reminding him of how much change he had made since he first came to the program, I asked him what in his estimation enabled him to make the transformation from an angry and spoiled teenager to a responsible and mature 16-year-old.

Paul thought for a moment and said, "I changed because I have learned to accept Jesus Christ as my personal Saviour. I am learning to make my attitude the same as that of Jesus."

Do you need an attitude change? Focus on Jesus.
Ask that His attitude will become yours.

83

THE
HOLY SPIRIT'S
"HEIMLICH MANEUVER"

"I tell you the truth, no one can enter the kingdom of God unless he is born of water and the Spirit. . . . You should not be surprised at my saying, 'You must be born again.'" John 3:5-7, NIV.

We were celebrating with relatives at a Mexican restaurant. Suddenly Oscar stood up, bent over the table, and moved his mouth as if to talk. His hand went to his throat and his eyes looked wild.

They call it a "café coronary." It's when someone gets a piece of food lodged in their windpipe and can't get a breath. At first glance it looks like a heart attack. But it isn't. And without prompt help, the person has only about four minutes to live.

Dr. Henry Heimlich in 1974 described the emergency treatment that would save a person who was choking, and today thousands all over the world owe their lives to this innovative physician. Oscar does too.

My husband recognized the problem immediately. "He's choking," he screamed. Jumping up, he slipped behind Oscar, grabbed him around his midriff, clutched his hands in a fist, and yanked upward toward his chest. Oscar coughed out a tiny piece of food, took a breath, and gratefully collapsed on the seat. It was a close call.

Jan used the Heimlich maneuver to save Oscar's life. It forces the diaphragm to curve upward into the chest, creating a rush of air pressure through the windpipe where the food has lodged, enabling it to be coughed out.

In a way it was like being born again. For a time Oscar had a desperate struggle that he was powerless to win by himself. Then with help—the Heimlich maneuver—Oscar received a second chance at life.

We're all in a desperate struggle for our lives—choking on sin. It doesn't matter what it is: murder, adultery, gambling, pornography, slander, gossip, envy, pride, overeating, selfishness. Any violation of God's moral or natural law is sin. Anything that takes priority in our lives above our allegiance and honor to God blocks our windpipe to salvation.

But God has a "Heimlich maneuver" to save us. It's called being born again. With the Holy Spirit's help, the sin we're choking on can be knocked out of our lives, and we can once again breathe God's lifesaving air.

Ask the Holy Spirit to convict you of your sins, repent,
and then enjoy the breath of fresh air the Holy Spirit
will bring to your life. You can be born again—
and enter God's kingdom.

"For I know the plans I have for you," declares the Lord, "plans to prosper you and not to harm you, plans to give you hope and a future. Then you will call upon me and come and pray to me, and I will listen to you. You will seek me and find me when you seek me with all your heart." Jer. 29:11, NIV.

Adelante, the lifestyle center of the University of Montemorelos, in Mexico, gives hope of a healthy future to many people. Here's a letter of appreciation I received from a man named Jose:

"I am 56 and am from Monterrey, Mexico. In my search for health, I heard of a program called Adelante. My wife and I came to this program with great interest and some skepticism. What we found was a group of health professionals who captured our attention because of their great hospitality and selfless service. They showered us with attention and gave us much encouragement in changing our lifestyles. To our surprise, thanks to God, we have experienced such dramatic changes in our 10 days here that we can only say, 'This is a miracle.'

"For 25 years I have suffered from bad circulation, blindness, and uncontrolled mature-onset diabetes. When I left the program, my blood sugar was normal (without medication), my blood pressure was normalizing, the edema in my feet and legs was gone, I no longer had urinary pain, and I was walking 5 kilometers [three miles] a day. I looked and acted like a different person.

"In only 10 days my body has so favorably changed that the inconveniences and sacrifices of waking early and walking an hour, a vegetarian diet, steam baths, contrast showers, Jacuzzi, and massage are more than worth the effort.

"At first the program seemed tedious and boring. I felt desperate when I did not receive medications for my many symptoms, just water, water, water, and more water—about seven to nine glasses each day and more if I exercised. I felt skeptical and disappointed. But surprise! I noticed a change in my body. In the evenings, just as I was going to bed, I would think, *I am not going to walk tomorrow!* But the next day as I looked at my feet and legs, now no longer inflamed as they had been for years, I realized how beneficial this program was.

"God bless you for your care and prayers, because a miracle of faith and hope has changed me."

Lord, bless all those who are learning about Your lifestyle at one of the hundreds of lifestyle centers around the world. Give them hope for a healthy future. Amen.

POPULATION DENSITY AND DISEASE

David J. DeRose

My people will live in peaceful dwelling places, in secure homes, in undisturbed places of rest. Though hail flattens the forest and the city is leveled completely, how blessed you will be, sowing your seed by every stream, and letting your cattle and donkeys range free. Isa. 32:18-20, NIV.

Does population density affect health? That was the question raised by researchers at the Bureau of Cancer Epidemiology in New York.

Dr. Philip Nasco and his associates divided the state of New York (except New York City) into categories based on population density.

Their findings were startling: the more rural the area, the less cancer among the residents. The increased risk experienced by the urbanites was in the range of 20 percent to upward of 70 percent. Many types of cancer also increased in frequency. They included cancers of the esophagus, mouth, colon, stomach, liver, pancreas, voice box, lung, bladder, and brain.

The general nature of the study made it impossible to determine the cause of the difference in cancer rates.

The authors suggested that smoking habits may provide one possible explanation. Many smoking-related cancers take decades to develop, and 20 to 25 years earlier the urban areas studied had more smokers. The urbanites may now be experiencing the consequences of long-term smoking habits.

Work-related exposures, pollution, more stress, less exercise, and poorer food choices may also help to explain why city dwellers have more cancer.

Years ago God spoke through Ellen White of the health risks of city living. Although she mentioned risks from the physical environment, such as pollution, she also raised concerns about the health risks of social factors, such as crowding and "bustle and confusion" *(Medical Ministry,* pp. 308-311), that contribute to stress and certain diseases. Could this be part of the secret of "the rural advantage"?

God's ideal was that His people would "live in peaceful dwelling places, in secure homes, in undisturbed places of rest" (Isa. 32:18, NIV). Sounds like healthy country living, doesn't it?

If you find yourself having a hard time hearing God's voice in the traffic, noise, concrete landscape, and rush of urban living, maybe it's time to accept the invitation Jesus gave centuries ago: "Come . . . to a quiet place and get some rest" (Mark 6:31, NIV).

How can I get some of the benefits of country living even if I believe the Lord has called me to minister in the city?

SEX, TWENTIETH-CENTURY STYLE

Walter Thompson

Will not the Judge of all the earth do right? Gen. 18:25, NIV.

S ome have argued that the Sodom and Gomorrah story is fiction—that the ancient cities were victims of a natural disaster arising from an accidental ignition of the oil and tars prevalent in the region. They claim that this whole bit about sexual immorality is just a threatening myth and nothing more. After all, are people so much different from the animals that sex must be regulated by law? Is God so picky that we can't use our own common sense about the way we live our lives?

Just for fun, let's assume that the Bible is nothing more than myth, and that the code of ethics that has come down to us through the centuries represents the cunning efforts of ancient strongmen to control the masses.

Now look at our society. Do you like what you see? Broken homes, broken people. Kids with a dozen sets of parents, yet no parents at all. Divorced people trying to pick up the pieces of a shattered relationship, devastated, never to be the same again. Nursing homes full of old, displaced persons whose families have scattered before the four winds. And each succeeding generation compounding the problems of the one before. Is it any wonder that self-esteem has reached an all-time low, and that drugs, perversion, and violence have come to rule our world?

No, it seems that the evidence speaks for itself. Things haven't gone too well since we have taken the law into our own hands. Perhaps the old Book is right after all!

But in a society that blatantly displays sex on every signpost, in which sexual innuendos dominate common conversation, in which dress and high fashion inflame temptation, how can anyone pass through unscathed? What hope is there of living godly lives when people in our own homes become the victims of adulterous relationships and sexual abuse?

There is none, except to place ourselves in the care of Jesus and let His strong arms protect us. Remember what happened to the crowd that rushed Lot's door? Is His arm now too short, so that it cannot save? "Will not the Judge of all the earth do right?"

What can you do to protect yourself from sexual temptations?

TAKE AN INTERNAL SHOWER

Jesus answered, "Everyone who drinks this water will be thirsty again, but whoever drinks the water I give him will never thirst. Indeed, the water I give him will become in him a spring of water welling up to eternal life." John 4:13, 14, NIV.

Are you drinking enough water? Forcing the body to work with limited amounts of fluid is a bit like trying to wash the dinner dishes in a cupful of water. When you don't drink enough water, the body must excrete its wastes in a more concentrated form, causing body odor, bad breath, and unpleasant-smelling urine.

Our bodies are about 70 percent water, and our kidneys process more than 47 gallons of it in a day. Without it we'd look more wrinkled than California raisins!

But why is this colorless, tasteless, calorie- and salt-free substance that has no nutritional value so absolutely necessary?

The answer lies in the physiological workings of the body. Water to the body is like oil to a car engine. It's the magic lubricant that makes everything else work. A drink of water is like an internal shower and is exactly what the body needs to carry out all its life processes.

But won't other beverages, such as fruit juice or diet soda, do the job? Beverages other than water pose special problems for the body. Many have calories that must be digested like food. Such calories may produce extra fat storage, swings in the blood sugar, and slowed digestion. Sugar in beverages requires extra water for metabolism. Most beverages increase acid secretion in the stomach. And many sodas contain phosphorus, a chemical that can help deplete the body's calcium supplies, contributing to brittle bones.

Drinking water eliminates these problems. It has no extra calories to slow down digestion or add unwanted fat. No irritants to stress the sensitive linings of the digestive tract, and fewer chemicals to threaten delicate body machinery.

How much do you need? The body loses about 10 to 12 cups of water a day through skin, lungs, urine, and feces. Food provides two to four cups of water, leaving you six to eight glasses of water to drink on your own.

Pure water is one of God's greatest gifts for your health. Help yourself. And when you do, remember to ask Jesus for the "water" He gave the woman at the well that will completely satisfy your spiritual thirst and become like a "spring of water welling up to eternal life" (John 4:14, NIV).

To get your quota for the day, drink a glass of water the first thing in the morning, another two glasses midmorning and midafternoon, one about a hour after supper—and never pass up a drinking fountain! And for your spiritual thirst, drink freely from God's Word.

NOT ALL CALORIES ARE EQUAL

When you sit to dine with a ruler, note well what is before you, and put a knife to your throat if you are given to gluttony. Do not crave his delicacies for that food is deceptive. Prov. 23:1-3, NIV.

You can't just cut your calories and expect to lose weight. Here's why: By nature, your body is highly efficient in storing fat calories. It uses only about 3 percent of the fat calories you eat to digest, transport, and deposit fat into your body's fat storage areas. That means you must exercise the vast majority out of the body if you don't want to gain weight.

In contrast, your body metabolizes protein calories and excretes the by-products rapidly. You can have problems with excess protein, of course, because it stresses your liver and kidneys by forcing them to work overtime. But excess protein doesn't usually add to obesity. You have no efficient metabolic pathway in your body by which you can turn protein into fat for storage.

Calories from carbohydrates also rarely get stored as fat, because the metabolic pathways that your body uses to convert extra carbohydrates into fat and then store them demand that you burn a lot of calories to do the job. It takes 24 percent of the calories in carbohydrates to do this—a highly inefficient use of the energy in the carbohydrates.

In studies in which researchers put radioactive carbohydrate markers in food, they learned that the body converted and stored less than 1 percent of the carbohydrate load as fat. Even when people ate carbohydrates excessively, they generally burned them up in "wasteful" metabolic processes that tended to increase the body's metabolic rate, not reduce it—as happens in calorie-restricted diets.

Another way to put this is that one gram of fat contains nine calories, while one gram of protein or carbohydrates has only four calories.

The moral of the story is: avoid fat calories—they stick to your bones!

There's an interesting bit of advice in Proverbs 23:3 about overeating. It says don't crave a ruler's delicacies, because that food is deceptive. How true! Most rich food is filled with fat calories that may be tough to get rid of.

Sin is deceptive, too. It may look and taste good, but the consequences of indulging may be even harder to get rid of than fat calories.

Watch your moral diet, "for the wages of sin is death" (Rom. 6:23).

GOD UNDERSTANDS OUR NEED

Lois (Rittenhouse) Pecce

Before they call I will answer; while they are still speaking I will hear. Isa. 65:24, NIV.

All her life Virginia had enjoyed the closeness and comfort of family and friends. Then her husband died, and her own disabilities worsened. Her son brought her north to live in a nursing home near him. Even though she helped choose the facility, she still hated it. She felt angry at her husband for dying, and angry at God for letting it all happen. Her only solace lay in corresponding with old friends and family.

One day, checking her calendar, she noted five birthdays were coming up. She had no cards—no way of buying any. It seemed the ultimate proof of God's abandonment. Angry and depressed, she cried out, "God, don't You even care? Here I am in this place needing just five birthday cards, and I can't even get those!"

The next day, still discouraged, she returned from lunch to find a large envelope from a woman she'd not heard from in more than 10 years. The woman had visited a mutual friend. From her she learned that Virginia was in a nursing home. "Thought maybe you can use these," she wrote.

Inside were five birthday cards and a book of stamps. "Shivers just went up my spine," Virginia said later. "Especially when I checked the postmark and saw they'd been mailed five days earlier!"

She accepted it as proof that God had not abandoned her or turned against her. He'd chosen the very thing she thought too small to ask of anyone to demonstrate that He, the Creator and Lord of the universe, does care.

That event did not take away all her loneliness or solve her physical problems. But it helped her accept her situation better just by realizing that God knows her needs and wants even before she realizes them herself.

"Keep your wants, your joys, your sorrows, your cares, and your fears before God. You cannot burden Him; you cannot weary Him. He who numbers the hairs of your head is not indifferent to the wants of His children" *(Steps to Christ, p. 100)*.

Have you felt as if God has abandoned you or turned
His back on you? Why not talk to Him about it?

CONQUEST OF CHOLESTEROL

February 28
Raymond O. West

Pay attention and listen to the sayings of the wise; apply your heart to what I teach, for it is pleasing when you keep them in your heart and have all of them ready on your lips. Prov. 22:17, 18, NIV.

Are you confused with all the discussion about cholesterol? Is it bad or good? The answer is both. Let me explain.

The HDL (high-density lipoprotein) cholesterol is good, and the LDL (low-density lipoprotein) is bad. What we eat and do, and to some extent even what we think, influence the relative amounts of each.

Just as in our automobiles we carefully guard the oil level, so in our bloodstreams we expectantly watch the cholesterol level. Our chief concern with the crankcase of our cars is that the oil level is full. But with cholesterol we urgently need to know how much is "full" and how much is "too full."

Our bodies require cholesterol. The liver continuously manufactures it, keeping our body's supply full. The problem comes when we ingest additional cholesterol in our food. This is akin to adding oil to our gasoline, a procedure that would foul the engine.

The ideal oil level in our car is simply full or nearly full. But what is the ideal cholesterol level in our blood? Our goal is lower than 200. Some say it should be much lower, perhaps in the 100-150 range.

The Japanese have little heart disease, and cholesterol levels that, by and large, range under 150. And the same is true of many developing cultures that follow low-fat vegetarian diets.

The famous Framingham heart study has scrutinized several thousand residents of that now-famous Massachusetts town closely during the past 35 years. It notes that individuals whose cholesterol levels were under 150 have had no heart attacks.

Would you like to know what could make heart disease as rare as leprosy is in our culture? Eat fruit, vegetables, whole grains, and nuts and legumes, and push away all meat, fish, fowl, and animal products. This may sound unrealistic, but it's commonsense nutrition!

"Pay attention and listen to the sayings of the wise." Doing so can mean the difference between death and life; heart failure and heart health.

What changes could you make in your diet to bring down your level of cholesterol to below 150? Why don't you make that your goal?

LIFE'S ESSENCE

March 1

Marjorie V. Baldwin

The wind blows wherever it pleases. You hear its sound, but you cannot tell where it comes from or where it is going. So it is with everyone born of the Spirit. John 3:8, NIV.

We can live weeks without food, days without water, but only minutes without air. Air conveys life, vigor, and electrifying energy to every cell of the body. The most vital element in air is oxygen.

How does the vitalizing power of oxygen get to every cell of the body? This is where the body's delivery system, the blood circulation, cooperates. The heart sends blood singing on its way filled with red blood cells, whose hemoglobin picks up fresh oxygen in the lungs, and delivers it to every cell. There it exchanges the fresh oxygen for the carbon dioxide produced by the normal living processes of the cell, transporting it back to the lungs for removal from the body. Meanwhile the fluid part of blood carries indispensable nutrients to satisfy every hungry cell.

It reminds us of the two essential aspects of the Christian's life—fellowship with Jesus and ministry to others. Constantly we receive the Holy Spirit's life-giving, energizing power. And constantly we should share it with all we come in contact with.

That's what life is all about. Fellowship with Jesus through the Holy Spirit, thereby receiving His strength, power, love, joy, and peace for the purpose of being more effective in our ministry to others. To others our lives can become God's vital life-giving oxygen that helps sustain them through trial and discouragement.

Take three deep breaths and praise the Lord for
the Holy Spirit—life's true essence!

DOING YOUR BEST, LEAVING GOD THE REST

Edwin Martin

> Let everyone be sure that he is doing his very best, for then he will have the personal satisfaction of work well done, and won't need to compare himself with someone else. . . . And let us not get tired of doing what is right. Gal. 6:4-9, TLB.

I've lived my life with a new goal every morning: to get up and do my best, and leave the rest to God. It's helped me live a very satisfying and fulfilled life.

A lot of things happen to us that aren't fair. It's easy to get caught up in feelings of self-pity, bitterness, and revenge. But I've learned if we just keep doing what we've got to do to the best of our ability, God works things out much better than you or I could.

I saw this happen when I was in military service. I made my first stripe and became private first class four months after I went into the Army. As it turned out, because of my Medical Cadet Corps, first-aid, and lab training, I had more experience than anyone else in my platoon, so they put me in charge.

When I got my first lab assignment, I worked to learn all I could and was put in charge of training others. About two months later I had a terrible stomachache and was nauseated. By Monday my white blood count was 14,000, and I ended up having my appendix out. Wednesday my fever went up; I became delirious and broke out with measles. After three weeks, when I got back to work, they had changed lab officers and given promotions to those who were there. One of the guys I had been training had been made corporal. "Hey," my friends complained, "Martin ought to get that rating!" But that's the way life is. Sometimes, because of circumstances beyond your control, others get the rewards you deserve.

Late one night I was working emergency, down on my knees scrubbing the floor with a brush, when the surgeon in charge of the hospital came in with some labwork. When I handed him the results, he asked, "Martin, what rank are you?"

"Buck sergeant, sir." I was soon promoted to staff sergeant. The other fellow who was already staff sergeant didn't get a raise.

I've learned that if you are just faithful in your work, doing your best, determining to learn all you can, and giving more to the job than required, God works things out.

*Are you giving your best to your work,
to your family, and to your God?*

93

THE PHYSIOLOGY OF VICTORY

March 3

Kay Collins

Do not conform any longer to the pattern of this world, but be transformed by the renewing of your mind. Then you will be able to test and approve what God's will is— his good, pleasing and perfect will. Rom. 12:2, NIV.

You determine your destiny by the choices you make each day. How you think and feel shape your moral character, for they influence all of your words and actions. It's a fact: "As he thinketh in his heart, so is he" (Prov. 23:7).

I was excited when I read Eldon and Esther Chalmers' book *Making the Most of Family Living* and learned that our choices actually make physical and chemical changes in our brain cells and nervous system. Each time we make a decision to think the same way, repeat the same words, or do the same things over again, a small protein molecule, called a bouton, begins to form at the end of the sending fiber of the brain cell being stimulated. This bouton enlarges and multiplies with each repetition. It also secretes a chemical that causes the message to be transferred along the nerve pathway. The boutons make it easier and easier to do the same thing. Repetition of anything, good or bad, causes the habit to become confirmed in our lives; and fixed habits determine our character.

The good news is that we can overcome old sinful habit patterns— those boutons don't have to fire! When we choose to give our will over to Jesus, and avail ourselves of His abundant provisions of grace to keep us from falling—daily study of His Word, heartfelt prayer, and practicing His presence—the Holy Spirit begins to form sanctified boutons that secrete gamma-aminobutyric acid, and this chemical puts the brakes on the firing action of the old sinful habit pattern. The boutons of new sanctified habits also increase and multiply with the choices we make—thus we are being transformed by a literal renewing of our minds. This is the physiology of victory and how we can develop a character like that of Jesus.

Through the full surrender of your will to Jesus, you can know the joy of victory over every inherited and cultivated tendency to evil and will be prepared to meet your Saviour face-to-face.

Jesus, I need Your sanctified boutons to put the breaks on my bad habits. I surrender my will to You.

94

BATTLING INFECTIOUS DISEASE

> "The days are coming," declares the Lord, "when I will punish all who are circumcised only in the flesh—Egypt, . . . all who live in the desert in distant places. For all these nations are really uncircumcised, and even the whole house of Israel is uncircumcised in heart." Jer. 9:25, 26, NIV.

Not too many years ago scientists thought that they were on the verge of conquering infectious illnesses. Advances in hygiene, nutrition, antibiotics, and immunization had apparently removed much of the serious threat of infectious scourges. In many countries it sounded like ancient history to talk of the ravages of such diseases as measles, mumps, rubella, tuberculosis, polio, or smallpox. Yes, it seemed to be a real triumph for humanity and medical science.

Today, however, humans seem particularly impotent when it comes to defeating infectious illnesses. For every success a new infectious threat seems to arise. Newly recognized infections keep raising their ugly heads. A dozen years ago who heard of the deadly hantavirus that not too long ago grabbed attention in the four-corners area of the U.S. Southwest? Who knew about the diarrheal illness called cryptosporidiosis, which in a single outbreak caused some 400,000 Midwesterners to develop prolonged diarrhea? What about the scourge of recently recognized tick-borne infections such as Lyme disease and Ehrlichiosis? And then there are the international tragedies of the human immunodeficiency virus (HIV) and drug-resistant tuberculosis.

E. coli 0157 h7 was unknown until 1982, but since that time it has caused multistate outbreaks and deaths from eating ground beef. Other infectious diseases relatively recently have become an important part of our vocabulary. They include Ebola virus, hepatitis C, Legionnaires' disease, and toxic shock syndrome.

Yesteryear's seeming progress of science against infectious disease is much like our individual human struggles against sin. Sometimes it may appear that we are getting the upper hand. By our ingenuity, determination, and effort we seem to be making ourselves into better people. But then reality confronts us. It is only through Christ that the power of sin can be broken in our lives.

"'Let not the wise man boast of his wisdom or the strong man boast of his strength or the rich man boast of his riches, but let him who boasts boast about this: that he understands and knows me, that I am the Lord, who exercises kindness, justice and righteousness on earth, for in these I delight,' declares the Lord" (Jer. 9:23-25, NIV).

Can you boast that you understand and know God?
What could you do today to get to know Him better?

BREAKFAST
WITH
THE KING

In the morning, O Lord, you hear my voice; in the morning I lay my requests before you and wait in expectation. Ps. 5:3, NIV.

I'm not a morning person. I wake up, doze, and put off getting out of my bed as long as possible. At times I've even mused that if God really wanted me to enjoy the morning hours, He would have created them later in the day! But I've learned that just because it's hard for me to get going in the morning is still no excuse to skip breakfast.

The Iowa Breakfast Study (from 1949 to 1961) found that those who ate breakfast could perform physical and mental tasks in the late morning more efficiently, with faster reaction times and less neuromuscular tremor, than those who skipped the morning meal. Students who ate breakfast had better attitudes and higher academic attainment. Children are far less able to tolerate long periods without food because of their higher metabolic rates. They quickly get tired, apathetic, and irritable.

It's a common saying that we should eat breakfast like a king, lunch like a queen, and supper like a pauper. How you treat your body the night before will determine whether you'll feel ready for a kingly breakfast. If you eat a big evening meal and hit the sack before your food has a chance to digest, your body has to work to digest that food instead of getting the eight hours of total rest it needs. That's why you wake up groggy and don't feel like eating and why some people advocate nothing but fruit for breakfast, because it's easier on a digestive system that has worked part of the night.

The fact is that the food you put into your body in the morning will affect your day—whether it's physical food or spiritual food. That's why you should not only eat breakfast like a king, but also have breakfast with the King.

Before you roll out of bed, spend a few minutes praising your King. Then get on your walking shoes and walk and talk with Him. Come back invigorated and ready to eat the "morning manna" of His Word.

When you start your day with breakfast with the King, I'll guarantee you'll feel more like eating breakfast like a king.

Try eating supper like a pauper, and see if it doesn't make you feel more like having a spiritual breakfast with your King and a physical breakfast like a king.

FIGHTING THE CIVILIZED WAR

March 6

DeWitt S. Williams

Then, because so many people were coming and going that they did not even have a chance to eat, he said to them, "Come with me by yourselves to a quiet place and get some rest." Mark 6:31, NIV.

As long ago as the Civil War people were aware of it. Back then palpitations of the heart were so common among military troops that the condition became known as "soldier's heart."

During World War I a crippling anxiety developed among soldiers. Physicians referred to it as "shell shock" because they thought it to be caused by heavy artillery.

By the time World War II came along, the symptoms were called "battle fatigue." Then veterans of the Vietnam War experienced "post-traumatic stress disorder."

We now know that all of these illnesses had a single cause. The soldiers succumbed to a constant barrage of stressful combat episodes. They could find no rest, no renewal. And in this unending fight-or-flight environment, their reserve systems eventually collapsed.

But you're not in a war—or are you? Chances are you're involved in never-ending battles with job pressures, finances, and family problems. If you sometimes want to run away from it all, you're a casualty of the modern "civilized" war.

Alvin Toffler's book *Future Shock* describes this civilized war as "the distress both physical and psychological that arises from an overload of . . . adaptive systems and decision-making processes. Put more simply, [it] is the human response to overstimulation."

Overstimulation equals overload. It's estimated that we are subjected to 100 times more stressors than were our grandparents. Toffler insists that the civilized war exposes us to too much input in three areas:

1. *Sensory overload.* The human body responds to noise as it does to fear and anger. Even pleasant sounds at too high a volume can trigger a fight-or-flight response in us, and since World War II noise levels in the United States have increased 32-fold.

2. *Informational overload.* We live in the midst of an informational explosion, bombarding us with jangling telephones, daily newspapers, weekly magazines, home entertainment units, AM-FM radios, paperback books, monthly magazines, and home computers.

3. *Decisional overload.* Toffler suggests we are assaulted with a minimum of 560 advertising messages each day!

Lord, help me to tune out life's stressors and tune in to You.

E-4

97

CHOOSING
THE LORD

March 7

L. J. Saxon

> You shall love the Lord your God with all your heart, and with all your soul, and with all your mind, and with all your strength. Mark 12:30, NRSV.

As Christians we are taught to believe in God, trust Him, lean on Him, and depend on Him for all our needs. We're to be a witness to others of God's love and never-ceasing care. I've known this and believed this since I was a child.

Then misfortune struck. In spite of a healthy lifestyle, I became a victim of chronic fatigue syndrome. My energy gone, my life became a series of trials. Pain, weakness, and ever-changing symptoms filled each day. I found myself complaining bitterly to God of the injustice that I couldn't make a living for my family or witness to others in all those ways God could have blessed us with. Mental and physical anguish were my constant companions.

With great consternation I wondered where all my faith and adoration for God's constant care had gone. I questioned, What do those verses mean: "All things work together for good for those who love God" (Rom. 8:28, NRSV) and "Whenever you face trials of any kind, consider it nothing but joy" (James 1:2, NRSV)? I struggled with lost dreams and growing doubts.

One day I realized the very words I had used to witness to others now condemned me. My faith was an empty shell of words that failed the test. Even my prayers were for those things I wanted, not what God desired for me.

I've learned that God places a test before each person. With the promise of unconditional love He gives us freedom of choice to "choose this day whom you will serve" (Joshua 24:15, NRSV). We are to accept God with our faith based not on circumstances, but on His Word.

No matter what trials come to us, they will strengthen our faith in our Father when we trust Him explicitly to sustain us. Hebrews 13:8 says: "Jesus Christ is the same yesterday and today and forever" (NRSV). We are the only variable.

In our lives of constantly changing circumstances we can survive in only one way—a complete trust in our heavenly Father.

Grasp God's steadiness when your life gets shaken up.
Emulate His steadfast character so you can always shine with
His love, regardless of earthly circumstances.

WHAT ABOUT GRANDADDY?

March 8

Gerri Bradley

Even when I am old and gray, do not forsake me, O God. Ps. 71:18, NIV.

Grandaddy came to live with us when he was 94 years old and stayed for two years, until declining health forced him into a nursing home. Some people think taking care of older people is a chore. If that's what you think, it will be. But Grandaddy wasn't a chore. He was family.

We had raised our kids within a stone's throw of Grandaddy's little house. He'd help care for our chickens and animals, and he loved to tell the children stories. We even took him on vacation to places he'd never seen before, such as Myrtle Beach or the Great Plains.

When our place burned, Grandaddy wanted us to rebuild. Instead we purchased 200 acres and built a number of miles away. That was tough on him, because his eyesight was failing. He needed us close.

My original plan was that he would stay with us at night, and then I'd feed him breakfast and take him to his house during the day. But when he moved into our house he became so depressed I couldn't leave him alone. I guess he decided he was going to die. He wouldn't eat or drink water. Although he could walk, he wouldn't, so I got him a wheelchair and pushed him around the house. After three weeks he decided that maybe he wasn't going to die after all, so he started eating and walking and grew to like our place.

Grandaddy was easy to care for, since he ate with us and fit into our routine. But trying to get Grandaddy to take a bath was a challenge. He thought twice a month was often enough! Sometimes he'd get mad at me and stomp his foot, but I didn't take it personally. When we needed to get away, we'd use his pension money to pay some friends to stay with him. They loved him as much as we did. Grandaddy was good company.

Life is what you choose to make of it. Sure, we gave up a little of our freedom when we chose to have Grandaddy move in with us, but we gained far more in return.

What can you do to make an elderly person's life more fulfilling without taking away that person's freedom?

THE MIND-BODY CONNECTION

March 9

Jan W. and Kay Kuzma

For as he thinks in his heart, so is he. Prov. 23:7, NKJV.

It's accepted knowledge that a strong connection exists between the body and the mind. Even a slight deficiency of 30 or 40 known nutrients can alter the biochemistry and function of the brain and result in such common emotional problems as irritability, fatigue, and depression. In order for the brain to transmit signals efficiently, it has to have just the right amounts of certain nutrients. *What we put into our bodies does affect our minds.*

But there is also a mind-body connection. As Mark Richliu, former executive editor of *Prevention* magazine says: "Your thoughts and feelings are the nutrition of your mind. Just as we need a certain balance of vitamins, protein, and other nutrients to help our bodies reach maximum health and energy levels, each of us needs a specific balance of mental 'nutrients' for a happy, tranquil, and creative mind. . . . People who have close ties to others, who share time and thoughts and worries and laughter with kindred souls, reap profound health benefits."

Although Richliu based his statement on recent scientific research, the idea of a mind-body connection is not really new. Here are a few amazing statements—amazing because they were published in 1905 when the rest of the world was oblivious to the influence of the mind on the body.

"The relation that exists between the mind and the body is very intimate. When one is affected, the other sympathizes. The condition of the mind affects the health to a far greater degree than many realize. . . . Grief, anxiety, discontent, remorse, guilt, distrust, all tend to break down the life forces and to invite decay and death. . . . Courage, hope, faith, sympathy, love, promote health and prolong life. A contented mind, a cheerful spirit, is health to the body and strength to the soul. 'A merry [rejoicing] heart doeth good like a medicine' (Prov. 17:22).

"In the treatment of the sick the effect of mental influence should not be overlooked. Rightly used, this influence affords one of the most effective agencies for combating disease" *(The Ministry of Healing, p. 241).*

When a negative thought flashes into your mind, push it out with a positive Bible promise.

SOCIAL GATHERINGS AND GLUTTONY

John A. Scharffenberg

When you sit down to eat with a ruler, consider carefully what is before you; and put a knife to your throat if you are a man given to appetite. Prov. 23:1, NKJV.

Socializing with others is an important part of a healthy lifestyle, whether it be at church fellowship meals, picnics, weddings, or fancy banquets.

But when you attend these special events, the counsel in Proverbs 23:1 is: *You don't have to eat everything offered.* Even at the highest levels of society ("when you sit down to eat with a ruler"), the advice is to "consider carefully what is before you." Just because you find an incredible variety of foods and everything tastes so good, it isn't a license for you to stuff yourself. In fact, Solomon says you should "put a knife to your throat if you are a man given to appetite." The New International Version says: "if you are given to gluttony."

Scripture gives this advice for two good reasons. First, if you eat everything and eat too much, it's not healthy. Second, think of the example you can be by choosing healthful items and eating in moderation.

Don't boycott a social event because the food served doesn't conform to your dietary standards. Consider the example of Jesus.

"While Christ accepted invitations to feasts and gatherings, He did not partake of all the food offered Him, but quietly ate of that which was appropriate for His physical necessities, avoiding the many things that He did not need. His disciples were frequently invited with Him, and His conduct was a lesson to them, teaching them not to indulge appetite by overeating or by eating improper food. He showed them that portions of the food provided could be passed by, and portions chosen.

"Christ went to these feasts because He wished to show those who were excluding themselves from the society of their fellow men how wrong their course of action was. He wished to teach them that truth was given to be imparted to those who had it not" *(Ellen G. White Manuscript Releases, vol. 7, p. 412).*

So enjoy socializing with others, but just remember: "A right example will do more to benefit the world than all our profession" *(Christ's Object Lessons, p. 383).*

*How can you be a positive example to others
at the next social event you attend?*

I CHOSE HOW
I WANTED
TO FEEL

E. John Reinhold

The wrong desires that come into your life aren't anything new and different. . . . And no temptation is irresistible. You can trust God to keep the temptation from becoming so strong that you can't stand up against it, . . . He will show you how to escape temptation's power. 1 Cor. 10:13, TLB.

A s executive director of a Christian ministry made up of thousands of members who take care of one another's medical bills, you would think I would have known better. I was 45 percent overweight, was on three heart medications, was taking pain medication for arthritis, had lower back pain, had reoccurring diverticulosis, was listless, and had shortness of breath. I had one criteria for eating, and that was "How does it taste?"

Finally I admitted that I was powerless in my own strength to change and desperately needed God's help. An acquaintance introduced me to some basic nutritional information that led me to eat only fruits and vegetables for 10 days so as to cleanse my body. My cravings totally changed in that time. Next I made a conscious choice between how I wanted to feel and how I wanted things to taste. Choosing how I wanted to feel, I later discovered new tastes with even greater fulfillment than the old.

Then a friend gave me *Counsels on Diet and Foods*. I found the book instructive and extremely advanced. I began to see my problem as one of lust of the flesh. I was enslaved to the first inch of my tongue.

Now, 17 months later, I am off all pain and heart medication, am 80 pounds lighter, and have more energy than any time since my college days (I am closer to 60 than 50). Last fall my son and I enjoyed hiking six to eight miles a day. I found myself praising the Lord for a new life and outlook.

Can you see the parallels? After we come to a point where we admit that we are powerless against sin, we turn to a gracious Lord who is ready, willing, and able to change us from the inside out. We repent, enjoy His cleansing, and launch a life based on choices pleasing to Him and best for us. He rewards us by giving us fulfillment and blessings. Then He brings people into our paths to touch us and help us on our way, while also leading us to those we can help.

God is the giver of new life. How can we not adore Him?

Are you choosing how you want things to taste
over how you want to feel? Give the 10-day
fruit and vegetable diet a chance to reeducate
your taste to the delights of God's original diet.

FAT CAT
FIGHTS THE
IMMUNE SYSTEM

And I will put enmity between you and the woman, and between your offspring and hers; he will crush your head, and you will strike his heel. Gen. 3:15, NIV.

The human body consists of several important organ systems, each of which carries on a special function. The one most extensively studied in recent years has been the immune system.

Like a nation's Department of Defense, our immune system protects against foreign invaders and helps maintain national peace. While the armed forces defend their country, the immune system employs B lymphocytes, T lymphocytes, phagocytes (neutrophils, monocytes, and macrophages), killer cells, and natural killer cells to do the same. Macrophages are the "national guards" stationed throughout our bodies, while the other types circulate in the blood to keep us healthy.

When we put harmful things into our bodies, we destroy God's temple. For example, in Leviticus 3:17, God says: "This is a lasting ordinance for the generations to come, wherever you live: You must not eat any fat or any blood" (NIV). Science now knows that a high-fat diet contributes to heart attacks, strokes, several types of cancer, as well as immune cell destruction. A simple way to illustrate destructive health habits is with the acronym FAT CAT. F stands for *fatty* and highly processed *foods,* A for *anxiety* and stress, and T for *toxicity*—unhealthy exposure to toxic chemicals and environment. CAT represents three legalized drugs: *caffeine* and caffeinated drinks, *alcohol,* and *tobacco.* All these factors harm our immune system, and as a result destroy our bodies.

To maintain a healthy immune system, we need to stay away from the FAT CAT and nourish the immune cells with wholesome, unrefined foods—fresh vegetables, fresh fruits, whole grains, and legumes—as close to their natural state as possible. We also need pure water externally and internally, and regular, meaningful, outdoor exercise. Above all, trusting in God, reading the Bible and inspirational literature, and sharing our faith will fill us with hope, joy, and direction in life.

Just as your body's healthy immune system combats disease, a healthy spiritual immune system fights off temptation and sin. What destroys your spiritual immune system? Lack of Bible study, prayer, and meditation, along with selfishness, pride, intemperance, and a negative attitude.

A great struggle is going on between Christ and Satan. What are you doing to make sure your spiritual immune system is strong and healthy?

Great are the works of the Lord; they are pondered by all who delight in them. Ps. 111:2, NIV.

've delivered thousands of babies, but I'm still amazed how God designed the wonderful process called birth.

When the fullness of time arrives, the baby is ready to leave its warm and comfortable home within its mother's body. The distance the baby must travel through the mother's birth canal is short, yet potentially dangerous. The relatively large head of the baby must pass through bony openings in the canal that are often narrower than would seem to be comfortable. The bony space is larger from side to side at the upper part of the birth canal, but larger from front to back in the lower part. Since the Creator formed both the baby and its mother, He designed them to meet together in an almost perfect fit! Through a careful series of slow-motion twists and turns of the baby's head, birth will usually take place smoothly.

God planned that as the baby starts down the birth canal, its head first tucks forward so its chin rests against its chest. This allows the narrowest part of the baby's head to lead the way. And to help the process, the back part of the baby's skull is still soft enough to mold to the shape of the opening. As the labor contractions gently but firmly push the baby along, its head then turns sideways so it can slip through the upper birth canal. Then as the baby dips down farther, its head rotates 90 degrees to allow it to pass through the middle part of the canal. Finally, as the baby emerges from the mother's birth canal, its head tips backward, making delivery easier.

These carefully orchestrated moves and twists occur without any effort on either the part of the mother or the baby. They take place naturally because of the shape of the baby's head as it meets the bones of the mother's pelvis.

What an example of an infinite architect and engineer who designed this marvelous performance. In the face of evidence such as this, it is hard not to believe in a loving Creator-God.

I praise You, my God, for Your wonderful creative power.

THE BREATH
OF LIFE

Come near to God and he will come near to you. James 4:8, NIV.

The day was one of those you dream about. The earth was fresh from the hand of God. "Let us make man in our image" He said (Gen. 1:26, NIV). Bending over, He carefully formed the first human being from the dust of the ground. He lay there. Fragile. Made of dust. There was no movement or life.

God bent again. And He breathed into that dusty form. Air flowed into the being's nose and down into his lungs. It brought life. What joy God must have felt as He witnessed that first breath of His new creature.

Air is the breath of life. We are fully dependent upon it to give us oxygen to operate the powerhouses in our cells. These powerhouses, called mitochondria, are the backbone of every activity carried on in our bodies. They use the oxygen to burn the food that fuels our cells.

There's also an air supply that provides power to our Christian experience. The power comes from air that's unpolluted by any smog. Martin Luther called this air the "breath of the soul," for just as surely as our physical bodies need air to survive, so our spiritual selves need the power of this air supply to continue to grow. The air that provides such a heavenly atmosphere is prayer.

"Prayer is the opening of the heart to God as to a friend. Not that it is necessary in order to make known to God what we are, but in order to enable us to receive Him. Prayer does not bring God down to us, but brings us up to Him" *(Steps to Christ*, p. 93).

God longs to be your friend. He wants you to talk with Him the same way you'd converse with your best friend. The only way you can do that is through prayer. Share your thoughts, your problems, your joys and successes. He listens. The Bible suggests that we should "pray without ceasing" (1 Thess. 5:17). That means becoming so comfortable with the fact that God is our friend that we have a continual open communication with Him. That's when prayer becomes as natural as breathing!

Are you looking for a life full of vitality, happiness, and joy?
Are you needing a breath of fresh air? Prayer is the air
your soul needs to breathe.

THE HAPPIEST
DAY IN
38 YEARS

"See, you are well again. Stop sinning or something worse may happen to you." John 5:14, NIV.

He had been by the Pool of Bethesda for 38 years with no one to help. Paralyzed in some way through a reckless lifestyle, he hoped that the magic waters would bring a quick fix to his problem.

That day began just as every other of the previous 14,000 or so. He peered into the water, hoping he would be the first to slide into its healing waves.

Then he saw a reflection of a Stranger's face distorted by the ripples. Before he could look up, he heard a strange question: "Do you want to get well?"

This man must be a newcomer, the paralytic mused to himself. *Everyone who's come to the temple has seen me here.*

"Sir, I have no man . . . to put me into the pool." Squinting his eyes to see the face of the Stranger haloed by the sun behind Him, the paralytic felt a surge of hope explode throughout his body. *Will the water stir while this Man stands here? Will He, the first who has ever shown an interest in me, be the one to restore my hope for healing?*

Then the Stranger made a command as strange as His question: "Get up! Pick up your mat and walk."

The paralytic gazed into the waters, his quick-fix solution. In that glance he saw the waters for what they were: powerless. The Stranger's words still rang in his ears: "Get up!"

Though the Stranger asked the impossible, the paralytic sensed the power attached to that command. He decided to try. What did he have to lose?

And at once the man was cured.

The paralytic's disease was primarily the result of his own bad habits. Telling the man to "stop sinning or something worse may happen to you," Jesus made the point that we have often brought disease upon ourselves by transgressing the laws of God. Health can be preserved only by obedience (see *The Ministry of Healing*, pp. 81, 82, 113).

Many who are sick today are "lying beside the pool," trusting in human beings for a quick-fix solution to problems they brought on themselves. But only Jesus can heal us as a whole. Treating the body and ignoring the soul is not enough.

Don't wait to feel that you are whole. Believe His Word,
and it will be fulfilled.

SIMPLIFY— SIMPLIFY

March 16
Larry Richardson

Whosoever believeth in him should not perish, but have everlasting life. John 3:16.

Several years ago I joined a group on a 10-day backpacking trip across the Sierra Nevada range. Everything we needed—food, clothes, cooking equipment, tent—had to fit in our backpack. Since the recommended load for a backpack is one third your body weight, I needed to keep mine below 60 pounds.

I had been on several weekend hikes before, but packing for 10 days is a far cry from packing for two days. I had to keep reminding myself to simplify. No fancy meals—only freeze-dried entrées that mix with boiled water. Not two coats to change into—just one. Not three pairs of pants—just the one pair to wear. Not six sets of underwear—just two. No extra shoes or towels. No books for evening reading. Every item had to pass the test: "Do I *really* need this item?" A friend of mine even cut off the handle of his toothbrush to eliminate excess weight. What a difference it all made while hiking on the trail. Every pound we left behind was a blessed relief those 10 days.

At times in my life I thought salvation was too complicated—at least the way some make it appear. It seemed as if reaching heaven depended on what I ate, how I dressed, where I went, how I interpreted Bible prophecy, how I chose to worship, and on and on. The simple formula of John 3:16 had become a 100-pound backpack.

But Jesus set the record straight. In a stern rebuke, He declared: "Woe to you, teachers of the law and Pharisees, you hypocrites! You shut the kingdom of heaven in men's faces. You yourselves do not enter, nor will you let those enter who are trying to" (Matt. 23:13, 14, NIV).

Simplify! Simplify! Salvation is not so complicated. The prophet Micah reduced it to three simple elements: "To do justly, to love mercy, and to walk humbly with your God" (Micah 6:8, NKJV). Ah! Now that's a load off my shoulders.

How could you simplify your life so the load
you are carrying doesn't weigh you down?

FRIENDS AND
THE QUALITY
OF LIFE

Therese L. Allen

> Some men came, bringing to him a paralytic, carried by four of them. . . . They made an opening in the roof above Jesus and . . . lowered the mat the paralyzed man was lying on. When Jesus saw their faith, he said to the paralytic, "Son, your sins are forgiven." Mark 2:3-5, NIV.

To say that I am a hockey fan is somewhat of an understatement. Even though I had been an avid hockey fan since I was a tiny tot, I had never seen a live National Hockey League game. Now I was on my way to the fabulous Forum in Inglewood, California, to see my first NHL game. To say I was excited was another understatement.

With seven of us jammed in a small car, we had to leave my wheelchair behind. Our plan was to carry me from the entrance of the Forum to our seats. Fortunately for me (and others) I weigh less than 100 pounds. Plans . . . do they ever go right?

When we arrived at the Forum, we could not even get inside the parking lot, let alone up to the entrance. My friends tried to tell the attendant our situation, but to no avail.

I began to worry that they were going to regret bringing me, or that I had ruined the evening. Not so. Don carried me from outside the parking lot all the way to my seat. What an entrance! And what friends!

I remembered this experience when I read about a paralyzed guy and his friends coming to see Jesus. When he and his friends reached the house where Jesus was teaching, they couldn't get to the entrance either. I wonder if he had any of the same thoughts I had.

Then the wild idea. Why not go up on the roof, cut a hole in it, and voilà! down we go? Insane . . . I love it! Friends add greatly to one's quality of life.

Because of his faith, not only was the man healed physically but also Jesus forgave his sins.

Unfortunately, Scripture does not tell what Christ thought of the friends and their little escapade. Knowing Him as I do, though, I believe He was as amused as I was. He knew the value of friends. And because of their faith, I tend to believe, the friends also had their sins forgiven and experienced that wonderful blessing of spiritual healing.

What could you do today to show someone
that you are a faithful friend?

PURE MILK
OF THE WORD

March 18
Betty M. Larson

Then away with all malice and deceit, away with all pretence and jealousy and recrimination of every kind!
Like the new-born infants you are, you must crave for pure milk (spiritual milk . . .), so that you may
thrive upon it to your souls' health. Surely you have tasted that the Lord is go.od. 1 Peter 2:2, 3, NEB.

No picture intrigues me more than one showing an infant looking
deeply into the eyes of its mother, and with the same tenderness, the
mother's searching gaze at her nursing baby. Studies have shown
stronger bonding between the breast-fed baby and mother than the bottle-
fed infant and mother.

Humanity has yet to improve on what God has made for the nourishment of human infants. Not only does illness decrease a great deal through
the baby receiving the mother's immunities through her milk, but also studies have now shown that intelligence and development increase.
Apparently the brain continues to develop in the breast-fed baby because
of chemicals found only in mother's milk. Scientists have discovered more
than 90 elements in mother's milk that change in strength according to the
developing child's needs.

The mother benefits from breast feeding as well as the child. Breast
feeding mothers seldom hemorrhage, because of the presence of a chemical
secreted during breast feeding. This chemical causes the uterus to contract
to its normal size and the now unused circulatory system to the uterus to
close itself off. Yet another chemical has a calming or tranquilizing effect
on the mothers. Breast feeding is convenient for the mother in that she has
no bottles to wash or formula to buy or prepare—thus the cost of breast
feeding is extremely small.

Ellen White says, "The best food for the infant is the food that nature
provides. Of this it should not be needlessly deprived" *(The Ministry of
Healing,* p. 383).

As I consider all the benefits of the milk that God provided for a baby,
I find my mind drawn to the phrase "pure milk of the word" in 1 Peter 2:2
(NASB). What a marvelous God we have, to have provided so well for the
needs of infants, whether they be babies sucking at their mother's breast,
or spiritual infants, such as you and I. The "pure milk" found in God's
Word is far superior to the most eloquent human words. Why is it then
that we drink so little of this spiritual nourishment?

*Are you daily drinking deeply from the "pure milk of the word"
for your soul's health? Why substitute human-made "milk"
when God's "milk" is abundant and free?*

CLIMBING INTO OLD AGE

Jan W. and Kay Kuzma

Even youths grow tired and weary, and young men stumble and fall; but those who hope in the Lord will renew their strength. They will soar on wings like eagles; they will run and not grow weary, they will walk and not be faint. Isa. 40:31, NIV.

Hulda Crooks first climbed 14,495-foot Mount Whitney, North America's highest mountain, in 1962 at age 66 and continued to climb it nearly every year after that until she was 91.

Also when she was 91 years old she climbed Japan's 12,388-foot Mount Fuji, reaching the summit on July 24, 1987, the oldest woman ever to do so. Six weeks later she again climbed Mount Whitney. Incredible as it may seem, between 81 and 90 years of age she climbed 97 peaks. When someone challenged her to climb the steps leading to the top of the Capitol Dome in Washington, D.C. (steps are sometimes more difficult than a mountain trail), Hulda Crooks accepted the challenge—and won. When she was 94 her doctor told her she had the heart and lungs of an 18-year-old.

She lives by the philosophy that "muscles, not used, atrophy. Bones, not put under stress, lose minerals and become weak. Joints, not moved sufficiently as in walking, working, or other forms of exercise, become stiff from disuse. The blunt facts are that your body needs intelligent care."

Hulda has proved that a lifestyle change can take place at any age. She describes herself in her teen years as being nervous, anemic, and perpetually tired. At age 31, when she was overweight and not physically well, her physician-husband encouraged her to become more physically active. She followed his advice, and it changed her life. Since then she has said that we can't separate diet and exercise. "The diet provides the materials for the body's functions. The exercise is absolutely essential in keeping up a good circulation. If we don't exercise, the circulation is sluggish, and that affects the entire body, the mental as well as the rest of the body."

Hulda's life is an inspiration to all, regardless of age, to get up and get going!

What lifestyle change do I need to make to be able to "run and not grow weary," or "walk and not be faint"?

EITHER
BURN OUT
OR DELEGATE

"Why do you alone sit as judge, while all these people stand around you from morning till evening?" . . . *"What you are doing is not good. You and these people who come to you will only wear yourselves out. The work is too heavy for you. . . . Select capable men . . . and appoint them as officials."* Ex. 18:14-21, NIV.

During the time that Moses was involved in the liberation of the Israelites from Egypt, he had left his wife and two sons with Jethro, his father-in-law. When Jethro heard that the Israelites were migrating near to where he lived, he took Zipporah and their boys back to Moses.

Soon Jethro noticed a problem. Moses didn't have any time for them—or for himself, for that matter. So Jethro spoke up and basically said that even though Moses was God's appointed leader of the children of Israel, that didn't mean he had to do everything himself. Read this fascinating story for yourself in Exodus 18.

For the first 40 years of his life Moses had been trained in the court of Egypt in matters of government and administration, so he had great ability in dealing with people. Now he had a divine mandate to educate and train God's people in loyalty to their Creator. A conscientious person, Moses felt a great sense of responsibility and urgency for those under his charge.

Jethro understood that Moses was unselfishly doing his best to fulfill his God-given commission. But he also recognized that Moses was in danger of burnout. Israel's leader was exerting himself in a most worthy cause, but that did not justify his being presumptuous in expecting the Lord's continued blessing.

So Jethro said to Moses, "Listen now to me and I will give you some advice, and may God be with you" (Ex. 18:19, NIV). He then outlined an administrative structure in which Moses would continue to be the people's representative to God, and God's representative to the people, but would also train others to administer groups of thousands, hundreds, fifties, and tens. "That will make your load lighter, because they will share it with you" (verse 22).

Then he said, "If you do this and God so commands, you will be able to stand the strain, and all these people will go home satisfied" (verse 23). And Moses too could go home at a decent time to his wife and children, who also needed him!

Are you trying to do more than your share? Ask the Holy Spirit and your family how you could cut down before you burn out.

THE STEWARDSHIP
OF HEALTH

Do you not know that your body is a shrine of the indwelling Holy Spirit, and the Spirit is God's gift to you? You do not belong to yourselves; you were bought at a price. Then honour God in your body. 1 Cor. 6:19, 20, NEB.

God's ownership of everything rests first on creation and second on redemption. It does not limit itself to material possessions—we human beings belong to Him because we are "bought at a price." God does not enforce His ownership—rather, He seeks to have human beings voluntarily recognize it. Such a recognition leads to the relationship between God and human beings called stewardship.

A steward controls the goods of the owner, but control is not ownership. Many have acted much like a rebellious teenager. They have confused God's purpose in making them stewards. Instead of learning to use life so they could be trusted with it for eternity, they have run away from God, saying, "My life is mine. I will use it as I please, eat what I want, and do what I want." Trouble, frustration, and eternal loss are the certain result.

Suppose someone gave you a beautiful cut glass goblet. Although it is very fragile, if you care for the goblet, it will last indefinitely. However, if you are careless with it, the chances are it will break and become useless.

On the other hand, suppose that you receive an equally beautiful silver goblet. That sturdy vessel can endure quite a bit of abuse without breaking. Even if you treat it roughly, it will probably last indefinitely.

The two goblets represent two alternatives of what a person might inherit in physical health. Some may have a more fragile constitution than others, but all will benefit from a careful preservation of the health resources entrusted to them.

Consider God's gift of health. He expects us, as stewards, to preserve that gift with every resource available to us. Health always faces constant assaults from factors over which we have no power. But we can control most of the influences that cause degenerative disease and premature death.

When men and women consider themselves God's steward they can rest in the assurance that regardless of circumstances, they are under the direction and protection of the owner of the world.

Am I caring for my body as a steward would, or as an owner would? What more could I do to be a good steward?

OLYMPIC
CHAMPION

"You have so little faith. I tell you the truth, if you have faith as small as a mustard seed, you can say to this mountain, 'Move from here to there' and it will move. Nothing will be impossible for you." Matt. 17:20, NIV.

Ever since I can remember, I have dreamed of being an Olympic champion. The feel of adrenaline flowing, the heart throbbing, and the sweat pouring as I strive for a gold medal for my country. Wow, what a thrill that would be!

As a child I would get all my neighborhood friends together, and we would pretend we were competing against each other in gymnastics. I would always try to be the one representing America. You should have seen us out in the backyard doing somersaults and cartwheels.

That dream came to a sudden stop the winter I was in fourth grade. I was sledding in the mountains of Colorado with friends and family. Eagerly I shouted to my dad, "Push me first." Then while speeding down the hill I hit a huge bump that tossed me through the air and onto my elbow. The impact badly broke my arm.

Although my arm did heal after the accident, it remained terribly crooked, and I soon realized that being an Olympic champion would probably never happen. I did not let that stop my interest in gymnastics and other sports, however, for I remembered a Bible verse that says "Be strong and very courageous" (Joshua 1:7, NIV).

I refused to let that accident prevent me from enjoying the sport I loved all through grade school, high school, college, and beyond. I may not lead my country to a championship, but I *can* still strive to become the very best I can be. And I *can* be a champion of strength and courage for others who experience setbacks—others whose dreams get shattered like my elbow.

If Satan has put hurdles in your life, I encourage you to claim Matthew 17:20, for with God's help, nothing is impossible. You may not be an Olympic champion, but God can change your attitude from one of disappointment to one of acceptance. With God you can be a champion and receive the gold medal of His kingdom.

If you are struggling with the thought that you cannot accomplish the things you would like to because Satan has put a boulder in your path, take that challenge and use the obstacle to climb your way to new heights.

A REST
FROM
STRESS

Nancy Newball (based on an
NAD Church Ministries article)

Come to me, all you who are weary and burdened, and I will give you rest. Matt. 11:28, NIV.

Imagine you're driving back home from a sight-seeing trip, and you find yourself in Amityville, New York. It's 2:00 a.m. You're alone. Having made a wrong turn, you find yourself in an eerie section of town. Just then you look at the gas gauge. It's on empty.

Pulling over to the side of the road, you step out into the darkness to look for a public telephone. Suddenly you hear heavy footsteps behind you. Your eyes dart back, then from side to side, but you see no one. The footsteps get faster, closer, and then a huge hand grabs your face, stifling your scream.

How do you feel? Science has shown that your body responds automatically to stressful situations. We call this response the "fight or flight" response. Stress causes certain changes to instantly take place in your body:

- Circulation, breathing, and muscle function speed up.
- More energy-rich sugar appears in the blood.
- Blood-clotting mechanisms accelerate.
- Blood cells enter the bloodstream from storage depots.
- Senses become keener.
- The digestive system goes into a temporary halt.

These responses help you deal with emergencies in life. But what would happen if these responses took place in your body 10 hours a day for 10 years and you never acted upon them? Some people go through life racing and battling as though a huge hand were grabbing at them all day long. We call it stress.

But it doesn't have to be that way. There's a way to find rest. Part of the solution lies in your perception of life. We usually cope with trouble better if we intersperse a couple breaks during the day.

And take God at His word when He says, "Remember the Sabbath day by keeping it holy. . . . On it you shall not do any work" (Ex. 20:8-10), and you'll find that your troubles aren't as heavy. One day a week you can rest from that stressed-out feeling you get as if someone were grabbing you. God has given you permission.

When you feel the pressure mounting today, take a little break.
And don't forget to rest on the Sabbath!

GIVING UP
WHAT
ISN'T GOOD

March 24

Therese Valin

Be strong and courageous. Do not be terrified; do not be discouraged, for the Lord
your God will be with you wherever you go. Joshua 1:9, NIV.

Don't let anyone kid you, caffeine is addictive.

As a child I didn't like water or milk, so I drank Kool-aid, Coke, or Pepsi. I drank so much Pepsi I started to crave it. By the time I was 25 it was my only drink—four to six cans a day. Yet I didn't know I was addicted.

In January 1989 a Seventh-day Adventist friend invited me to church. I had breakfast and my usual glass of Pepsi before we left. She didn't tell me she had the whole day planned, so by late evening, with no Pepsi since breakfast, my caffeine addiction was more than I could bear. I abruptly got up to leave. Unable to concentrate, I couldn't even carry my Bible, and almost fell down the steps. My friend stopped at a gas station and got me a Pepsi, which I drank in 20 seconds. Immediately I felt better. It was then I realized I had a drinking problem.

She took me to her place, made popcorn and smoothies for me, and listened and held me while I cried out in pain and confusion. She told me about God's concern for my total well-being and how He doesn't want me to be caught up in an addiction cycle. Not wanting me to be alone in my condition, she told me to stay at her house for the night. Although she made me a wonderful nutritious breakfast the next morning, I still had a Pepsi when I got home.

After that night I prayed to God to help me cut down gradually so I wouldn't go through intense withdrawal. I told God the weekend I wanted to stop completely. I wanted to be alone with God if I had withdrawal symptoms.

To my surprise, God helped me, so when the day came to stop completely I didn't have any cravings or withdrawal symptoms. Today I drink only water or juice. I am grateful to God, for He hears and answers our cries for health and healing.

*Are you addicted to a drink or food? I challenge you to pray
about it, cut down, pick a day to stop, and spend
that day with God. He will help you through it.*

GRIEF: AN EXPERIENCE IN LEARNING AND LEANING

Those who know your name will trust in you, for you, Lord, have never forsaken those who seek you. Ps. 9:10, NIV.

When my father passed away two years ago, I was angry with God. Why did it have to be my father? There were other fathers He could take; why mine? I felt God had deserted me. Who was going to look after me? Who was going to help me provide funding for my school fees? Who was going to stand beside me through my adolescence? Who was going to teach me how to change my car oil? Who would give me away when I got married?

On Father's Day I had no reason to go to the Hallmark store for a card. Neither would I have any reason to go to the men's department store for a gift. Most of all, I missed having my father around and was furious with God. I couldn't face the world alone! *Why me?* I wondered.

Jesus asked God, when He was nailed to the cross, why God had forsaken Him: "Eli, Eli, lama sabachthani? that is to say, My God, my God, why hast thou forsaken me?" (Matt. 27:46). And I asked the same question.

These past two years have been a learning and leaning experience. Learning that God allows trials and tribulations to attack us so that if we choose to let God help us, we can be stronger. And it's been a leaning experience. In God I have found my solitude, peace, and hope. God has not forsaken me. He has always been my friend and partner.

I began reading the Psalms, because David had many of the same doubts I had. He could tell God exactly how he was feeling, get it out of his system, and turn around and praise God. I've learned that that is the answer to getting rid of the bitterness and finding healing. And the result is an intimacy with God that I never had before.

Currently I am working with hospice patients. I have had the opportunity to share my experiences with my patients and their families. God is using my personal experience to help my faith and be a witness for Him. And I can praise Him for that.

Have you been feeling that God has forsaken you? Tell God how you're feeling, read His Word, and experience His healing.

WAKE UP YOUR HAPPY HORMONES

Thus you will walk in the ways of good men and keep to the paths of the righteous. Prov. 2:20, NIV.

D o you feel tired? blue? anxious? stressed out? If so, what you need is to exercise the 10-step plan and walk it off!

Our bodies have an amazing hormonal system of morphinelike chemicals called endogenous opioids, or more commonly, endorphins. It appears that exercise activates these hormones, helping people feel better.

The Perrier Survey of Fitness in America found that those who had a deep commitment to exercise reported feeling more relaxed, less tired, and more disciplined, had a sense of looking better, greater self-confidence, and increased productivity, and in general felt more at one with themselves.

This information wouldn't surprise your grandmother. She knew that scrubbing the kitchen floor when she felt upset really helped. But today, with our tiny kitchens and easy-to-clean floors and so little time for family or God, what you need is a 20-minute brisk walk in the fresh air—together with your family or God or both.

If you have tried exercise programs before and just couldn't stick with them, try the 10-step plan. All you do is make a commitment to the first 10 steps of a daily walk. That's it. Set the alarm for a certain time, and when it rings, get out of your easy chair, turn off the TV, put on your walking shoes, open the door, and take at least 10 steps. Once they are behind you, you can turn around and go home, if you wish. Or you can continue around the block.

The 10-step plan works because it eases you past those difficult first steps. It gets you up and going, and if you are like most people, once you get going you will finish the entire walk.

Why wait until fatigue, depression, and stress get the best of you, when with the 10-step plan you can exercise those happy hormones, talk to God, enjoy His nature, and perhaps memorize a meaningful passage of Scripture—all at the same time!

Lord, may I walk in the way You would have me go.

GOD'S
INCREDIBLE
SUN

Jan W. Kuzma

and Cecil Murphey

Light is sweet, and it pleases the eyes to see the sun. Eccl. 11:7, NIV.

D o you realize the incredible freebie that God has given us in the sun? Just think of it—without the sun we wouldn't have any green plants. Chlorophyll, the green pigment in plants, traps the energy of the sun and stores it, mainly in the form of glucose. This simple sugar is the building block for more complex carbohydrates and is the body fuel that gives animal life most of its energy.

Sunlight provides the environment needed for our existence by enabling plants to create oxygen and carbon dioxide, and its rays regulate temperature and humidity at life-supporting levels.

Plus, sunlight is good for us!

1. *The sun helps heal certain diseases.* It kills germs. Sunlight has been used to treat tuberculosis successfully, and it has a healing effect on infections such as strep throat, pneumonia, puerperal fever, and even leprosy.

2. *When the sun touches your skin, your body makes vitamin D.* That's why vitamin D is sometimes referred to as the sunshine vitamin.

3. *Sunlight that enters your eyes improves body function*, stimulating the pituitary, hypothalamus, and pineal glands, as well as the neurotransmitters of the brain.

4. *Moderate sunlight gives you healthier skin.* Some medical personnel suggest that tanned skin is three times more powerful in killing germs than untanned. However, too much sunlight can damage the skin. Sunburn is associated with skin cancer and wrinkles, so don't overexpose yourself to sunlight.

5. *Sunlight is good for your nerves.* It elevates your mood and probably increases the endorphins your brain manufactures to give you a feeling of well-being.

6. *Sunlight strengthens your heart.* Just like exercise, sunlight lowers the resting pulse rate, tones up the heart muscle, increases cardio output by improving your heart's efficiency, and normalizes blood pressure.

7. *Sunlight enhances your immune system* by increasing the oxygen-carrying capacity of the red blood cells.

Sunlight to the body is something like thanksgiving to the soul. It gives one an incredible feeling of well-being—and it's free.

Bask in God's incredible sunlight for at least five minutes today, and let God know how thankful you are for this freebie!

THE ADVENTIST
ADVANTAGE

March 28

Neal C. Wilson

What advantage, then, is there in being a Jew, or what value is there in circumcision? Much in every way! First of all, they have been entrusted with the very words of God. Rom. 3:1, 2, NIV.

In Romans 3 the apostle Paul said, in effect, What is the advantage of being one of God's chosen people with advanced knowledge, hope, and guidance? (In the King James Version it says, "What advantage then hath the Jew?") Then he goes on to describe how they were the recipients of God's oracles. They had that divine advantage of knowing, of understanding. But it does nothing for us at all unless we put it into practice, unless it becomes a part of our life.

I believe there is an "Adventist advantage." More than 130 years ago God gave the Adventist pioneers special health information. But the Adventist advantage won't do Adventists any good unless they are a living testimony that demonstrates the superiority of God's lifestyle to the world, both physically and spiritually.

When I was a young man I spent several years at Vincent Hill School up in the foothills of the Himalayas in North India. Because of the favorable climate at 10,000-foot altitude, a number of schools existed in that area. Ours, however, was the smallest and the subject of ridicule because we had a vegetarian diet. The others would challenge us in all kinds of sports, but we always declined because of school policy. They said it was because we were afraid of them.

There came a time when a few of us were tired of the ridicule. Annually the area schools held a competitive run to a mountain about 20 miles away that required traveling over difficult terrain with huge gorges spanned by little rope bridges, and scrambling steep mountainsides. We were really not supposed to compete in it. However, three of us decided that we would enter to demonstrate to all our critics that there was an Adventist advantage.

It was a privilege to return from that three-day ordeal and be at least a quarter of a mile ahead of the next competitor! And the two others from our school took the third- and fourth-place positions. After that there was never any question about the "grass eaters" and the Adventist advantage.

Are you a living demonstration to the world
of the Adventist advantage?

FOR GOOD?

Connie W. Nowlan

*And we know that all things work together for good to them that love God,
to them who are the called according to his purpose. Rom. 8:28.*

None of us ever planned our lives exactly as they are. But real life is never packed in neat boxes with labels to be unloaded at the end of the journey like the contents of a moving van. Our second son, Terry, has a wheelchair, which we call his "purple Porsche," so he can keep up with the rest of us.

Terry has been part of our family for 25 years. Years of love, hope, tears, joys, frustration—as well as lessons in patience and dependence that have slowed us, his family, down.

My morning prayer for "strength just for today" has become so natural, I can't imagine beginning the day any other way. For having a person with a long-term disability in one's family is an everyday challenge, not just once a month or for a weekend. And God's strength has sustained us all, daily, weekly, monthly throughout those 25 years.

The word "good" and "for good" are poles apart. God's original plan did not include families having sons or daughters with disabilities. Having such a son or daughter is not "good," but personal reactions to circumstances can work "for good" when God's children allow Him to mold us despite less than perfect circumstances. For God waits patiently, His arms outstretched toward His hurting children, desiring to be their comforter, their strength, and their guide.

I can understand my own inability to "work my way to heaven" better as I care for my son, doing for him things he cannot do for himself. It reminds me that I cannot be "good enough" for heaven without my Saviour's sacrifice. This fact has transformed my self-sufficient tendencies into grateful acceptance of Jesus' earthly sacrifice.

I look forward to the time when we move from earth to our heavenly mansion, for Terry will be leaving his purple Porsche, and we will enter heaven with our fellow Christians labeled "perfect in Christ." Together we'll walk the golden streets. Memories of the purple Porsche will fade as we, with all heaven's inhabitants, praise God for Christ's death for us that entitles us to our heavenly home.

*What are you looking forward to leaving behind
when Jesus comes and labels you "perfect in Christ"?*

EXERCISING
YOUR FULL
POTENTIAL

Karis Osadchuck

Now we see but a poor reflection as in a mirror; then we shall see face to face. Now I know in part; then I shall know fully, even as I am fully known. 1 Cor. 13:12, NIV.

Six months pregnant is an exciting time in a couple's life, especially with the first child. Together my husband and I are experiencing the development of our new little person. The intensity of our relationship with the baby is growing as the baby exercises its expanding capabilities each day.

The first several weeks and months of pregnancy are a blur of emotions, hormones, and questions. Next one eagerly awaits the unknown moment of first detectable movement. Finally it happens, and with each passing day the sensation of life within becomes stronger.

The baby must continue to explore its little cocoon of a world in order to develop its muscles, nerves, circulatory systems, and other body parts fully. In essence it must experience itself fully, completely at every stage of its maturation.

Just as our baby can't control much of its world—what I eat or drink and how much rest and activity I get—we may feel limited by our circumstances, especially as we think about reaching out and witnessing to others. But just as the growing baby in the womb has an opportunity to stretch its arms, legs, feet, and fingers and to discover itself with all its potential, so do we as Christians. What will we do in our environment, our little sphere of service? Will we reach out our arms and legs and touch others, or will we maintain the status quo?

Just as my husband and I thrill to feel and see the baby growing stronger every day, I wonder if it's anything like God feels as He watches and experiences with us our spiritual exercise and growth?

Let's each exercise not only our bodies every day but also our chance to be born of the Holy Spirit. Only then can we reach out, stretching beyond our comfortable routines and cocoons, touching lives for the kingdom, and in so doing realizing our fullest potential as humans.

Here's the challenge: Reach out to someone
today and share God's love.

ALHAJI

Jerre St. Clair

With a mighty hand and outstretched arm; His love endures forever. Ps. 136:12, NIV.

One encounters many wonderful stories at a mission hospital, but those in which hope and function are restored to a child are perhaps the most heartwarming. Alhaji, a little 9-year-old boy from Freetown, the capital of Sierra Leone, is one of God's miracles.

One day when Alhaji was playing outside, he saw that the room in which he lived with his mother and little sister was on fire. He ran in to save some of their possessions, but unfortunately a burning curtain fell down on him. Although he was able to get out of the room, he was in terrible condition. The left side of his head, arm, and trunk had severe third-degree burns, and his ear had been completely burned off.

His mother took him to the government hospital in Freetown, where he stayed for 11 months. There most of the wounds healed, but his arm grew to his body. It looked as if he had no arm—only his hand was sticking out. The doctor told him that the only thing he could do was to cut off the hand so that it wouldn't look so ugly. The boy and his mother were terrified and refused.

They had heard about Masanga Leprosy Hospital and decided to come for advice. Alhaji was lucky to meet Dr. R. Kazen, who performed the first surgery, cutting the skin and separating the arm from his body. Then the tedious, time-consuming process of skin grafting and exercises started to restore its function. Later a visiting hand surgeon, Dr. Robert Horner, performed an operation that made his left hand more functional.

Alhaji's mother and little sister stayed with him all through his ordeal and encouraged him greatly. After a whole year at Masanga he was able to use his arm again. Although not perfect, he felt like a human being again, instead of a deformed monster.

When I see Alhaji with his arm stretched out and functional, I think of how good God is to stretch out His arms, through dedicated health workers, to people who otherwise would have no hope.

We can all be recipients of God's "surgery"! God has promised
to cut away our sin and restore us to an abundant life,
if we will submit to the unavoidable pain.
Oh, how grateful we should be for His outstretched arms to us.

THERE'S HEALING IN A GOOD JOKE

Our mouths were filled with laughter, our tongues with songs of joy. Then it was said among the nations, "The Lord has done great things for them." Ps. 126:2, NIV.

I awakened in the early-morning hours feeling really sick. As I lay in the darkness, I could hear the strange night sounds of the African village nearby, still new to me six weeks into our mission term in Nigeria. I knew this pain was something new, for I was experiencing what seemed like those last excruciating pains before childbirth, and I definitely was *not* pregnant.

Creeping out of bed, I quietly made my way to the refrigerator, where we kept a bottle of malaria pills. We had been told that at the first sign of malaria a person should take six pills to make the attack less severe, but alas, I found only one pill. Swallowing the tablet, I headed back to our bedroom, where my husband lay sleeping. Finally I awakened Gary, told him what I thought was happening, and asked him to put a blanket over me. In the darkness he tossed a cover over me, but that only created a new problem. For the first time in my life, I could feel every wrinkle. When I asked him to smooth out the wrinkles, he too knew I was in trouble.

At sunrise my husband went to get the doctor. A few minutes later Elena arrived, and as Gary greeted her, she asked, "What can I do?"

Without missing a beat, he replied, "I think you should shoot her." He immediately laughed when he saw Elena's horrified face. Realizing the double meaning behind his words, she promptly gave me the necessary treatment to endure and survive my first bout with malaria.

During our years in Nigeria, Elena often laughed at Gary's jokes. Gary's ability to see a funny side in almost every situation has helped make many strangers become friends. His humor not only draws people, but it has helped bind our family together. Humor has added enjoyment to our everyday life and has often lifted our spirits during rough times. God wants us to enjoy life to the fullest, and I'm thankful to have a special dose of humor in our home.

Can others see that the Lord has done great things for you?
Try to sprinkle a little more humor and laughter
into your life, and maybe they will.

DIET FOR THE YEAR 2000

Marilyn Renk

> Then God said, "I give you every seed-bearing plant on the face of the whole earth and every tree that has fruit with seed in it. They will be yours for food." Gen. 1:29, NIV.

The diet that scientists in the field of nutrition are advocating for the year 2000 is incredibly similar to the one God gave to Adam and Eve: fruits, grains, seeds, and nuts, plus the vegetables added at the time of the Fall. Eating this diet, even without access to the tree of life, human beings lived close to 1,000 years.

After the Flood people added clean meat, which resulted in a drastically shortened life span (Gen. 9:2, 3). This flesh-food diet has been the accepted human diet since!

Then in 1863 Ellen White began to speak out against meat. In 1864 she wrote: "Many die of disease caused wholly by meat eating; yet the world does not seem to be the wiser" (Counsels on Diet and Foods, p. 385). At the turn of the century, between 1902 and 1905, she made the following comments: "I am instructed to say that if ever meat eating were safe, it is not safe now" (ibid., p. 384). "Flesh was never the best food; but its use is now doubly objectionable, since disease in animals is so rapidly increasing" (ibid.). In 1902 she predicted, "It will not be long until animal food will be discarded by many besides Seventh-day Adventists" (ibid.).

Now, almost 100 years later, the prediction is coming true. In 1977 the scientific community finally admitted they were wrong to recommend meat and animal products as a primary source of good nutrition. And in 1992 they issued, based on scientific evidence, a new food guide, the Food Guide Pyramid, that looks amazingly similar to the eating plan recommended in the Bible. The foods they suggest that we should eat most frequently are low in fat and provide fiber, complex carbohydrates, vitamins, and minerals. These foods come from grains and plants; breads, cereals, rice, pasta, fruits, and vegetables.

God told us what to eat in the beginning, and although it has taken us thousands of years to realize that fact, we're finally coming around and accepting God's diet as the diet for the year 2000.

Challenge: take a look at your current eating pattern. Choose
one small change you would be willing to make
immediately to move closer to the plan of eating as
God intended for optimal health.

THE GIFT OF THE SABBATH

If you keep your feet from breaking the Sabbath . . . , if you call the Sabbath a delight and . . . honorable, and . . . not going your own way and not doing as you please or speaking idle words, . . . I will cause you to ride on the heights of the land and to feast on the inheritance of your father Jacob. Isa. 58:13, 14, NIV.

The Sabbath is a special day—a time to put aside work, schedules, and daily commitments. It's a time to *rest, relax, refocus* and *remember* that God created you, and to *recount* all His blessings. The Sabbath offers us opportunity for *re-creation* for our battle-weary bodies, our muddled minds, and our starved souls. It provides fellowship with our Creator and with each other. Each Sabbath is a 24-hour celebration of life.

To really get the health benefits God created this day for, you've got to make it different, special, and stress-free. That's why it's important to avoid such things as newspapers, radio, TV, video games, or any business involvement. When you put aside secular pursuits, the pressures and job tensions decrease or even disappear. Sabbath is a moral battery-charging time—a time to gain spiritual insights and inspiration.

If you want to live a healthier lifestyle, you can't afford to overlook or ignore what the Sabbath can do for you. On this day you can seek solitude in the outdoors and avoid stress-producing noise. It's a day to avoid jammed freeways, shopping malls, packed stadiums, competitive sports. By doing this you'll be able to maintain healthier blood pressure levels. Worshiping God, instead of your work, frees you from the pressure to perform, produce, and compete. Taking a weekly vacation from stress can rejuvenate your entire system.

The Sabbath is a day to cease from work, but it's far more than that. It's also a time to cease from accomplishment, from worry and tension, and to stop trying to control your own life. For six days you have been in the driver's seat and have tried to shape the world by your wit, creativity, brains, and brawn. But on Sabbath you receive permission to slide over and let the God of the universe take the driver's seat while you enjoy a chauffeured, no-hassle trip. A 24-hour free ride with the One who created it all. Wow! So, sit back, relax, and enjoy the trip.

The Sabbath is a weekly gift with incredible blessings attached.
Don't forget to open it each week and experience
God's promises in Isaiah 58:13, 14.

RUNNING THE GOOD RACE

Larry Richardson

> Let us throw off everything that hinders and the sin that so easily entangles, and let us run with perseverance the race marked out for us. Heb. 12:1, NIV.

Several years ago I started jogging for exercise. While it has brought me many wonderful health benefits, I can see why many folks avoid it. The sore muscles, tired joints, weary lungs, and everyday aches and pains that jogging can produce discourages the easily disheartened.

However, I have decided that avoiding such pain may not be in my best interests. As a jogger I've learned to listen to my body's signals and learn from them rather than hide from them. While I am out running I look for pain: on the inside of my leg, the outside, the heel, the arch, the hip, the knee, wherever it may occur. Is it a true warning, or a trick my body is playing on me to get me to stop? If I move or turn differently, does it help or hurt more?

While most people feel that to seek pain is illogical, to endure it irrational, and to extend it insane, those who exercise regularly see things differently. Pain teaches, shapes, strengthens, and develops the athlete. It is the only means we have for knowing and doing our best. While most people see no reason to live with pain, athletes believe the opposite. They cannot live without it. As the popular saying goes: "No pain, no gain."

It is interesting that the apostle Paul compared the Christian experience to running a race, and the analogy seems quite fitting. As the runner endures pain, so the Christian suffers trials and tribulations. But in neither case are they to be shunned. The biblical writer James advises: "Consider it pure joy, my brothers, whenever you face trials of many kinds, because you know that the testing of your faith develops perseverance" (James 1:2, 3, NIV).

My jogging experience has taught me the blessings, benefits, and necessity of tribulation for refining the body and mind, and for the Christian it is no different. Discipline, commitment, faith, and perseverance are all shaped in hardship, difficulties, and failure. "So run, that ye may obtain" (1 Cor. 9:24).

What is hindering you from running the race and obtaining the prize of both good physical health and good spiritual health?

THE HEALING TOUCH OF MUSIC

Jimmy Rhodes

And whenever the evil spirit from God was upon Saul, David took the lyre harp and played it with his hand; so Saul was refreshed, and was well, and the evil spirit departed from him. 1 Sam. 16:23, RSV.

 King Saul was troubled, his conscience pricked. As he tossed upon his bed, sleep evaded him. There was no Nyquil, Sleep-eze, or Nytol in those days. So in the late hours of the night he would call for David, the young shepherd, to play soft melodic cadences on his stringed instrument, and sleep would come. Music refreshed him, calmed his nerves, and made him feel better.

The noted philosopher Friedrich Nietzsche wrote in 1889 that "without music, life would be a mistake." Music has a tremendous impact on the human psyche. In fact, it's now an accepted healing agent in modern medicine.

As a result of graduate study a few years ago at the University of Southern California, I became extremely interested in using music as a way of changing behavior in people. In my work at Life Care Centers I've seen how music in its many facets has changed the moods of people within minutes. Some older individuals who mostly sleep through the day, or perhaps just sit and stare vacantly, will begin tapping their toes and clapping their hands when they come to music therapy. Music reaches them when no person can.

Whitcomb reports that music is a "battery charger for the brain, and some people will frequently begin to reminisce, and verbalize thoughts and feelings in ways thought to be long dormant."

Satan, that musical genius, knows the effect music has on people. But instead of soothing them, he delights in just the opposite. Studies have shown that sensory overload can increase anxiety. He causes this with a fast-pulsing beat and loud, chaotic sounds. Music with less than 72 beats per minute (normal pulse rate) has a calming effect. Faster, loud, clashing sounds increase anxiety.

I can testify to the truth of Ellen White's words: "When turned to good account, music is a blessing; but it is often made one of Satan's most attractive agencies to ensnare souls. When abused, it leads the unconsecrated to pride, vanity, and folly. When allowed to take the place of devotion and prayer, it is a terrible curse" *(Testimonies,* vol. 1, p. 506).

The next time you have trouble sleeping, don't pop a pill.
Relax and fall asleep with God's beautiful music.

BITTER
WATER

April 6
David J. DeRose

> When they came to Marah, they could not drink its water because it was bitter. . . . So the people grumbled against Moses, saying, "What are we to drink?" . . . The Lord showed him a piece of wood. He threw it into the water, and the water became sweet. Ex. 15:23-25, NIV.

In December 1993 water treatment facilities for Washington, D.C., experienced serious problems. Because of the great possibility of contracting infection, local authorities told residents to avoid drinking tap water. Similar problems have occurred in other cities and towns.

In addition to water treatment facility problems, natural disasters such as floods, earthquakes, hurricanes, and tornadoes will threaten water quality. Campers and backpackers in North America as well as travelers drinking tap water in certain countries abroad may become ill from contaminated water.

Even crystal-clear water can harbor serious illness. For example, giardia, a parasite, often inhabits seemingly pristine running streams.

How can we guard against becoming infected from contaminated water? Do we need some advanced antibiotic or other drug? The U.S. Centers for Disease Control and Prevention tells us that we can kill all dangerous organisms by bringing water to a rolling boil for one minute. (Increase the boiling time if you live at elevations significantly above sea level.)

The remedy for microbially contaminated water is simple and inexpensive. It is the same with the remedy for life's trials. In fact, God used the illustration of impure water to teach this lesson:

"For every trial, God has provided help. When Israel in the desert came to the bitter waters of Marah, Moses cried unto the Lord. The Lord did not provide some new remedy; He called attention to that which was at hand. A shrub which He had created was to be cast into the fountain to make the water pure and sweet. When this was done, the people drank of the water and were refreshed. In every trial, if we seek Him, Christ will give us help. Our eyes will be opened to discern the healing promises recorded in His word. The Holy Spirit will teach us how to appropriate every blessing that will be an antidote to grief. For every bitter draft that is placed to our lips, we shall find a branch of healing" *(The Ministry of Healing,* p. 248).

Think of a time when you came to the "bitter waters of
Marah" and recall how God brought blessings out of bitterness.
Praise the Lord, for He is good.

128

YOU CAN
CHOOSE LIFE
OR DEATH

*Take heed, you senseless ones among the people; you fools,
when will you become wise? Ps. 94:8, NIV.*

Many years ago I worked for a worldwide finance company. At the
time I was not a Seventh-day Adventist, and in fact knew very little
about spiritual things.

My job involved contacting customers delinquent in paying their ac-
counts. One day I visited the home of such a customer. The wife, who obviously was not having a very good day, greeted me at the door. My
appearance on the scene only added to her unhappiness.

The husband, who was our customer, had just learned that he was going
to have some of his toes amputated from one foot. Poor circulation had led
to the problem. The doctor told him that he must quit smoking and drinking, and that he must change his lifestyle, or the other foot would be next.

The toes were amputated, and he went right on smoking and drinking. Several months later I contacted the family again, only to find that
our customer was back in the hospital having his foot amputated. Did he
quit smoking and drinking? No! He continued his habits and later had
his leg amputated.

Continuing to smoke and drink, he lost the other leg about a year later.
A few months after that, he died! He ignored all the warnings and continued his habits until his body could no longer take the punishment.

"Extreme case," you say. Hardly! This kind of thing goes on every day.
I personally know people who have suffered heart attacks and have been
warned to change their lifestyle, but have kept right on with their unhealthy habits. Their ignoring of their doctors' advice will eventually cause
them even greater pain and suffering.

Unfortunately we humans tend to violate good counsel more than we
follow it. God has given us information about how to keep our bodies
healthy and live righteous lives, and He has asked us to be obedient to His
will. When we do it, we will be healthy physically and spiritually. His ways
are always the best. Isn't it time to stop our foolish unhealthy lifestyles and
do what He says?

*Dear Lord, help me not to foolishly live the way I want to live.
Give me wisdom and willpower to live according to Your will. Amen.*

ARE YOU AT RISK OF ACQUIRING AN EGYPTIAN DISEASE?

April 8

Henry C. Martin

> I pray that you may prosper in all things and be in health,
> just as your soul prospers. 3 John 2, NKJV.

Seven million Americans have diabetes. The typical high-fat (40 to 47 percent), high-sugar standard American diet (SAD) contributes to adult onset diabetes. Thirty-four centuries ago God urged us to avoid fats (see Lev. 7:23-25), but most of us still ignore this important counsel and reap the results of age-old diseases such as diabetes.

Archaeologists have discovered 3,000-year-old mummies that show the evidence of diabetes and atherosclerosis, the same diseases we have today. At that time the wealthy Egyptians had Hebrew and other Asiatic slaves to do their work, while they enjoyed a rich diet and the sedentary lifestyle of a couch potato.

"If you diligently heed the voice of the Lord your God and do what is right in His sight, give ear to His commandments and keep all His statutes, I will put none of the diseases on you which I have brought on the Egyptians. For I am the Lord who heals you" (Ex. 15:26, NKJV).

By choosing a plant food diet and getting plenty of regular exercise it is possible to reduce dramatically the risk of adult onset diabetes and in many cases eliminate the need for medication. God knew the nutrition humanity needed, so at Creation He offered an abundant variety of plant foods: fruits, grains, nuts, and vegetables.

After a two-day Reversing Diabetes Seminar at Arrowhead Springs Christian Conference Center, one grateful wife said, "My husband stopped using his 85 units of insulin on the second day. Now, five months later, he has lost 50 pounds, and I have lost 34 pounds. We are praising the Lord."

God promises health rewards for those who are obedient. "So you shall serve the Lord your God, and He will bless your bread and your water. And I will take sickness away from the midst of you" (Ex. 23:25, NKJV).

And finally, for ultimate health, God sent Jesus Christ: "I have come that they may have life, and that they may have it more abundantly" (John 10:10, NKJV).

*If you haven't done so already, begin today living a
healthier lifestyle. Choose to avoid the diseases of the Egyptians.*

POISON IN
THE AIR

The Spirit of God has made me; the breath of the Almighty gives me life. Job 33:4, NIV.

It happened one Sunday when I decided to go scuba diving with my fellow student missionaries, Matt, Monica, and Julian. We'd been down about 30 minutes to a depth of 60 feet exploring the wall that rises from the ocean floor and eventually surfaces as the Majuro atoll in the Marshall Islands.

Beginning to feel strange, I motioned to my buddy, Julian, that I was going up. During the trip up I kept checking my gauge so I wouldn't surface too quickly and end up with the bends. Then at about 30 feet I couldn't see my gauge or concentrate. Julian realized I was in trouble and grabbed my arm. At 10 feet I was breathing extremely fast and felt I wasn't getting any air. We finally broke surface, and I spit out my regulator and gasped the fresh air. I inflated my buoyancy compensator and started to float.

Freaking out, I exclaimed, "I can't see!" Everything was blurred. I concentrated on Julian's goggles long enough to finally read the word "tempered" on the glass. I had a headache and felt light-headed. Julian towed me in to shore, and I just sat there on the reef while he went to find our friends.

Later, back at our room, Mr. Lane, the principal, came by and said we shouldn't use our tanks because two tanks had accidentally gotten filled with carbon monoxide when the compressor broke. The man filling the tanks switched to another compressor to finish filling them, not realizing that the tanks held lethal gas. The mistake was discovered when the guy using the other tank passed out in 20 feet of water. His dive buddy brought him up, but he was unconscious for four hours in the hospital. That's when I realized I was lucky to be alive.

And that's when I thought about how lethal the consequences of a little mistake can be. The broken compressor nearly killed two people! Sin is like that. It might not be something others can see or smell, but it can cause death just the same. The fact is, Satan kills, and "the breath of the Almighty gives me life."

Don't wait until sin is choking you to breathe freely from God's Word. It's the only protection against Satan's poisonous gas!

JEALOUSY CAN DESTROY YOUR HEALTH

Harold Shryock

Do nothing out of selfish ambition or vain conceit, but in humility consider others better than yourselves. Each of you should look not only to your own interests, but also to the interests of others. Phil. 2:3, 4, NIV.

Throughout earth's history jealousy has been one of the devil's most effective means of producing trouble. At the time of the wilderness wandering of the Israelites, Miriam and Aaron became jealous of their brother Moses, and the Lord sternly rebuked them, striking Miriam with leprosy for seven days (Num. 12:1-14).

Solomon wrote, "Anger is cruel and fury is overwhelming, but who can stand before jealousy?" (Prov. 27:4, NIV).

Jesus found it necessary to reprimand His disciples because they jealously wanted to be the greatest (see Mark 9:33-35).

The apostle Paul lists jealousy among the "acts of the sinful nature" in Galatians 5:19, 20.

Jealousy affects one's emotions. The emotions, through the autonomic nervous system, influence the functions of the body's various organs. In the case of jealousy, one's intellect loses control of the emotions, thus allowing illness to develop.

In one of the classics of medical literature, Dr. Edward Weiss tells about a young woman who complained of persistent headaches. Dr. Weiss performed a thorough physical examination and arranged for a series of laboratory tests, but found no explanation. Meanwhile other symptoms developed, including intestinal disorders. The patient finally became bedridden. Discouraged because of lack of improvement, she discharged Dr. Weiss and called in the old family doctor who had known her from childhood. In casual conversation he discovered that her brother had married and that she was overwhelmed with jealousy toward the woman. Once she was convinced that her emotional upheaval had caused her symptoms, her symptoms lessened and she eventually recovered.

Here are two important points that Ellen White makes: First, "the condition of the mind affects the health to a far greater degree than many realize" *(The Ministry of Healing, p. 241).* And second, "if the mind is free and happy under a consciousness of rightdoing and a sense of satisfaction in causing happiness to others, it will create a cheerfulness that will react upon the whole system, causing a freer circulation of the blood and a toning up of the entire body" *(Medical Ministry, p. 105).*

> *Clean up your emotional garbage—jealousy, envy, anger—and you'll feel better.*

132

BREAD
FOR LIFE

April 11

Velda Nelson

I am the living bread that came down from heaven. If anyone eats of this bread, he will live forever. This bread is my flesh, which I will give for the life of the world. John 6:51, NIV.

This cool spring morning I stand at my kitchen counter measuring ingredients into the big brown bowl. It is breadmaking day, a time to replenish my store of plump brown loaves of the staff of life, as my father always called bread. No meal was complete to him without a slice of the bread my mother made.

Mother taught me to make the wholesome wheat bread our family relished, often quoting: "It is a sacred duty for those who cook to learn how to prepare healthful food. . . . It takes thought and care to make good bread; but there is more religion in a loaf of good bread than many think" (*The Ministry of Healing*, p. 302).

And so I carry on the tradition, although now my family is grown, and I could easily buy wholesome bread at the market. To me it is almost a spiritual exercise to knead the soft dough, to shape it into loaves and put it in the pans, then to wait for it to rise. And as the bread bakes, the mouthwatering aroma of fresh bread fills the whole house.

With pleasure I share the brown, crusty loaves with a busy young mother and her lively youngsters next door, or my retired friend whose wife is no longer able to bake and cook as she once did.

As I measure and mix the ingredients, I challenge my imagination to devise symbolic spiritual metaphors. Flour—the whole kernels of God's word. Leavening—the working of God's love in my life. Salt—Jesus said, "Ye are the salt of the earth" (Matt. 5:13, NIV). Honey—the sweet spirit of love for God, for family, for all I meet. Oil—the Holy Spirit. Water—the living water Jesus offered (see John 4:10, 14). Bread—the completeness of Jesus' life and His sacrifice when He called Himself the Bread of Life.

Give me, dear Lord, this bread of life that I may live thereby, now and eternally.

Challenge: you can learn to bake bread. Ernestine Finley from
It Is Written has a great video, called Natural Lifestyle Cooking:
Homemade Breadmaking Made Easy, *to inspire you and get you*
started. Call 1-800-522-4234 or contact your
local SDA church for instruction.

Is any one of you sick? He should call the elders of the church to pray over him and anoint him with oil in the name of the Lord. And the prayer offered in faith will make the sick person well; the Lord will raise him up. James 5:14, 15, NIV.

Doctor Bland walked into my husband's hospital room and announced with tears in his voice, "Dan, there's nothing else we can do for you. Your liver has ceased to function!"

My husband bravely asked, "Well, Doctor, how long do I have to live?" The doctor responded that they did not have time to attempt a liver transplant, with all that would be involved in that process. Unless he was able to tolerate the massive intravenous dosage of a drug that might possibly shock the liver back into function, he could expect to live only eight to 10 days, depending on his endurance. We knew, with his history of drug reactions, that the medication might end his life even sooner!

Dan looked up and said, "God has given us the counsel that when we're faced with illness, we should have the leaders anoint us with oil and intercede in prayer. Let us have an anointing service, then proceed with the intravenous drugs. The Great Physician is able to heal me, if it is His will, and He can keep me from reacting adversely to the medication."

As the anointing service proceeded, Dan prayed: "Father, if You see fit to heal me, don't just patch me up. I want to be filled with more of Your Holy Spirit's power, for the finishing of Your work, than I have ever yet experienced." God heard and answered that prayer!

Nearly four years have passed since Dan received that "death notice." His liver has been completely healed, and he is preaching with more of the Holy Spirit's power than ever before. God has intervened to spare my husband so that he and I could continue reaching people for Him. Yes, I believe in miracles.

Some folk don't believe in miracles, but I most surely do;
For if God didn't intervene, how could I make it through?
When others have lost their lives, somehow mine was spared;
It surely speaks to my heart: My heavenly Father cared.
Yes, I believe in miracles; I serve the God above,
Who watches o'er His children with a tender Father's love.

*God can work a miracle for you. To increase your faith,
go through the Bible and put your name in the promises
for healing. Then ask, believe, and claim.*

MIRACLE
HEALING

> Confess your sins to each other and pray for each other so that you may be healed.
> The prayer of a righteous man is powerful and effective. James 5:16, NIV.

Why don't we see more miracles of healing? I have pondered that question. Not believing that it was because of a lack of prayer for one another, I began to study deeper into the question. I believe I have found a partial answer from some statements that Ellen White made.

In *Medical Ministry* Ellen White indicates that a major factor preventing healing in response to prayer is the sick individual's health practices. "Many have expected that God would keep them from sickness merely because they have asked Him to do so. But God did not regard their prayers, because their faith was not made perfect by works. God will not work a miracle to keep those from sickness who have no care for themselves, but are continually violating the laws of health and make no efforts to prevent disease" (p. 13).

She further says: "It is our duty to study the laws that govern our being, and conform to them" *(Healthful Living, p. 13)*.

Finally, "when we do all we can on our part to have health, then may we expect that the blessed results will follow, and we can ask God in faith to bless our efforts for the preservation of health. He will then answer our prayer, if His name can be glorified thereby; but let all understand that they have a work to do. God will not work in a miraculous manner to preserve the health of persons who are taking a sure course to make themselves sick" *(Selected Messages, book 2, p. 464)*.

Working with sick people, I can verify the above statements. I have seen healing occur as miraculous as answers to prayer when people start following the laws of health. The return to good health has been far out of proportion to what we would expect medically from the lifestyle changes the individual has made. It is as if God is giving an A for effort to such individuals!

My experience indicates that when we make a decision to follow God's laws of health and act on it, He delights in giving us more health benefits than we medically deserve.

Would you like a miracle? Is there anything in your lifestyle
habits that might be preventing God from working
a miracle in your behalf?

HAVING A HEALTHY
ARGUMENT
WITH GOD

April 14

Jacalyn Nosek

> If you accept my words and store up my commands within you, . . . applying your heart to understanding, and if you call out for insight . . . and search for it as for hidden treasure, then you will understand the fear of the Lord and find the knowledge of God. Prov. 2:1-5, NIV.

For five years I watched my mother slowly die from amyotrophic lateral sclerosis (ALS), a disease that gradually degenerates the motor neurons, causing paralysis. Although the motor (movement) nerves are dying, the sensory (feeling) nerves continue to function, so every movement someone makes with their body causes excruciating pain. There is no cure. For the person with ALS it is like living in a glass coffin. Their mind is sharp, but their body becomes completely paralyzed, until they finally die of suffocation when the diaphragm stops functioning.

Watching my mother die this hideous death made me so angry. I prayed for her healing. When that didn't come, I prayed for God to take away her pain. And when that didn't happen, my faith faltered. How could a "loving" God permit such suffering? My mom had done so much good, especially for blind children, so how could God arbitrarily strike her down? Then I thought of Uzzah. He was only trying to stabilize the ark. Why did God strike him dead when he touched it?

One day when I was desperate, broken, and unable to go on, I opened my dust-covered Bible and read Isaiah 43:25, 26, in which God says, "I . . . am he who blots out your transgressions, for my own sake. . . . Review the past for me, *let us argue the matter together*" (NIV).

I began searching the Scriptures for answers and arguing with God. Then I thought about the parent who tells a child, "Don't touch the stove; you'll get burned." When the child disobeys and gets burned, is it the parent who burned the child? No! And then it became clear to me. God didn't kill Uzzah. God knew His glory would destroy sinful human beings, and because the ark was filled with His glory, He in love warned them not to touch the ark. Uzzah disobeyed and suffered the natural consequence.

As I began to see pain and death as a consequence of sin, and not something caused by God, I began to trust. Now I know that God has the answers to our pain and confusion, if we'll just reason with Him as He asks us to do.

If you're confused about what has happened or what is happening to you or to someone you love, argue with God. His Scriptures and His Holy Spirit can provide incredible healing insight.

WORRY-FREE MONEY MANAGEMENT

> Keep your lives free from the love of money and be content with what you have, because God has said, "Never will I leave you; never will I forsake you." Heb. 13:5, NIV.

The New Testament author of Hebrews in a few final words of fatherly advice quotes from Deuteronomy 31:6 some of the last words of encouragement Moses gave to God's people: "Never will I leave you; never will I forsake you." The grand old leader was 120 years old and full of experience and wisdom when he basically said, Don't put your trust in perishable things. Unlike money, fame, possessions, and other substitutes, the God of heaven will never leave you nor forsake you.

Yet most of us spend about 80 percent of our waking hours in the pursuit of money—thinking about it, earning it, or spending it! Money has become our god, or at least one of our gods. And what does this do to our health? The pursuit of money too often comes packaged with stress, worry, frustration, jealousy, and discontent.

Charles Caleb Colton once said: "Wealth, after all, is a relative thing since he that has little and wants less is richer than he that has much and wants more." The producers of goods and services through the advertising industry spend more than $40 billion a year hitting us with about 300,000 advertising messages each day to make us unhappy with what we have so that we will use money or credit to purchase their products that promise illusive fulfillment. Is it any wonder that money has become our god and the pursuit of money our passion?

The result is often increased debt. The *Wall Street Journal* reported that the average middle-aged American couple had only $2,600 in net financial assets. Translated, that means that because so many are not content with their pay, they are borrowing heavily on their future earnings. The result is no savings, few available assets to donate to the Lord's work, and heavy debt.

By way of contrast, the Walden Pond philosopher, Henry David Thoreau, once said: "We make ourselves rich by making our wants few."

Trusting in the God of heaven, not in money and what it can buy, is the coin of contentment, a key to healthful, fulfilled living in this world and for eternity in the world to come.

Lord, let me be content with the richness of Your blessings and not the world's money.

A CONTENTED
MIND

And now, my friends, all that is true, all that is noble, all that is just and pure, all that is lovable and gracious, whatever is excellent and admirable—fill all your thoughts with these things. Phil. 4:8, NEB.

While working as an Army physician, I noticed that near the end of the year many of the wives, especially those of servicemen on extended duty away from home, would come to the dispensary looking for tranquilizers.

However, one woman, a nurse, always had a smile on her face and a bubbly personality. Since this was quite unusual, I asked how she could keep such a sunny disposition while everyone around her was so nervous and depressed. Here was her response:

"Frequently people share gossip and other negative information about what is going on around the base. But when someone comes to my house, I invite them to have a seat while I continue working and listen to their chatter. But if they begin talking about who is having problems, whose children are getting into trouble, or whose husband or wife is unfaithful, I stop them and say, 'I have enough problems of my own, so I don't need to hear about others. If you want to talk happy, you are free to stay, but if you want to talk negative, you will have to leave.'

"As you can expect," she said laughingly, "I don't have many close friends, but those I have are positive.

"The second thing I do is keep my mind fresh and alive. Whenever I read about something in the news or the papers that I don't understand, I run to the library and ask the librarian if she can help me find books that I can understand to explain the problem area, so I always keep my mind filled with new information and positive thoughts. That's why I don't need medicine to keep me happy."

Two points that will help you keep a contented mind:

1. Avoid negative input—from anyone.
2. Keep improving your mind.

Paul said the same thing in our text for today. The secret to the successful Christian life lies not so much in what we do as in what we choose to let into our minds. Positive, kind, excellent, admirable, and praiseworthy thoughts breed the same kind of mind in us as was in Christ Jesus.

What will you fill your mind with today?

SHARING
YOUR GIFT
OF MERCY

Kay Kuzma

The wisdom that comes from heaven is first of all pure; then peace-loving, considerate, submissive, full of mercy and good fruit, impartial and sincere. James 3:17, NIV.

The Bible speaks of many spiritual gifts. Take, for example, those in Romans 12:6-8. Some are more noticeable, such as the gifts of prophecy, service, teaching, giving, and administration. Even those individuals with the gift of encouragement, who lift people up with their optimism and joy, tend to be seen and appreciated. But at the tail end of the list is a gentle, quiet gift that few notice and appreciate, but which I consider the greatest of all: the gift of mercy.

Kari is a dictionary definition of mercy: kindness in excess of what may be expected or demanded by fairness; kind or compassionate treatment; relief of suffering.

Jogging along a road near Andrews University, Kari came upon a little old man with his head bowed down, slowly walking back home from the cemetery where his wife lay. Kari slowed her pace and walked with him to his house. He was so grateful that someone had showed interest. She stayed in touch with him. Sometimes she would stop to admire his immaculate garden, or she would drop him little notes of encouragement.

She met Grandma Lois at a prayer meeting. Kari was with two other girls. When they broke up in pairs to pray, Kari looked around for someone to pray with and spotted a woman sitting by herself. Surprised that Kari would approach her and be so interested in her, she started crying. She had lost her husband, and things were kind of hard. They struck up a friendship. Kari would go over and visit, and Lois would write her postcards. They became family. Grandma Lois even traveled more than 600 miles to attend Kari's wedding.

Kari is a physical therapist now, but her errands of mercy continue. A little note here, an extra minute to sit and listen there, a flower, a phone call, a smile, and the life of pain and disability that many must endure doesn't seem so bad.

You may not have the gift of mercy naturally, but with God's grace you can practice it. All you have to do is look for someone who's hurting and go out of your way to show them how much you care.

Think of someone you know who could use a little cheering up.
Why not write them a note or give them a call right now?

THE PRESENCE
OF THE LORD

The Lord stood at my side and gave me strength. 2 Tim. 4:17, NIV.

My husband and I heard our oldest son, Chuck, scream and then shoot himself to death. It was 7:10 p.m. on a dark night, physically and spiritually, in December. But I want to share with you something that even to this day I believe is remarkable: the Lord stood at my side and gave me strength! We talk of miracles and of throwing out our fleeces, and we moan that we no longer live in the age of miracles. I don't believe that. Miracles happen all the time, and I consider what happened that lightless and desperate night one of the greatest sensations of my life, even as we stood there appalled and disbelieving that such a thing could happen.

I actually felt a Presence beside me as the various thoughts raced through my horrified mind. I can't explain it, but I know I felt it. As the sad months went by and we tried to gather the fragments of mind and spirit, I would think about that Presence and give thanks that He was—and still is—there. Otherwise, I don't know how I could have kept going that night. Psalm 110:5 declares: "God stands beside you to protect you" (TLB). I thought of this verse, too, that night, when I remembered the article I had recently read about the young man who killed his mother and father before he killed himself. God protected us that night—another miracle.

One of the greatest statements of faith appears in Daniel 3:17, 18: "If we are thrown into the blazing furnace, the God we serve is able to save us from it. . . . But even if he does not . . ." (NIV). But if He does not . . . ! I recall begging God to not let this horror happen. But it did happen. Sometimes what we pray for doesn't happen, but God compensates, of that I am sure. Several months after Chuck's death I wrote a booklet, literally on my knees, that was eventually published and went into a worldwide ministry. Chuck lives in those hearts that have been comforted!

If you're going through tough times, remember, the Lord is standing by your side and will give you strength.

YOU CAN
BEAT THE PAIN

Edwin Krick

Because of your wrath there is no health in my body; my bones have no soundness because of my sin. . . . My back is filled with searing pain. Ps. 38:3, 7, NIV.

Practically everyone, if they live long enough, will have some arthritis. It can be caused by something external that gets into the system, such as a virus or a bacteria, and affects the body by damaging the tissues. That's why keeping your immune system healthy is crucial.

Rheumatoid arthritis is the crippling type. It can create swelling in any of the 200 synovial joints in the body, half of which are in the back. When the joints become inflamed, the joint lining swells. Fluid pours out, disrupting the normal function of the joint as well as causing quite a bit of pain, tenderness, and the sensation of heat. Treatment for arthritis involves physical therapy, appropriate rest, splints, devices to assist the joints to keep them from being stressed, hot and cold compresses, and gentle exercise. Judicious use of medication can also be of help.

Rheumatism differs from arthritis, because it affects surrounding tissues outside the joint itself, including muscles, tendons, ligaments, and the bursas, the lubricating sacs around joints. Four lifestyle factors trigger it: overstress, overweight, underexercise, and the most important one—lack of sound sleep.

You can prevent the most common type of arthritis, osteoarthritis, to some extent through the following approaches. Lose weight—the extra stress on the joints doesn't help. The health of the cartilage is the next most important thing, and that, of course, is related to its use. Cartilage (the pad between the bones) doesn't have a blood supply, so it has to get its nutrition from the joint lining, which occurs only when we use the joint. So we need exercise. Normal daily activities are adequate for most people, but we recommend that patients work up to 20 minutes of brisk walking four times a week. In addition, watch your diet, especially avoiding high fat and protein consumption.

Just as moving painful joints is important in reducing the pain, so it is in the spiritual realm. Dealing with guilt, bitterness, and anger, although painful, is the only way to experience true spiritual health. Don't let pain keep you from doing what you know you should!

Challenge: If you're bothered by arthritis, try a radical change in lifestyle: lose weight, eat fresh fruits and vegetables (eliminate fat and too much protein), lower stress, exercise, and get plenty of sleep!

THE ELIXIR
OF DEATH

April 20

Auldwin T. Humphrey

> Do not get drunk on wine, which leads to debauchery. Instead,
> be filled with the Spirit. Eph. 5:18, NIV.

It was 1981 in one of the Midwest's major metropolitan areas. A five-week evangelistic seminar had led more than 50 converts into the Adventist lifestyle. One of these individuals was Larry, a young college-age man who had not known of the Seventh-day Adventist faith. One of the most profound impacts on Larry's life was the health message. Its influence would later save his life.

During the 10 years following his baptism he took many turns that led him in and out of the church. However, some of his Adventist lifestyle habits never faded.

By the early 1990s Larry had settled into a steady job managing an apartment building in the heart of the city.

One of the tenants in Larry's building was a very intelligent, soft-spoken man who owned a computer. Larry was invited to use the computer from time to time and frequently visited the tenant's apartment. On each occasion the tenant would offer Larry a beverage that the Adventist lifestyle frowned on. Larry's convictions about health caused him to decline the drinks.

One day Larry observed the man on the street near the apartment complex. He had a scowl and seemed despondent. Larry passed it off as a youthful mood swing. Later, when he watched the evening news, it became clear why he was depressed. The police were closing in on him.

The city was Milwaukee and the tenant was Jeffrey Dahmer, the notorious serial killer who had gained control over his victims by drugging their drinks. Larry shuddered when he thought that he had escaped the fate of others because he, like Daniel of old, refused to drink the forbidden.

How many people, young and old, have lost their lives because they left the avenues of appetite unguarded? How many victims partook of the king's drink and the elixir of death?

Today Larry gives God the glory for allowing him to be exposed to the Adventist lifestyle. Unlike addictive substances, being filled with the Spirit has no negative side effects, and the Spirit satisfies.

*Keep the health principles you have been taught. You never
know when they might save or prolong your life.*

THANKS FOR
THE THORNS

Antonio M. Rosario

Weeping may remain for a night, but rejoicing comes in the morning. Ps. 30:5, NIV.

An ancient legend tells of a woman who comes to be ferried across the river Styx to the land of departed spirits. The ferryman, Charon, offers her a potion that would cause her to forget the life she is leaving. In the end she doesn't drink it. She chooses to remember life's pains, sorrows, and failures rather than to forget its joys, triumphs, and loves.

We discover the significance of life when we enjoy its pleasures *and* gladly accept its pain, suffering, and disappointments.

The famous Scottish preacher George Matheson, who found it hard to praise God when things went wrong, learned this lesson. When he began to lose his sight, he struggled with his burden until he was able to pray, "Oh, my God, I've never given Thee thanks for my thorns in the flesh. Thousands of times I've given Thee thanks for my roses, but not even once for the thorns. I've looked forward to a world where I'll be recompensed for my cross, but I've never thought of my cross as a present glory. Teach me the worth of my thorn" *(Our Daily Bread,* April 14, 1990).

All of us have thorns we must live with. We can pray for deliverance and acceptance as David did. In his anxiety and anguish he often cried out to God, "O Lord, do not rebuke me in your anger or discipline me in your wrath. Be merciful to me, Lord, for I am faint; O Lord, heal me, for my bones are in agony. My soul is in anguish" (Ps. 6:1-3, NIV). But he was also able to accept the thorns and sing, "Your rod and your staff, they comfort me" (Ps. 23:4, NIV).

As we read God's Word we can be comforted by how Jesus' presence and His words "I am the resurrection and the life" transformed Mary and Martha's pain and grief (John 11:25, NIV). And we can say with apostle Paul: "My grace is sufficient for you" (2 Cor. 12:9, NIV).

When bad things happen to you, pray the prayer of George Matheson:
"Teach me the worth of my thorn," and praise the Lord.

HEALTHY
COMMUNITIES

If you have faith as small as a mustard seed, you can say to this mountain, "Move from here to there," and it will move. Nothing will be impossible for you. Matt. 17:20, 21, NIV.

There is a mountain of illness out there," said the nurse.

"There is a mountain of ignorance out there," said the teacher.

"There is a mountain of crime out there," said the judge.

"There is a mountain of poverty out there," said the social worker.

"Yes, there is," said the wise one, "and it's all the same mountain."

A national telephone survey published in 1994 by the Daniel Yankelovich Group asked 1,000 adult Americans, "What creates health?" They concluded:

● People are discouraged about the health of their communities.

● The public has a new concept of what creates health, one that shifts away from the idea of mere disease avoidance and toward the active pursuit of wellness.

● Family security dominates perceptions about healthy communities.

● The public is ready to play a more proactive role in the health of their communities.

According to a 1994 statement by the U.S. Health Corporation, "the concept of a healthy community is a simple one, rooted in the recognition that the major determinants of health have little to do with the health-care system. Rather, health is determined by equitable access to such basic prerequisites for health as food, shelter, clean air and water, adequate resources, education, income, a safe physical environment, social supports, and so on."

The question is Are we as Christians ready to get involved in making our communities more healthy places to live? Jesus said that faith as small as a mustard seed could move a mountain.

But moving the mountain of illness, ignorance, crime, and poverty will require active faith. We must work together with everyone interested in the health of our communities—educators, law enforcement agencies, local governments, business leaders, and others—to address the fundamental issues affecting our communities. Together we can move mountains and build healthy communities—places where people care for each other, education is valued, work and play are honored, children are loved and the elderly are esteemed, and where neighbors laugh and cry together. Such communities will provide protection for the weak, opportunity for the strong, healing for the ill and infirm, and growth for all.

What can you do today to build a healthy community where you live?

144

WIPING
AWAY TEARS

He will wipe every tear from their eyes. There will be no more death or mourning or crying or pain, for the old order of things has passed away. Rev. 21:4, NIV.

The door burst open as Eric's panic-stricken scream shattered the calmness of the Thursday afternoon. "Mama, come quickly. Richard's dying!"

Eric did not wait for any response from me, but quickly turned around and headed back into the orchard. I followed closely behind him. As we moved deeper into the orchard, I called after him, "Eric, what happened?"

"Richard fell off the tractor and it ran over him!"

"No, Lord, not this way," I prayed as I stopped, struck by the words Eric had said. "Lord, give me peace. Help me to know what to do!" In a moment I was beside Richard.

As we were waiting for the paramedics to arrive, 7-year-old Richard in a calm voice said, "Mama, I'm going to die."

As I prayed for the wisdom to respond, strength and courage welled up inside me as God spoke: "I will never leave thee, nor forsake thee" (Heb. 13:5).

Bending over his small, boyish frame, I asked, "Richard, you love Jesus, don't you?"

"Yes, Mama, I do," he said.

"You know Jesus loves you, Richard, don't you?" I asked.

"Yes, Mama. He loves me."

I began praying aloud for healing and God's mercy. The child repeated after me, "I'm sorry, Jesus, for all the wrong I ever did." Peace and tranquillity engulfed my son and me as we prayed there in the orchard. Never again would he speak after that heart-searching dialogue with me.

By faith my husband, Tim, and I know that Richard's prayer was heard and answered by Jesus, that all his sins were forgiven. We know that Richard sleeps resting in the arms of Jesus, and yet that does not take away the physical, mental, and emotional pain of missing him from day to day. And that is the beauty of a loving God who is willing to physically hold us in His arms and wipe away all our tears when we are hurting and suffering.

One day there will be no more death, sorrow, crying, or pain. Oh, what a blessed hope to look forward to!

Can you feel God holding you in His arms? He'll carry you over grief and pain and will never leave you or forsake you. Hold on to that promise.

GREEN
GARDEN
GOLD

> Now the Lord God had planted a garden in the east, in Eden; and there he put the man he had formed. And the Lord God made all kinds of trees grow out of the ground—trees that were pleasing to the eye and good for food. Gen. 2:8, 9, NIV.

Growing a garden is good for your health.

It may sound like work, but pruning some trees and sowing some seeds out in the fresh air might be just what you need to lower stress in your life, clear your mind of worries, and help you get the exercise you need to feel better. In fact, just viewing beautiful landscapes can alter blood pressure, heart rate, and muscle tension!

Joel Flagler, an agricultural agent at Rutgers University, says more people garden than any other leisure activity because "it's a wonderful way to counteract stress, refresh yourself, and become more productive."

Studies on people in prisons and mental hospitals report that working with plants releases nurturing instincts and makes them feel useful and renewed. "Role reversals occur when patients who require constant care become caregivers for living things," says Flagler. It makes them feel better about themselves.

But a garden offers more health benefits than just stress-reduction. If you eat fruits and vegetables grown in good soil, without pesticides, you have the best possible chance of getting all the vitamins and minerals your body needs.

For example, low trace mineral levels have been correlated with such problems as allergies, diabetes mellitus, hypertension, and arthritis. We get such minerals primarily from our food. In an attempt to determine how commercially grown food compared with homegrown or organically grown food, it was found that in most instances the organic food won, with 240 percent more iron, 120 percent more manganese, and 100 percent more zinc than commercial foods.

All these health benefits from gardening are enough to keep me pruning and planting. And as I look at my Goldcot apricots and rose-blushed Gala apples, and bite into that incredibly sweet, juicy Belle of Georgia peach, I have no doubt in my mind that it was all worth it.

I think God knew what He was doing when He planted a garden for Adam and Eve. It doesn't say He spoke it into being—it says *He planted it!* For the sake of your health, maybe it's time you followed your Creator's example!

Think about what you could plant this season. Maybe a patio tomato, a cucumber vine, and some radish seeds, and enjoy God's green garden gold.

AN OLD BUT INCREDIBLY EFFECTIVE REMEDY

April 25

Agatha Thrash

Is there no balm in Gilead? Is there no physician there? Why then is there no healing for the wound of my people? Jer. 8:22, NIV.

Charcoal has amazing healing properties. In fact, if I were stranded on a desert island and could take only one thing along to protect me from disease, infection, and injury, I would choose charcoal.

My little grandchild accidentally sat down on a hill of fire ants. Instantaneously hundreds of ants bit her. She screamed hysterically from the intense pain. We grabbed her, stripped off her clothing, and ran for a bathtub. Filling it with water, I added charcoal. In less than two minutes submerged in that charcoal bath, she stopped her crying. The charcoal neutralized the poison, and she was pain-free.

Charcoal has incredible adsorption capacity. The total surface area of the sum of the particles in a small cube of charcoal only two fifths of an inch on each side is 1,000 square meters, a field about 35 yards square! Once a substance is adsorbed onto charcoal, washing it with blood plasma or gastric juice will not cause the adsorbed material to desorb. That's why Bertrand in 1913 survived after swallowing five grams of arsenic trioxide mixed with charcoal, and Touery in 1831 survived after swallowing 10 times the lethal dose of strychnine with an equal amount of charcoal.

Charcoal will even adsorb cancer-producing agents such as methylcholanthrene and benzopyrene, which, when free on the skin, are capable of producing skin cancer.

Ellen White extols the virtues of charcoal poultices for fever and inflamed wounds. Then she adds, "I write these things that you may know that the Lord has not left us without the use of simple remedies which, when used, will not leave the system in the weakened condition in which the use of drugs so often leaves it" *(Selected Messages,* book 2, p. 296).

God has also provided us a balm for the wounds of sin—His blood. It has such incredible "neutralizing" qualities that there is no sin wound so bad that it can't be healed. But just as with charcoal, its incredible healing power won't do much good unless you apply it to your own life.

Accept Jesus' sacrifice today, and experience God's incredible healing for your wounded heart.

BE HAPPY AND LIVE LONGER

DeWitt S. Williams

Rejoice in the Lord always. I will say it again: Rejoice! Phil. 4:4, NIV.

Science has documented that happiness prolongs life. Drs. Belloc and Breslow conducted a study of approximately 7,000 people in Alameda County, near San Francisco. It asked simple questions regarding health habits and observed causes of death. The study found age of death to be associated with certain health habits. Surprisingly, diet and exercise, although important, were not the greatest contributors toward longevity. During a nine-year period 57 percent more unhappy people died than did happy people.

Ellen White makes two interesting statements about "perfect" health. One is that "perfect health depends on perfect circulation" *(Testimonies,* vol. 2, p. 531). But the second statement has nothing to do with exercise or what we eat. She says, "In order to have perfect health our hearts must be filled with hope and love and joy" *(Counsels on Health,* p. 587).

Could it follow that a happy smoker might outlive a gloomy, depressed vegetarian? And could it be possible that a happy nonexerciser might be better off than a gloomy vegetarian marathoner?

Joy and happiness can get flabby if you neglect to exercise them. Joy is a habit. Don't let circumstance, no matter how morbid and distressing, kill your joy and contentment. Happiness is more than that little yellow smiley face we stick on envelopes. It's an option that we must choose and use or it will shrivel away, just as muscles atrophy when they receive no exercise.

Considering the circumstances under which the book of Philippians was written—while the apostle Paul was incarcerated in a Roman dungeon—the book is an amazing piece of work. Instead of the gloomy, depressing tone one would expect from a prisoner, Philippians is called the Joy Epistle. In fact, the idea of joy or rejoicing appears more than a dozen times in this short letter. Paul says, "I have learned how to get along happily whether I have much or little. I know how to live on almost nothing or with everything. I have learned the secret of contentment in every situation" (Phil. 4:11, 12, TLB). Can you say the same?

When you get discouraged, read the Joy Epistle,
and rejoice in the Lord always.

I'M THANKFUL
FOR MY LEGS

Therese L. Allen

My God will meet all your needs according to his glorious riches in Christ Jesus. Phil. 4:19, NIV.

I am thankful for my legs—for the strength in my legs and for my feet. You might think this rather strange, since I have been a quadriplegic for 25 years.

For the first few years after my accident, I was able to do standing transfers, and I wasn't bothered by pressure sores, since I was able to contract my quadriceps. I like looking "normal."

But the following year I took a bad spill, and my left foot became seriously infected. After it turned various shades of blue, green, and purple, I went to the hospital for five weeks.

I thought my doctor had a crazy sense of humor, because he kept saying he was going to have to take my foot. I didn't realize until after I was released (with both feet) that he really thought he would have to amputate. The tumble left me unable to do standing transfers, but I could still use my quads, and *I looked normal.*

Unfortunately, six years later I had a really bad fall. It fractured my femur, and I had to be put in a full-length leg cast. My doctor was concerned because of the location of the break and began planning for an amputation "just in case." I was not too concerned, since God had already seen me through a neck injury. But after a short time a sore began to develop. I tried hard to go on, but it got worse. Soon I entered the hospital with a full-blown pressure sore, since I had not been able to use my quads.

I was in the hospital and bedridden at home for a total of six months. But my sore and leg healed without surgery.

Jesus has said He will supply all our needs. He has taken care of needs I never knew I had! Now you can see why I'm thankful for my legs and for my feet. He has given me a very special gift—*I still look normal.*

Sometimes we don't realize how much we have to be thankful for until we meet someone who has less! God is so good. What special gift has He given you? Thank Him for it today.

DON'T BE SO GENEROUS

Good will come to him who is generous and lends freely, who conducts his affairs with justice. Ps. 112:5, NIV.

Believe it or not, there is a time when we are better off not being so generous. It all has to do with calories, sugar, salt, alcohol, and other things that destroy health. More is not necessarily better!

Some estimates suggest that in India the daily caloric intake is in the range of 1,400 calories per person, and in Africa, 1,200-1,900 calories. By comparison, Americans recommend approximately 2,400 calories per day per capita, and many eat far more. Is it any wonder that obesity has reached epidemic proportions?

Many Americans eat their body weight in sugar annually. The average sugar consumption per person each year is 125 to 130 pounds. Many of today's youth eat sugar as though they had a sugar deficiency. Yet we know that sugar clogs the system, causes tooth decay, and depresses the immune system.

The body requires as little as a half teaspoonful of salt per day. Yet we tend to consume 10 or more times that amount.

America has 18 million adults with alcohol-related illnesses. And among youth, some estimate that three out of every 10 have problems with alcohol. It's frightening to learn from the 1989 FBI reports that alcohol was involved in 70 percent of murders, 66 percent of fatal accidents, 60 percent of crimes against children, 60 percent of child abuse, 56 percent of fights and assaults in the home, 55 percent of all arrests, 53 percent of fire deaths, 50 percent of rapes, 41 percent of assaults, and 37 percent of suicides.

We are a generous people, eating too much, especially too much sugar and fat. We drink too much. And we salt too much. It's a part of our self-indulgent "generous" nature!

It's about time we quit partaking so generously of things that aren't good for us and exercised a little more generosity in wholesome practices, such as drinking water, exercising, eating fresh fruits and vegetables, *and in sharing our blessings with others.* Generosity is a wonderful trait when exercised in behalf of others instead of self!

Lord, help me to have the willpower to say no to things
that aren't good for me, and yes to generously sharing
the good things I have with others.

MOBILIZE
YOUR
DEFENSES

Jan W. and Kay Kuzma

Don't you know that you yourselves are God's temple and that God's Spirit lives in you? If anyone destroys God's temple, God will destroy him; for God's temple is sacred, and you are that temple. 1 Cor. 3:16,17, NIV.

The invaders stealthily surround the sacred temple. Silently they take up their positions and wait. At the right opportunity they will attack. In the meantime, they continue their surveillance patrols and strengthen their offensive. They don't realize they will lose the upcoming battle because of *one* significant factor. The temple has an incredible defense team. It's the IS, better known as the immune system.

This highly trained team consists of cells known as lymphocytes, including T cells, killer cells, and natural killer (NK) cells. They watch for the first sign of invasion and stay ready to mobilize their forces. The paratroopers, NK cells, patrol the sacred temple daily. They know they can't stop invaders from taking up their positions, but they can throw off their attacks. The T cells prepare to identify the invaders, then give orders to the killer cells to wipe out the invaders. If they fail to destroy the invaders, the message goes to the B cells—the artillery of the army.

If you can visualize this situation, then think of yourself as that sacred temple. Around you and inside you is the battlefield. Every day enemies seek to destroy your temple. You can win each time only if your immune system with its killer cells stays vigilant. Your enemies—bacteria, viruses, cancer cells, fungi—assault your body through any possible opening, such as mouth, eyes, nose, or even your skin. Anything that weakens your energy, health, alertness, and perception gives the invaders an advantage.

You have other enemies as well. Pollutants, chemicals, and stress continually attack your body. How will you handle the next onslaught? Will you lose the battle to a flu bug? get felled by a nasty cold? let a bronchial infection knock you out of action for a week? Or will you take charge and fight?

Just as God has given us the IS (immune system) to fight off physical disease, God has given us the HS (Holy Spirit) to combat spiritual disease. You are the temple of God. Use your IS and HS defenses and protect God's property.

Pray for the Holy Spirit to give you power to keep your immune system strong and healthy.

CHOICES AND OUTCOMES

April 30

C. A. "Bill" Oliphant

So whether you eat or drink or whatever you do, do it all for the glory of God. 1 Cor. 10:31, NIV.

A simple diet pared of rich foods is the ideal for health of body, mind, and spirit.

Two examples: Sometime in 605 B.C. the Babylonians captured Daniel and took him to Babylon, where he had to make a decision about his diet.

And in A.D. 1635 an English farmer, Thomas Parr, whom King Charles I invited to live at his palace, also had to make a decision about diet.

A relative of the defeated Jewish monarch, Daniel, with other Hebrew captives, was placed in a three-year training program to prepare for Babylonian government service. As a specific benefit, Daniel and his companions were entitled to food from Nebuchanezzar's table.

Daniel, however, was determined to adhere to his customary dietary practices. He "resolved not to defile himself with the royal food and wine" (Dan. 1:8).

You know the story. After 10 days on a vegetarian diet and water, Daniel and his companions "looked healthier and better nourished" (verse 15) than any of the young men who ate the king's food.

According to the Scripture, Daniel became prime minister of the Babylonian Empire, a towering example of what a man steadfast in his integrity can be.

The farmer, Thomas Parr, was allegedly 152 years old when he came to the attention of King Charles. Church and legal records appear to confirm that he was quite elderly.

Because Parr was such a lively fellow, such an amusing wit with endless stories to tell, King Charles had asked him to move into the royal palace in September 1635. As a member of the king's household, Thomas Parr abandoned the simple lifestyle that had sustained him for so many years and began enjoying the rich food and drink served during the king's four-hour banquets.

In November 1635, in the middle of one of the feasts, Parr toppled from his chair and died. An autopsy performed by the royal surgeon, William Harvey, decided that "acute indigestion brought on by indulgence in unaccustomed luxuries" had been the cause of death.

King Charles ordered Parr buried in Westminster Abbey, where today he lies, a self-indulgent curiosity, among England's kings and queens.

Two men. Two choices. Two outcomes.

When faced with a choice between what tastes good and what's good for you, which will you choose?

CREATING A NEW HEART

Elizabeth Sterndale

Cleanse me with hyssop, and I will be clean; wash me, and I will be whiter than snow. . . . Create in me a pure heart, O God, and renew a steadfast spirit within me. Ps. 51:7-10, NIV.

Twice I had gone to the emergency room to treat a pulse rate of more than 160 beats per minute that had lasted several hours each time. Each time it took intravenous medications to slow the too-rapid rate. Treating my problem required careful monitoring and other specific medications and emergency equipment. The cardiologist said it could be cured. The treatment was a procedure called ablation.

In just a few days my doctor had me scheduled for the ablation. I checked in at the hospital early in the morning. Two physicians, a nurse, and a technician attended me.

They threaded four electrodes into the large vein of my groin that carries blood to the right atrium of my heart. One electrode went into my jugular vein and on into my right atrium. One cardiologist manipulated the five electrodes while the other cardiologist, with the aid of a computer, monitored my heart's reaction as the electrodes searched the inner surface of the heart chamber for the misfiring circuit of my heart. Once the team located the culprit, the technician with a second computer applied heat to burn out unwanted tissue.

As the technician applied the heat, I felt a very warm sensation in the area I thought my heart occupied. The warm heart made me feel good all over. The team did the burnout of unwanted cardiac tissue two more times. Each time I savored the warm glow. I wanted to keep that wonderful warm feeling forever. In five and a half hours they had completed the procedure, and the cardiologist gave me the good news. I would not need a pacemaker.

What about the sin in my heart? To remove it will not need two physicians, one nurse, a technician, and two computers with monitors and five electrodes. *Only Jesus.* He is the creator of clean hearts—instantly, as soon as you invite Him in.

Jesus doesn't take five and a half hours, nor is scheduling necessary. Simply invite Him in. The warm glow of His presence is a warmth that never goes away.

O God, create in me a clean heart. May I feel the healing presence of Your Spirit! May Jesus' love fill my soul this day and every day. Amen.

SELF-DISCIPLINE: THE KEY TO MENTAL HEALTH

My son, do not make light of the Lord's discipline, and do not lose heart when he rebukes you, because the Lord disciplines those he loves, and he punishes everyone he accepts as a son. Heb. 12:5, 6, NIV.

Scott Peck begins his book *The Road Less Traveled* with the thought that "life is a series of problems." He then suggests that "discipline is the basic set of tools we require to solve life's problems" (p. 15). "Problems," he continues, "do not go away. They must be worked through or else they remain, forever a barrier to the growth and development of the spirit" (p. 30). That's why self-discipline is the key to mental health.

Unfortunately, our lives sometimes resemble Todd's undisciplined life. An only child, indulged and spoiled, he was, at 14, hanging around with the wrong crowd and beginning to violate the law.

One Saturday night after his parents went to bed, he took his father's car keys. He and his friends rolled the car out of the garage and down the street, started it, and went for a joyride.

Another time Todd stole a gun. After he was caught and arrested, the judge was lenient and sent the boy to the Advent Home Youth Services, but told Todd that if he failed the program he would be sent to juvenile detention.

Todd spent nine months in the program and was doing well. One day at public school he met a girl who talked him into running away with her. They spent several days and nights on the beach. One night during a storm they broke into a beach house for shelter. The owner caught them. Arrested, Todd found himself sentenced to three years in juvenile detention.

Eighteen months later I received a letter from Todd. In it he said, "I have found Christ and am learning to love Him. . . . I realize the wrongs I have done and I am sorry for them. . . . When I get out of jail I will be completing high school and going on to college to become a psychologist and help teenagers who are like me."

Todd didn't want the discipline of being sent to a juvenile detention facility, but it taught him that if he didn't discipline himself, another authority would.

None of us likes discipline, but for our own good—for our mental and physical health—God sometimes has to discipline us with the consequences of our actions so that we will learn the importance of self-discipline.

God disciplines you because He loves you and wants you to learn to discipline yourself. Thank Him for that, and then ask yourself, "In what area of my life do I need more self-discipline?"

NOR ANY DROP TO DRINK

> Everyone who drinks this water will be thirsty again, but whoever drinks the water I give him will never thirst. John 4:13, 14, NIV.

Hiking the trail along the Na Pali Coast on the island of Kauai is a rare and breathtaking experience. The narrow ribbon of dirt hugs sheer cliffs that drop hundreds of feet to the Pacific Ocean below, and the lush tropical vegetation adds to the visual delight. Many streams flow along the 11-mile trail.

On a trip to Hawaii several years ago my wife and I set out to hike the Na Pali Coast, a 22-mile round-trip, all in one day. Since the trail guide promised lots of water along the way, we left our canteens behind to lighten the load. However, once into the hike we learned the truth. Bold signs posted beside every stream warned us: "BOIL WATER BEFORE DRINKING."

Since we hadn't brought any cooking equipment or matches, we were out of luck. Stream after stream presented the same dreadful warning, and soon our scenic day hike turned quite desperate. The intense heat and humidity made the trail a virtual sauna, and our water loss from sweat was rapid.

At one point the trail turned inland, where a vigorous roaring stream rushed along, with the same warning sign. We decided that if we couldn't drink the water, at least we could cool off in it. So very carefully we submerged ourselves in the stream up to our necks. It was wonderful relief from the heat of the day, but remembering "The Rime of the Ancient Mariner," we mused, "water, water, everywhere, nor any drop to drink."

Like my parched throat on the Na Pali Coast, my parched soul longs to be filled. Water has an amazing rejuvenating effect. When we finally found drinking water at the end of the 11-mile trail, my headache departed, my arms and legs felt invigorated, my whole body felt new again. So when I read that Christ promises everlasting water for the spirit and soul, I imagine its restorative properties. Like the Samaritan woman at the well, I too pray, "Sir, give me this water" (John 14:15, NIV).

Fill my cup, Lord, with Your pure water of life.
Fill me to overflowing with Your Holy Spirit.

I CLIMBED TO
THE CAVE
OF EN-GEDI

May 4
Norma J. Collins

Choose my instruction instead of silver, knowledge rather than choice gold, for wisdom is more precious than rubies, and nothing you desire can compare with her. Prov. 8:10, 11, NIV.

I had alarmingly high blood pressure and a cholesterol count that was frightening, and I easily ran out of steam. So when Weight Watchers brought a class to my workplace, I decided now was the time to do something about my condition.

Eight months later and 40 pounds lighter, I felt better, looked better, was more cheerful, and felt good about myself. I followed the program, but there was one thing I resisted. At the close of each class period I was asked to commit to an exercise program. For a number of weeks I refused, because it meant getting up early. Finally I promised to walk around the block one or two days a week.

To my surprise, I enjoyed it. The scenery was pleasant, I encountered friendly people, and when vacation time came I increased my walking distance to a mile. I bought earphones and listened to tapes of Robert Delafield reading the New Testament, exercising my mind at the same time. Walk time now is the favorite time of my day.

As my weight came down, so did my blood pressure. The exercise program brought my cholesterol down as well. After a few weeks I began to feel really terrific. I had more energy, pep, and vitality than I could remember. For the first time in a long time I could walk up those three flights of stairs to my apartment without huffing and puffing.

I had been walking about three months when I went on a trip to the Holy Land. It had mountains to climb, camels to ride, seas to swim in, and I was ready and able to do them all. I even made the three-hour climb to the Cave of En-gedi, where David hid from Saul! I took the snake path up to Masada, where Herod built a palace. And I rode a camel partway up Mount Sinai, hiked the rest of the way, and then hiked down. But I would not have been able to do all these things a year earlier.

I am not a young person; I regret that I did not start an ongoing exercise and self-improvement program when I was much younger.

Ellen White counsels: "Eat sparingly, thus relieving [the] system of unnecessary burden, . . . encourage cheerfulness, and give [oneself] the benefits of proper exercise in the open air"
(Counsels on Diet and Foods, p. 419).
Will you make a commitment to follow this prescription for healthy living?

BIBLE

CANDIDATES FOR

Harold Shryock

HIGH BLOOD PRESSURE

When the donkey saw the angel of the Lord, she lay down under Balaam, and he was angry and beat her with his staff. Then the Lord opened the donkey's mouth, and she said to Balaam, "What have I done to you to make you beat me these three times?" Num. 22:27, 28, NIV.

When a person becomes angry, the organs of the body respond by preparing for combat. Blood pressure rises to increase the circulation and provide the muscles with the extra oxygen and energy-producing nutrients. It is a normal reaction. In healthy persons the blood pressure returns to its usual level once the anger subsides. But some people have such a sensitivity to stressful situations that the blood pressure rises to high levels frequently and tends to remain there. The condition is called hypertension (chronic high blood pressure). The high blood pressure has a destructive effect on the body's various organs and, if it persists, may even cause death.

A number of individuals in the Old Testament could have been candidates for high blood pressure. Balaam, for example, on his way to curse the Israelites, got mad when his donkey refused to budge (Num. 22-24).

Jonah apparently had a habit of being angry. When God spared Nineveh, the prophet bemoaned the fact, and God asked him twice, "Do you have any right to be angry?" (Jonah 4:4, 9). Anyone who gets angry often is a likely candidate for hypertension.

Jacob gave vent to anger when he bargained for Rachel, the woman he loved, and found himself tricked into marrying Leah (Gen. 29:25). The way he favored Rachel's children over Leah's indicates his anger continued to smolder for years.

But among those who got angry in the Old Testament we find no mention of hypertension. Hypertension is a relatively modern condition. The human race has been deteriorating generation by generation ever since Adam and Eve sinned. In our generation we have only a fraction of the stamina that enabled the antediluvian people to live for hundreds of years. Therefore, we are susceptible to forms of illness unknown in Old Testament times.

What should we do about it? Realizing that hypertension comes in response to one's sensitivity to life's anxieties and fears, we must wait patiently on the Lord and "refrain from anger, . . . it leads only to evil" (Ps. 37:8, NIV).

When do you get angry? What could you do at such times so you could "wait patiently" on the Lord (verse 7, NIV) instead of harboring angry feelings and risking hypertension?

DON'T LET THE
DEVIL KILL YOU
WITH FAT

Jan W. Kuzma

The thief comes only to steal and kill and destroy; I have come that they may
have life, and have it to the full. John 10:10, NIV.

The cancer statistics for the U.S. are grim. In 1993 physicians diagnosed 1.9
million new cancer cases, and about 530,000 people died from the disease. Cancer causes more than 20 percent of all U.S. deaths. The rate has
been rising steadily during the past 60 years, from less than 150 deaths per
100,000 population to around 200. Adventists can take some comfort, since
their rates are about 40 percent lower than those of the national population,
according to the Adventist Mortality Study, but it's still a major problem.

Based on today's rates, one out of three Americans will eventually develop cancer. According to the National Cancer Institute, the overall cost
is staggering—$104 billion. This amounts to about 10 percent of the total
cost of disease in the U.S.

Dr. Richard McGinnis, an expert on cancer prevention, attributes more
than 85 percent of the cancer cases to three factors—smoking, a low-fiber
diet, and a high-fat diet—and to a large extent, one can consider cancer a
self-inflicted disease. This would imply that if we would be willing to
change our bad habits, our chances of getting cancer would greatly drop.

Smoking is not the major problem in the church that it is outside it, and
most Adventists eat a variety of fresh fruits, vegetables, and nuts, so they
have a reasonable fiber intake. But it's that third area that trips most of us
up: a high-fat diet. The clever packaging, the advertising, and the good
taste of so many products, which conceal the fat, make this a subtle and
complex problem. We may avoid meat, or feel guilty if a church member
sees us pull up to KFC for finger-lickin' chicken, but we think nothing of
ordering a chocolate shake, brownies, french fries, or apple dumplings
loaded with fat—and calories!

Isn't it about time to take a closer look at what we eat, and instead of just
asking "Where's the beef?" so we can avoid eating it, ask "Where's the fat?"

When it comes to cancer, why be just two-thirds protected by not
smoking and by eating fiber when, according to Dr. McGinnis, we could
be 85 percent protected by avoiding the fat as well?

*Read the labels on your favorite products and add up those grams of fat.
You'll be shocked at the amount of fat in even "low-fat" products. How
can you lower your fat intake? Don't let the devil kill you with fat!*

158

THE DAY I CRIED OUT

*In the day when I cried out, You answered me, and made me bold
with strength in my soul. Ps. 138:3, NKJV.*

We had been in the emergency room only minutes, but it seemed like hours since Carol and I had received a phone call 45 minutes earlier that our son, Jimmy, had been accidentally shot.

Our hearts pounded and we held each other tight as we waited and prayed. It was one of those times when one realizes how human and helpless we are.

The doctor came into the room and with tears in his eyes said, "I'm so sorry. We couldn't save him." No words can express how we felt at that moment. The pain was unlike any other a human can experience.

At the time I had 20 years' experience in the ministry, but none of it seemed relevant. I was absolutely lost as to what to do or say. In another room a family grieved the loss of a mother. I knelt with them and prayed that God would comfort them.

How I longed for someone to come and minister to Carol and me. It was then that I remembered Psalm 138:3: "In the day when I cried out, You answered me, and made me bold with strength in my soul."

Since that night we have cried many times together or alone. Crying is healing! We have reached out to God for courage and strength, and He has not failed us. Had it not been for our faith in God, I know our loss would have overwhelmed us.

As a pastor and a police chaplain I witness every day the results of a godless life. I see drug addicts and alcoholics, the broken and sick. I have looked upon the dead forms of people who have died as a result of their habits. My heart has ached for survivors of loved ones who could go no further and took their own lives.

In a world filled with broken hearts, broken lives, and broken bodies, I thank God for His healing grace. His grace truly is sufficient for us. He surely will answer us when we cry out for help. He really will strengthen us so we can carry on.

*Thank You, Lord, for Your healing grace, and for giving
me strength to carry on when bad things happen.*

HORMONES
AND HAPPINESS

May 8
Kathy Corwin

Do not cast me from your presence or take your Holy Spirit from me. Restore to me the joy of your salvation and grant me a willing spirit, to sustain me. Ps. 51:11, 12, NIV.

During my early 30s I struggled with a terrible, hopeless depression, combined with crying spells, tiredness, a grouchy disposition, paranoia, nightmares, and lower-back pain. My period came as often as two weeks apart, and I felt as if I were in a deep black hole.

At times I wanted my life to be over. I had seen a number of doctors—they wanted to write me prescriptions for Valium and told me to contact a psychiatrist. Finally, in confused desperation, I cried out, "Lord, if You are there, please help me! Bring joy and balance back into my life."

The very next day another minister's wife from a distant town called me. She said, "Kathy, I understand you are going through some real depression. I want to recommend a doctor."

I didn't want any more doctors, but she persuaded me to go anyway. After the doctor listened to my symptoms, his response amazed me. He said, "I can help you. I believe you have endometriosis. This means that when you have your period it affects your ovaries in such a way that they do not produce enough estrogen and progesterone."

He immediately scheduled me for a laparoscopy that proved his diagnosis correct. With a hysterectomy and estrogen therapy my symptoms disappeared, and God restored joy to my life.

I share this story because it may help others who suffer with such a disease that has been neglected or misdiagnosed. Before my experience I had a close friend with similar symptoms who took her own life. She didn't see any way out of that dark hole.

I'm so thankful that God led me to a health professional who understood my condition. When we lose balance and joy in our lives, we need friends and professionals to help. But most of all, we need to realize our dependence on God.

I know from personal experience that the Great Physician understands what it takes in each of our lives to restore and sustain us with His healing touch of balance and joy.

What healing do you need today to restore the joy and balance in your life and that of your family?

MOMS' CLUB
—DEPRESSION'S
CURE

Dawna Sawatzky

These older women must train the younger women to live quietly, to love their husbands and their children, . . . to be sensible and clean minded, spending their time in their own homes, being kind and obedient, . . . so that the Christian faith can't be spoken against by those who know them. Titus 2:4, 5, TLB.

I had always considered depression to be a condition others experienced; but not me. And I had prepared for the year when both of our children went away to school by finding a full-time job to keep myself busy. It didn't work. I had "lost" my two good friends, my two funniest acquaintances, and a big chunk of my favorite full-time job—mothering. It left me depressed!

"God, what would You have me do?" I prayed. Then two statements I had read repeatedly came to my mind: "Let the older women teach the younger" and "let the sorrowful . . . help someone" *(Testimonies,* vol. 6, p. 266).

Who needed more help than the mothers of young children? Why not share what I was good at—homemaking? The result was a club for community moms to have a time for themselves while someone else cared for their children.

Moms' Club met one morning a week at our church. Sharing time and general conversation followed a short program on anything from haircutting to bread baking. "Grandma's Corner" cared for the children and repeated the Sabbath school kindergarten program. Church women and girls from the church school helped.

My depression "cure" worked. I was the one rewarded for all the effort, as I enjoyed new friends and being in touch with young women and little children.

Of all the many health outreach programs we have had in our congregation, this one paid the richest dividends. Several of the young families were baptized, while others are sending their children to church school. The club met each winter for seven years before "Grandma" wore out in her "corner." It has now been three years since our last meeting. At Vacation Bible School this summer one sixth of the children who attended were Moms' Club kids, some of them only infants when their mothers brought them to the meetings.

"Our work for Christ is to begin with the family in the home. . . . There is no mission field more important than this. . . . Christian homes, established and conducted in accordance with God's plan, are among His most effective agencies for the formation of Christian character and for the advancement of His work" *(ibid.,* pp. 429, 430).

Have you made your home and the homes of others your mission field?

A MOTHER'S DEDICATION

Steven L. Haley

A wife of noble character who can find? She is worth far more than rubies. . . .
Her children arise and call her blessed. Prov. 31:10-28, NIV.

Napoleon once said, "Let France have good mothers, and she will have good sons. The future destiny of the child . . . is always . . . the work of the mother."

She married Ken when they were 17 and both high school dropouts. Ken was good-looking, played backup guitar in a local band, and had a job at a lumber hardware store. What more could you ask for? Never mind that he swore a little and drank a lot.

Life was OK. But things changed when she joined the Seventh-day Adventist Church. Now, instead of Friday nights in a local tavern with the band, she spent them reading the Bible and in trying to teach three squirming, mischievous boys their memory verse.

Ken didn't mind his wife's religion, but he made it perfectly clear that Friday night, as every night, would be spent with Budweiser and his friends at the tavern. And so for a dozen years or more this struggling new Christian mother spent the beginning of the Sabbath hours singing "Jesus Loves Me" as she knelt with her boys. Every Saturday morning, while Father went to work, Mom brought her energetic sons to Sabbath school and church. She sacrificed to put them in church school and took them to Pathfinders, church campouts, and Saturday night socials. The young mother taught them the dangers of substance abuse and the importance of a healthy lifestyle. All this she did alone.

At times it must have been discouraging, hard, unrewarding, and thankless work. But the prayers and commitment of mothers work miracles . . . because I'm that mother's son.

The fact that I'm a pastor today and not at a neighborhood tavern is to a large degree a result of a mother's resolve that her children would grow up with a knowledge of and a love for the Lord. I agree with Theodore Roosevelt, who said: "The mother is the one supreme asset of the natural life. She is more important, by far, than the successful statesman, businessman, artist, or scientist."

Today is the day to arise and call your mother blessed.
Or why not just call her and tell her how much you appreciate
what she has done for you?

LET THE
SUN SHINE IN

> For you who revere my name, the sun of righteousness will rise
> with healing in its wings. Mal. 4:2, NIV.

Sunshine has so many healing properties that it is really one of God's best preventive medicines. Medical science has found it to aid in the reduction of high blood pressure, the normalization of blood sugar and cholesterol levels, and even to help in reducing obesity by stimulating the thyroid gland, which regulates the rate in which the body burns calories. Many years ago medical science discovered that the sun's healing rays helped to cure tuberculosis by destroying disease-producing bacteria. Sunshine lifts our spirits. It truly is one of our God's natural stress reducers.

How fitting that the God who created the sun and gave it all its wonderful healing characteristics should Himself be called the Sun of righteousness. To those who love God and choose to invite Him into their hearts each morning, Jesus arises with healing in His wings.

Just as the sunshine dispels all the shadows and darkness of night and sends healing rays onto every living thing, causing them to grow and flourish, Jesus comes to rid the darkness and gloom from our lives. He arrives with a new supply of physical, mental, spiritual, and emotional energy for the challenges we will meet each day.

If you find your strength waning and long for courage and fortitude to meet life's difficulties, or if you want to be successful in sharing the love of Jesus, just open up your heart—and let the Sun shine in!

Jesus, Sun of righteousness, come into my soul;
Dispel the shades of dismal gloom; touch and make me whole.

Jesus, Sun of righteousness, there's healing in Your wings;
As You shine upon my life, my heart, my voice just sings!

Jesus, Sun of righteousness, take the dark of night;
Give me strength to share Your love; fill me with Your light.

Jesus, Sun of righteousness, I long to see Your face;
May I live like You today by Your amazing grace.

*What three things can you do today to open up your heart
to the Sun of righteousness?*

FEED MY
SHEEP

---

*"Simon son of John, do you love me?" . . . He said, "Lord, you know all things;
you know that I love you." Jesus said, "Feed my sheep." John 21:16, 17, NIV.*

Peter is my kind of person—a crash-and-burn type! In the early days of
every church the leaders have the burning passion essential for the success of the little band of believers. My family's roots are in the mission
work of the Seventh-day Adventist Church in South America. Knowing the
real people and hearing stories of their courage and bravery bring a lump
to my throat. Those men and women were modern Peters—nothing was
too much for them.

A few years later as the church became well established, fewer places
remained for the Peters. The Matthews, the Jameses, and other types of
personalities now prevailed. In fact, the church let it be known that if you
wanted to succeed you needed to demonstrate the qualities of steadiness,
order, and position. Yes, there was a place for the caring Johns, but the
only place the Pauls were welcome was at a seminary!

Hippocrates, the ancient Greek physician, noted the differences in personalities among the people. He called some phlegmatics, people who care
and thus might choose as their model John the Beloved. Some the ancient
Greek saw as melancholics—people who need rightness and position; people who, like Matthew and the Pharisees, make the social order, but who
can be teachable or obstinate, depending on their walk with the Master.
Hippocrates identified the cholerics, such as Paul, who always, even as children, ask why and how and must organize everything around them and finish the task. And finally he defined the sanguines, those who, like Peter, set
out with passion to do what needs to be done.

Many different personalities. Many different talents. What has the
church done with them? Do we force all people into one mold? Do we classify some as good and others as bad?

Jesus valued all the varied persons among His disciples. He got to
know them in order to serve them. Through grace He gave them what they
needed, not what they deserved. Our Saviour put them to work in service
in the way their talents best fit. If only we could learn to do the same!

*Are you more like John, Matthew, Paul, or Peter?
How accepting are you of those with
different personality characteristics?*

NO CHOICE

Kenneth I. Burke

And now these three remain: faith, hope and love. But
the greatest of these is love. 1 Cor. 13:13, NIV.

A college friend of mine, seriously searching for a "one and only,"
went out with a number of young women. "I'm really trying to love
her, Burke," he'd confide about first one and then another. "I'm
really trying!"

He reminds me of Christians who, understanding that love constitutes
the highest motivation for healthful living, concern themselves with questions such as "Am I loving yet? (I'm really trying!)"

How much better to consider Jesus' love! (After all, it's His love that
saves, not ours.) His Spirit will then fill us with grateful love and encourage us in wise choices. Observe with me the way He worked in the life of
a young sea captain on board the *Empress,* bound for Brazil—a story told
by D. E. Robinson in *The Story of Our Health Message.*

One day the young man copied from a book a covenant with God that
he felt exactly expressed his purpose in life: "This day do I with the utmost
solemnity surrender myself to Thee. I renounce all former lords that have had
dominion over me, and I consecrate to Thee all that I am, and all that I have."

Not hurriedly, but carefully considering each choice, he began to make
changes in his lifestyle. First he dispensed with wine and tobacco as he became convinced of their harmfulness. Later, noticing that they had the
power to keep him awake at night, he left off coffee and tea. A number of
years later, in "heart-searching preparation for the expected return of
Christ," he resolved to eat no more meat. Still later he decided he would be
healthier without rich foods.

Let's imagine an acquaintance chiding the retired sea captain as he
passes up some rich delicacies on the table.

"What? You don't want any of these treats?"

Captain Joseph Bates smiles benignly. "I've eaten my share of them,"
he replies, and leaves it at that.

Thoughtfully, gradually, and without urging his lifestyle on others, the
old sea captain had pursued fitness. The love of Christ left him no choice.

We do well to follow his example.

Is God loving you into a better lifestyle? It's your choice.

SWEET
AND
WEAK

It is not good to eat too much honey. Prov. 25:27, NIV.

A few years ago a nutrition student, Judy Reeser, conducted a study in the laboratory of Dr. Benjamin Lau at Loma Linda University looking into the effect of sugars on the ability of neutrophils (a type of white blood cells) to engulf bacteria. Her subjects ate different kinds of refined sugars, one at a time, on different days. She had blood samples taken to determine neutrophil activity. Her research found that 10 teaspoons of white sugar, equivalent to that in one can of soft drink, decreased neutrophil activity by 50 percent, and it persisted for five hours. After 30 teaspoons of white sugar the neutrophils completely lost their ability to engulf bacteria. On the other hand, starch (a complex carbohydrate) had no effect on neutrophil activity.

We now know that sweets of any kind lower our resistance and make us vulnerable to all types of common infections. Children often catch colds after eating rich desserts or candy. When we eliminate sugar from their diet, youngsters no longer suffer frequent colds. Many mothers have learned that the best treatment and prevention for colds is a good diet with no junk food and sweets.

The Loma Linda researchers also studied the effect of fasting on neutrophil activity. They found that fasting (subjects ingested only water but no food) enhances neutrophil activity at least up to 60 hours. Furthermore, the research discovered that fasting with fresh fruit or vegetable juice enhances the activity of both neutrophils and natural killer cells for several days. Ellen White wrote in 1905: "In many cases of sickness, the very best remedy is for the patient to fast for a meal or two, that the overworked organs of digestion may have an opportunity to rest. A fruit diet for a few days has often brought great relief to brain workers" *(Counsels on Diet and Foods,* p. 189).

The bottom line message is this: When you don't feel good, don't force yourself to eat. A juice fast may well be just what your body needs.

What could you do to increase your neutrophil activity?
Is it time to consider reducing the amount of sweets you eat?

STOP
THE
BUSYNESS

Jan W. and Kay Kuzma

These are the things the Lord has commanded you to do: For six days, work is to be done, but the seventh day shall be your holy day, a Sabbath of rest to the Lord. Ex. 35:1, 2, NIV.

For too many of us the Sabbath is a busy day—just a different kind of busyness. We rush to get dressed, rush to get to church on time, and rush home to get a meal prepared for company. Perhaps we worry about the lesson we are to teach or about what people will think of our new hairstyle, worry about the kids sitting still in the pew, or worry about whether the guests we invited over for lunch will stay the whole afternoon so we won't be able to take a nap.

If on weekdays you seldom have any "down" time because of your hectic schedule, if you rush from one activity to another without taking time to enjoy them, then it is doubly important to *stop your busyness on the Sabbath.*

The root of the word *Sabbath* means "to stop, rest, cease." The rest refers to God's acts of creation. After bringing the world into being, God stopped, not from tiredness, but because He had finished His work, the reasoning behind the command to observe the Sabbath. God intended us to "finish" our work in six days so we too could celebrate with Him on the Sabbath.

But for most of us our work never gets "finished." So when the sun sets in the west on Friday evening, God gave us permission just to drop it, walk away from it, forget it, and take a vacation from it for 24 hours. You may not think you have the time. But the busier you get, the more important the Sabbath becomes. After a day of rest from your regular routine, you'll feel refreshed and ready to return to your job with renewed interest and energy, and will be able to work smarter, instead of longer.

Ceasing work on the seventh day isn't an arbitrary command. God sanctified (set apart) that day for the good of humanity. He had you in mind when He ceased His work and declared the seventh day of each week a holiday in His honor.

What busy things are you doing on the Sabbath that are robbing you of experiencing a Sabbath day blessing? What are you going to do differently next Sabbath?

A MODERN-DAY
EUTYCHUS

Linda Barton

For I am the Lord, your God, who takes hold of your right hand and says to you,
Do not fear; I will help you. Isa. 41:13, NIV.

A boy just fell out of the window!" The scream got my attention. As camp nurse I sprang to my feet, only to realize the boy in a pool of blood was my own 4-year-old son, Eric. He went into convulsions. The wait for the ambulance seemed to take hours.

Eric, looking for his daddy, had climbed onto the table and leaned against the window screen. The screen had popped loose, and he had fallen, striking his head on the sidewalk 15 feet below.

After the doctor in the small McCall hospital had examined him, the Life-Flight helicopter was dispatched from Boise. The doctor wanted him at a larger hospital with a neurosurgeon available.

The skull X-rays showed a fracture of the right side extending approximately seven inches in length from front to back. His vomiting in the emergency room at Saint Alphonsus Hospital was worrisome, but after a CT scan showed no depressed segments or obvious brain injuries, the neurosurgeon admitted him to the intensive-care unit for close observation. The long hours ticked by with hourly vital signs and "neuro" checks.

The next morning, however, Eric opened his eyes and clearly spoke his first words: "Mommy, I'm thirsty." Since the physician had ordered that Eric be given nothing by mouth in case he needed surgery to release intracranial pressure, I offered Eric a sponge stick dipped in water.

"No, Mommy, I want a drink out of a cup" was his reply as he pushed my hand away.

"Praise God!" I exclaimed. His speech was clear, and he was using his hands and legs normally.

Just 48 hours after the accident the hospital discharged him. As the neurosurgeon stood beside Eric's bed reviewing his chart, his comment, "I never would have predicted this outcome," brought tears to my eyes.

The Bible story of Eutychus falling out the third-story window, and of how Paul's faith raised him from the dead, now has new meaning (Acts 20:7-12). A modern-day Eutychus lives in our home, alive and healthy because of the faith of so many who were praying for him that fateful day in 1986.

Miracles still happen. Ask for a miracle, and experience
God's healing power.

KISSING AWAY OUR "OUCHIES"

Heal me, O Lord, and I will be healed; save me and I will be saved,
for you are the one I praise. Jer. 17:14, NIV.

Acute pain—none of us wants to experience the sudden, often-excruciating sensation. Yet all of us have bouts with it over the course of our lives. The intensity varies. Sometimes it's minor, such as when we were small and skinned our knees, and other times it's more intrusive, the result of a serious accident or disease.

Despite the degree of pain, two common reactions occur. First, we become focused on the pain itself. And second, at some point we seek care and comfort. When we were children, we often ran to Mom for reassurance and care of our "ouchies." Usually she washed out our wound, put on a bandage, and kissed the "ouchy" away.

Unfortunately, all acute pain is not so easily taken care of, and invariably we experience the other end of the pain spectrum, one that demands medical attention. Our pain has now become a signal of a more serious problem and alerts us to our need for more definitive care and treatment. We must seek a physician.

Our emotional and spiritual pain is not unlike our physical pain. It helps us focus and realize the need to attend to some problem. To regain health we need to heed this signal. We must seek treatment from the Physician. And only when we acknowledge our pain and seek help from the Source of health and life can we receive the appropriate treatment, care, and compassion that will lead to the restoration of our spiritual health.

Like Job, though, we may need to persevere. We must continually cling to our relationship with Christ even though we don't understand the reason for the pain. We may even cry out and question God, as did Job.

God may not intervene in the outcome of our physical condition, but He does promise to treat and restore our spiritual health. For it is His heart's desire that not one of us be lost. He, more than even our mothers, wants to kiss away our "ouchies" and make us whole.

Make this your prayer today: "Heal me, O Lord, physically,
emotionally, and spiritually. Kiss away my 'ouchies'
and make me whole."

WEAK
EYES

Now Laban had two daughters; the name of the older was Leah, and the name of the younger was Rachel. Leah had weak eyes, but Rachel was lovely in form, and beautiful. Gen. 29:16, 17, NIV.

L ike so much else, if the eye does not get exercised, it will become weak and not develop. What caused Leah to have weak eyes (also translated "delicate") Scripture does not explain. It certainly was obvious, and as a result she had to vie with her sister for Jacob's affection. Possibly Leah suffered from not having her eyes straight, properly called strabismus. Perhaps it might also explain why her father, a herdsman, had chosen his daughters' specific names: Rachel means "ewe" and Leah "cow." A cow's eyes are set widely apart, appearing divergent.

Unfortunately, strabismus is not merely a cosmetic problem, but may indicate something serious such as a brain or eye tumor. Tragically, even if nothing else is wrong, strabismus by itself often results in severe and permanent visual loss from amblyopia, or "lazy eye." Strabismus developing during adulthood causes severe double vision, but in a child the developing brain can suppress one eye. Over time this eye weakens and after a critical period remains irreversibly damaged.

Amblyopia was first noticed in donkeys bred and raised in dark coal mines. Although they had normal eyes, their brains never developed vision. Amblyopia can also develop from an uncorrected blurry image or significant opacity in the eye. Approximately one person in 50 has preventable amblyopia.

When the condition is recognized early, as simple a treatment as patching the good eye forces the lazy eye to exercise and thus develop normally. The relatively simple operation to straighten the eyes will make them look good and, more important, continue to see well! If the amblyopia is neglected, an injury to the good eye can result in total blindness.

Neglecting Leah's eyes may have caused much needless suffering, and its baleful influence marred the history of God's people. Neglected abilities and talents will also atrophy, resulting in permanent deficiencies and limitations. Blunders during the critical formative years will have long-term consequences that could have been completely avoided.

Is there anything in my life that if not corrected early could cause permanent physical, psychological, or spiritual damage?

WHAT IS NORMAL AGING?

Gregory R. Wise

Moses was a hundred and twenty years old when he died; his eye was not dimmed, nor his natural force abated. Deut. 34:7, RSV.

Americans are growing old. By the year 2020 an estimated 20 percent of the population, or 52 million Americans, will be 65 years of age or older. Women more than 85 have become the fastest growing segment of the U.S. population. The social and economic consequences of the "graying of America" are enormous. Many of my elderly patients have commented, "Doc, if I'd known I was going to live this long, I would have taken better care of myself!"

Our text gives us an example of normal aging. Moses was 120 years old and had spent the past 40 years leading the children of Israel through the wilderness. Before being laid to rest, Moses had the physical strength and vigor to climb the 2,600-foot Mount Nebo and with his still keen eye received a vision of the Promised Land. Now, that's the way to go!

For many of today's elderly, their greatest fear is not dying, but becoming increasingly feeble, frail, and dependent on others. The average 65-year-old woman in the United States has a life expectancy of 19 years. For far too many, these additional years will bring both physical and mental deterioration.

Such was not the case for one very remarkable woman. Hulda Hoehn was born on a farm in Canada on May 19, 1896. Raised on meat and potatoes by her German father, she became a Seventh-day Adventist when she was 18 years old, and since that time she has been a vegetarian. She earned a B.S. degree in dietetics at a time when few women attained advanced education. It wasn't until later in her life that she added vigorous physical exertion to her good nutrition and strong faith in God. On the encouragement of her husband, Dr. Samuel A. Crooks, she began climbing mountains. Hulda climbed Mount Whitney, the highest peak in North America outside Alaska, 23 times—the first time when she was 66, and the last in 1987 at 91! Crooks Peak, just two peaks south of Mount Whitney, was named for her.

Hulda, like Moses before her, is a perfect example of normal aging.

If time should last, what would you like to be doing at 91 years of age? If you want to be able to climb mountains like Hulda and Moses, what should you be doing today?

WITH WINGS
AS EAGLES

Wallace "Buddy" Blair

But they that wait upon the Lord shall renew their strength; they shall mount up with wings as eagles; they shall run, and not be weary; and they shall walk, and not faint. Isa. 40:31.

In August I received a clean bill of health after my annual physical. In October I had gotten an "I see no real problem" from the vascular specialist who inspected my swollen leg. But by November I started having occasional back pain. The swelling in the leg was still evident in December, when my sister eyed it with concern and made a doctor's appointment for me. The physician's words, "prostate cancer," sent a chill down my spine!

A few days later, back home in Tennessee, I was feeling somewhat tired. My usual optimistic attitude was failing. I thought of the words "They shall run, and not be weary." Then the pain hit, and I begged to be taken to the emergency room. Three days later the surgeons performed an orchiectomy and predicted I had six months to live.

During the next four and a half years I tried treatments ranging from herbs to experimental chemotherapy. By the fourth year I had sold my accounting business, since the pain was getting too great to hide, and I began an experimental chemo program at Vanderbilt. My courage was bolstered one day when I overhead another man on the same protocol telling his nurse that he was "back on the golf course again!" "They shall walk, and not faint."

For six months I took treatments and felt wonderful. My wife and I began traveling. I did odd jobs around the house and played with my grandson. "Run with me, Papa," he would say. Around and around I pulled him in his little red wagon, laughing and telling him stories. Then one day four months after the experimental chemo ended, the pain suddenly returned. I stubbornly tried pulling the red wagon with its special load, and I got sick—very, very sick.

I'm still in bed, too weak to function. My hospice nurse says she is "absolutely amazed" that I have been able to hang on so long. Maybe there will be a miracle yet. I keep that ray of hope. Then I think again of Isaiah: "They shall mount up with wings as eagles." Smiling, I am looking forward to that, too, in case the miracle doesn't happen!

Hang in there. God can use you regardless of your circumstances.
And that is a miracle in itself!

A WOUNDED HEALER'S PRAYER

> Praise be to the God and Father of our Lord Jesus Christ, the Father of compassion and the God of all comfort, who comforts us in all our troubles, so that we can comfort those in any trouble with the comfort we ourselves have received from God. 2 Cor. 1:3, 4, NIV.

Loving Lord God:

In these quiet moments before I begin another day with ill and hurting people . . .

May it be that out of all of the thoughts, the words, the silences of where I walk and out of the mystery and wonder of being a health professional, Your voice will speak to me in ever-deepening ways to help me know how much a tired and very sick but wonderful world needs what You can do through me.

Help me to know that there are words of truth and healing that may never be spoken unless I speak them; and acts of compassion and care that may never be done unless I do them.

Help me never to mistake success for victory, or failure for defeat.

Help me to tolerate those times of not knowing, not curing, and not healing.

Help me to face the reality of my sometimes powerlessness and my need of Your strength and power.

Help me to remember that behind every smile lurks a tear; in every hug, loneliness; in every friendship, distance; and in all forms of light, darkness. That without You and without love there is only the tear, the loneliness, the distance, and the darkness.

As I go now to be with my patients, may my heartbeat be warm and my own, may my hopes not be crushed or wasted, may my love not be shattered, may my commitment not be broken.

And may the day come soon when my patients and I stand before Your throne all healed and whole and praising Your name forever.

Amen.

Is there someone you know who could benefit from your healing touch?
Pray this prayer, and may God give you Holy Spirit
energy and wisdom to comfort the wounded.

GOD'S ORIGINAL "PILL BOTTLE"

Crystal Whitten

My God will meet all your needs according to his glorious riches in Christ Jesus. Phil. 4:19, NIV.

I went to visit a friend the other day and noticed her breakfast table covered with small white bottles—a home pharmacy of vitamins, minerals, and other substances.

Picking up a bottle labeled bee pollen, I asked, "What does this do for you?"

"It gives me energy," she replied. When I held up another bottle, she explained, "This helps control my blood sugar." After my cross-examination, I realized she was convinced of the need to take a handful of pills every day.

In His original plan God planted a garden and told Adam to eat from it freely. A garden supplied all the nutrients he needed for his well-being. It's still true.

Scientists have identified an eating pattern called the Food Guide Pyramid that will supply our daily needs. It recommends five to nine servings of fruits and vegetables per day. But a recent government survey of households found that only 23 percent of Americans eat at least five fruits and vegetables per day.

Following the Food Guide Pyramid recommendations would meet our daily nutrient needs. But many of us would rather eat refined, processed foods that lack many of the nutritive substances found in fruits and vegetables, and then we take a handful of pills to make up for the deficiency.

Fruits, grains, nuts, and vegetables have thousands of substances, mostly unidentified, that contribute to our health. They are God's "pill bottle" for us! By eating refined and processed foods, we limit our intake of phytochemicals and other helpful substances God designed that we get in our food, and thus have to take human-made supplements.

By participating in daily devotion and prayer we can tap into the incredible power God gives us to make clear, distinct, right decisions regarding our diet. If we subject our wills to God's desires, He will give us the ability to choose a diet that does provide all our daily needs.

Lord, the Creator of all living things, please give me the power to make right choices today that will promote my health and well-being. Help me eat the food You created to meet my nutritional needs, for I know that is Your will for me. Thank You for the wonderful variety of sensory pleasure You provide for sustenance and health. Amen.

SING
IN THE
MORNING

May 23
Georgia E. Hodgkin

Sing to the Lord a new song; sing to the Lord, all the earth. Sing to the Lord, praise his name; proclaim his salvation day after day. Ps. 96:1, 2, NIV.

Imagine starting each new day with a smile on your lips and a song in your heart. Can you imagine a better jump start for the day? Such an attitude makes all things possible, and the day will indeed be a delight.

Some choose as their jump start a jolt of caffeine. How often have you heard, "I can't start the day without a cup of coffee"? But as far back as the 1800s Ellen White told us that the influence of coffee is "exciting, and just in the degree that it elevates above par, it will exhaust and bring prostration below par" (Counsels on Diet and Foods, p. 421). Should we be surprised, then, that so many feel they have lost steam and need a coffee break by midmorning? They are just counteracting the letdown from their morning jolt.

Researchers have discovered that the withdrawal from the usual consumption of just one or two cups of coffee per day may lead to headaches. What the coffee ads never say is that the reason you later have that depressed, let down, headachy feeling is the coffee you drank earlier!

Coffee and tea lack vitamins, minerals, or any other health-supporting nutrients. The best beverage on either side of our meals is simply water, "the best liquid possible" (ibid.).

Begin each day with a helpful, health-filled beverage—such as water! And while you are at it, choose positive thoughts. Choose an attitude of gratitude that brings a smile and a song at the beginning of each new day. "It is good to praise the Lord and make music to your name, O Most High, to proclaim your love in the morning and your faithfulness at night" (Ps. 92:1, 2, NIV).

Lord, my gratitude overflows in singing this day. May my choices lead to a life energized by Your Spirit of faith, love, peace, gentleness, and joy.

175

MILK
AND
HONEY

Dick Duerksen

You will possess their land; I will give it to you as an inheritance, a land flowing with milk and honey. Lev. 20:24, NIV.

I wonder how many children rushed into Canaan hoping to see rivers of milk and honey. Could you imagine it? Just above Jericho, someone might say, there's a stream of milk flowing from a flower-filled meadow. And by the city gates it merges with a river of golden honey that comes from the forest at the edge of town. Then the two, now a mighty torrent of pearl and gold, rush . . .

Actually, the picture is not that attractive. So what was God promising?

Milk? Happy cows produce sweet milk that tastes great on Special K. And happy cows are most content when delectable grasses and small, clear streams carpet their pastures. That happy picture is also one that farmers conjure up in their fondest dreams. A picture of Paradise—a land flowing with milk.

And honey? Zillions of honeybees hum around the cows, reveling in the feast offered by multiflavored flowers in the pastures, in the orchards, in the gardens, and on the cliffs. Bees that take the pollen home and transform it into golden goodness with the taste of apples, lilies, and wildflowers. Sweet, distinctive nectars that bring a special flavor to Grandma's bread.

But milk and honey together? My wife, Brenda, has taught me that the two actually do go together well—in healing. Whenever my voice starts sounding like a lawn mower motor, she brings out the milk and honey. One mug of "almost hot" milk with a giant tablespoon of honey mixed in brings relief and healing to my singed vocal cords. It's a concoction I'm sure Joshua used every morning before addressing his troops.

Milk and honey together? We know that the much later Egyptian queen Cleopatra used a milk-and-honey mix for her special royal baths. "Take at least one milk and honey bath each week and your skin will always stay lovely and soft and clear, and you'll always have a complexion like a queen." No, I do not know if it works, but I do know God used an illustration that would bring smiles of understanding from former Egyptian slaves. Milk and honey. The promise of Paradise!

Are you looking forward to a land flowing with milk and honey?
What should you do to get ready for that wonderful day when
Paradise is no longer a promise but a reality?

REMOVING
THE PLANK

May 25

Raymond O. West

---

*Do not judge, or you too will be judged. For in the same way you judge others,
you will be judged. Matt. 7:1, 2, NIV.*

He was just a little guy, barely 6 years old, and he was afraid. Who
wouldn't be with a BB pellet embedded in his eye? Equally fearful
were the young parents, who had rushed him at dusk to our inner-city
emergency department.

As I examined the injured eye, I noted behind the lower lid an ugly
round blot in the delicate membrane, as if someone had poked him with a
nail. Here was the pellet's portal of entry. Somewhere in the depths lay the
errant and malignant sphere of metal. X-rays could locate it precisely, and
perhaps a skilled eye surgeon would later dissect it out and still preserve
the vision. Maybe.

But first, to complete the examination. As the mother sat in her corner
and sobbed softly and as the father white-knuckled her hand, I averted the
lower lid. With thumb and finger I sought a better look at the ugly point
of entry. Perhaps I could determine the direction that the pellet had taken
as it bludgeoned its way through the delicate tissue. While comforting my
little patient, and holding steady my position, I placed my opposite index
finger well below the margin of the lid and squeezed gently. Suddenly,
miraculously, the shining metallic orb welled up to the surface, squeezing
through the hole and into my eager hand. Placing it on a white square of
sterile gauze, I passed it to the happy parents.

BB guns fired indiscriminately at dusk by a careless neighbor boy can
be a scourge on defenseless eyes. And removal is rarely so sure or so simple. Yet how easy it is to remove the proverbial mote from a neighbor's eye
and fail miserably at finding it in our own! Jesus says, "You hypocrite, first
take the plank out of your own eye, and then you will see clearly to remove
the speck from your brother's eye" (Matt. 7:5, NIV).

Today let's opt anew for introspection—to see ourselves as others see
us, and to refrain from judging others.

*Lord, don't let me be a hypocrite, judging and criticizing others
when I have so much in my own life that needs to be cleaned up!*

177

EXERCISE ISN'T AN OPTION

Jan W. Kuzma

You must teach what is in accord with sound doctrine. Teach the older men to be temperate. . . . Train the younger women . . . to be self-controlled. . . . Similarly, encourage the young men to be self-controlled. In everything set them an example by doing what is good. Titus 2:1-7, NIV.

Since I've been gathering information and writing scripts for the daily *Got a Minute for Your Health?* radio program, I have become overwhelmed by the scientific evidence for the health benefits of exercising.

Exercise is no longer an option; it's a necessity for good health. It's at least as important as good nutrition in feeling and looking good. Besides helping the heart, it strengthens immunity, controls weight, promotes mental health, and lowers the risk of developing diabetes, osteoporosis, and some cancers.

Dr. Ralph Paffenbarger, Jr., a professor emeritus of epidemiology at Stanford University, has researched the effects of physical activity in several long-term studies begun in 1960 on large numbers of Harvard University graduates. Based on his findings, he says, "Starting to exercise is comparable from a health-benefit standpoint to quitting smoking."

The excuse "I don't have time to exercise!" is something like saying, "I don't have time to eat or sleep!"

People find the time to do what they really want to do. After all, you enjoy eating and sleeping enough to work them into your schedule. You've got to do the same thing with exercise—*it's just as important!*

Besides, exercise doesn't have to take that much time! Use the staircase instead of the elevator, park your car in the farthest parking place instead of the closest, get up from your desk every hour and walk to the drinking fountain, or go to the lounge and jump rope. All this adds up. When you arrive home, play basketball with the kids and then take a 20-minute moonlight walk with your spouse before bed. Make exercise a fun part of your daily schedule, and you can find the time!

But are people getting the message? Apparently not, for a 1995 survey of 15,000 households found that 60 percent of Americans do not exercise regularly. Ellen White challenges us to "take the living principles of health reform into the communities that to a large degree are ignorant of these principles" *(Testimonies, vol. 8, p. 148).*

Help spread the message, won't you? Exercise isn't an option—it's a necessity!

What are you doing to spread the message of good health to others?

ON BEING "LIVING STONES"

Walter Thompson

> As you come to him, the living Stone—rejected by men but chosen by God and precious to him—you also, like living stones, are being built into a spiritual house to be a holy priesthood, offering spiritual sacrifices acceptable to God through Jesus Christ. 1 Peter 2:4, 5, NIV.

We were sailing from San Francisco out across the vast Pacific to our first mission appointment. Our ship was a cargo vessel, but its crew had been host to many Adventist missionaries before us. According to custom, crew and passengers ate meals together. Our first mate treated us like royalty. He knew what "good" Adventists could and could not eat, and conscientiously worked to make sure we were well accommodated with a vegetarian diet.

Why have Adventists become known better for the things that they can and cannot eat, rather than for the living gospel that they profess to believe? Why have some become so fanatical about preserving their health—at almost any cost? What was God's real objective in making health such a central part of His message for the last days?

Adventists live longer than almost anyone else in their society. Is long life God's purpose? They have a lower incidence of most cancers, and their heart attacks come later in life. Is this the reason? Or is there some benefit provided by good health that assures passage through the pearly gates into the heavenly city?

I think not.

The health message is God's multipotential gift to our hurting world. Through it people can find a bit of relief from pain. It can open doors of interest to people's hearts to receive the full gospel, and faithful followers of Jesus might find opportunity for spiritual growth through ministry to their fellow human beings.

While compliance with the laws governing our being often provides a whole host of benefits to those who practice them, their real goal is to make of us a living sacrifice to be offered upon the altar of the world's needs. As such, whether we live or die as martyrs for the gospel, ours has been the special honor of sharing in the work of God and giving glory to His name. Could there be any greater possible reason to practice health's broad principles with diligence and balance?

Why do you keep (or why don't you keep) the biblical "laws of health"? Ask God to give you not only the willpower but also the correct motive to live healthfully.

DOING
GOD A
FAVOR

Richard Winn

Fathers, do not provoke your children to anger, but bring them up in the discipline and instruction of the Lord. Eph. 6:4, RSV.

The following fact is both good news and bad news! Almost everything our children will come to believe about God will be powerfully shaped by what they see in their parents. And most of a child's feelings about God will be formed when parents are fulfilling what some regard as our most Godlike responsibility: teaching them to obey.

Unfortunately, we as parents don't get any children to practice on. We have to make all our parenting mistakes, all our test runs and learning labs, on real children—even as our parents learned so much by watching what happened to us when they made some blunders.

Quite likely the apostle Paul had this in mind when he cautioned fathers about making their children angry. But let's face it—it's almost a given that when fatherly authority comes head-to-head against the high energy and freewheeling curiosity of youth, someone's going to get angry. Dad has to say no long before the children can understand why—which doesn't prevent a three-foot-tall challenge to adult dignity from insisting "Why?" At this point, anger is often just a blink away.

We face no more delicate task than that of helping human beings, who sense that they are free moral agents, learn to live within the boundaries of reality. When parents believe that they can accomplish this by their power, by their ability to "make them obey" through the threat of pain or physical force, they not only make their children angry, but also give God a black eye.

Though we use big Latin words such as "omnipotent" and draw images from notions of royalty such as "King of kings" to celebrate God's great dignity, our God simply does not stoop to the use of power and force to win the free, thoughtful loyalty of His friends—His created beings! Rather, He helps us understand the built-in benefits of choosing to live by His principles. And who can be angry about that?

*Are you giving God a black eye by the way you treat
your children and others?*

BETTER
ADVICE

Patricia K. Johnston

Now see to it that you drink no wine or other fermented drink and that you do not eat anything unclean, because you will conceive and give birth to a son. Judges 13:4, 5, NIV.

It has been more than 20 years since medical science first used the term *fetal alcohol syndrome* (FAS). But that was not the first time someone had described the condition. Classical Greek and Roman mythology suggested that maternal alcoholism at the time of conception could result in serious problems for the baby. Indeed, ancient Carthage prohibited the bride and groom's drinking on their wedding night so they would not conceive a defective child.

Reports in Great Britain during the mid-1800s described infants born to alcoholic mothers as having a "starved, shriveled, and imperfect look." Yet, more recently, few gave little credence to the possibility of damage from alcohol consumed during pregnancy. In fact, in the mid-1940s a report to the U.S. Congress dismissed the idea that maternal alcohol consumption during pregnancy caused any problems for the infant. As recently as the 1960s a major pediatric textbook said that alcohol crossed the placenta to the fetus, but that it did no harm.

It was these attitudes that caused one medical writer to say that the advice given so long ago to Samson's mother was "better advice" than people were then receiving (F. L. Iber, "Fetal Alcohol Syndrome," *Nutrition Today*, September/October 1980). Now medical textbooks no longer consider alcohol consumption during pregnancy harmless.

The surgeon general recently reported that in the U.S. at least 5,000 infants are born with FAS each year, and for every child with FAS, 10 more suffer from alcohol-related problems. FAS is the nation's leading cause of preventable mental retardation.

Although alcohol affects every fetus differently, certain facial abnormalities and other forms of physical damage recur. FAS children often experience seizures, have impaired judgment, and lack the ability to discern right from wrong.

Science recognizes no safe level of alcohol during pregnancy, and nursing babies can also be affected by the alcohol their mothers drink. Words penned in 1910 are still true today: "Every drop of strong drink taken by her [the mother] . . . endangers the physical, mental, and moral health of her child" *(The Ministry of Healing, p. 373).*

God's advice is always best. Is there any advice God has given in His Word that you feel convicted to follow? Why not start today?

THE PRAYER
OF FAITH

Is any one of you sick? He should call the elders of the church to pray over him and anoint him with oil in the name of the Lord. And the prayer offered in faith will make the sick person well; the Lord will raise him up. If he has sinned, he will be forgiven. James 5:14, 15, NIV.

In January of 1993 I thought I had the flu with stomach pains, bloating, and vomiting. My doctor had me hospitalized, and when things didn't improve, I had surgery. The surgeons found a blockage from carcinoid cancer in the small intestine. They told me I had from six months to 15 years to live.

I know God can heal, and I believe anointing should not have to wait until you are on your deathbed. So in May I was anointed at a mountain campout surrounded by my church family. Six months later I went in for more exploratory surgery, believing I was healed. When I found out there was more cancer, and it was in the lymph nodes, so it would probably spread, it really tested my faith. My hopes were crushed.

By now I needed major cheering up, especially when family and friends weren't around. I made a tape of songs that really spoke to my soul, and played it over and over. As the words of comfort became a part of me, I understood why the Pathfinder law says to "keep a song in my heart."

The bird feeder I could see from my bed, a simple daffodil on my bed stand, and the sun catchers dangling in my window all began to remind me of God's love. But my biggest comfort came from the Bible. Psalm 6 was my prayer of faith: "Heal me, for my body is sick, and I am upset and disturbed. My mind is filled with apprehension and with gloom. Oh, restore me soon. Come, O Lord, and make me well. In your kindness save me. For if I die I cannot give you glory by praising you before my friends. I am worn out with pain; every night my pillow is wet with tears" (verses 2-6, TLB). The psalm ends with a strong statement of faith: "The Lord has heard my weeping and my pleading. He will answer all my prayers" (verses 8, 9, TLB).

I claimed this promise. Although I don't know God's plan for my healing, I do know I am in His hands and can feel His peace.

If you're worn out with pain and worry, hold on to the prayer of faith in Psalm 6. Believe the Lord has heard your weeping and pleading, and He will answer your prayers.

HELP GOD
PUT OUT
THE FIRE

Then Judah came near to him and said: "O my lord, please let your servant speak a word in my lord's hearing, and do not let your anger burn against your servant. Gen. 44:18, NKJV.

Anger is like a volcano. It's unpredictable. Underneath, things boil and tension mounts, and either it vents its fury a little at a time, or it blows. Either way, watch out!

For example, consider the 15-year-old boy with no father and a mother who doesn't know how to handle him. He picks on his younger brother, gets in fights at school, and has failing grades, even though he has no learning problem. Dealing with anger that has built up over a lifetime of pain and frustration is like trying to hold the lid on a pressure cooker.

Anger is fairly common in people who have experienced a less-than-ideal home life. When a marriage breaks up, children feel as if they have been robbed of what life should have given them, and they are angry at those they think caused it. "If Mom hadn't screamed at Dad, he wouldn't have left." Or "Everything was fine until junior came along and the folks started fighting."

The longer such smoldering anger remains, the more chance that it will spill over into other relationships. If that happens, it can cause conflict, rejection, or alienation.

A person may express anger overtly, by yelling or hitting, or covertly, by rebelling, destroying things, or refusing to speak. Talking the anger out is better than acting it out. That's why counseling is so important.

Give God a chance to work. I have seen children healed from anger by Mom or Dad going into the child's room at night, placing their hands on that sleeping child, and praying in the name of Jesus. Ask God to send His spirit of peace upon children, to put a hedge of protection around them and fill their minds with love, replacing the bitter anger that has burned there so long.

Too often we get discouraged and give up too soon. We forget that God can heal the mind as well as the body. Remember the demoniac (Matt. 8:28-34)?

Why put up with a smoldering volcano when you, along with professional help *and God*, can put out the fire?

Think of someone you know (perhaps yourself) who shows signs of smoldering anger. What could you do to help put out the fire?

CHANGING YOUR THINKING

Search me, O God, and know my heart; test me and know my anxious thoughts. See if there is any offensive way in me, and lead me in the way everlasting. Ps. 139:23, 24, NIV.

A fundamental law of psychological well-being is that *you become what you think you are.* Your thoughts are incredible motivators as your thinking shapes your behavior. Therefore, it is vitally important to guard the avenues of your mind so you don't allow Satan to flood you with guilt, discouragement, anxiety, and depression.

Here's a five-step plan to safeguard your mind from Satan's attacks.

First, develop the habit of thinking of good things—interesting things: your successes, achievements, opportunities for service, people in need whose lives you can brighten.

Second, develop the habit of looking at every problem and difficulty as a stepping-stone to victory. I have never forgotten the cartoon of a boy with a saw looking with dismay at a piece of board with a notch he had just cut out to fit around a post. It was obvious he had cut out the wrong side of the board, but I'll never forget the caption: "Even a mistake shows you've tried!" Look at every mistake as something you can profit from—a stepping-stone to victory.

Third, feel yourself toughening up the muscles of your character as you tackle the unpleasant tasks, the mundane chores, the messy jobs. And then take as your motto, "I'll always be true to my conscience."

Fourth, make a habit of smiling at people from the inside. Practice feeling your happy thoughts toward the people you meet.

Fifth, memorize key scriptural promises that can carry you through periods of discouragement or despondency. Here are three:

● "The righteous cry out, and the Lord hears them; he delivers them from all their troubles. The Lord is close to the brokenhearted and saves those who are crushed in spirit" (Ps. 34:17, 18, NIV).

● "Blessed is the man who perseveres under trial, because when he has stood the test, he will receive the crown of life that God has promised to those who love him" (James 1:12, NIV).

● "Be strong and courageous. Do not be terrified; do not be discouraged, for the Lord your God will be with you wherever you go" (Joshua 1:9, NIV).

Ask God to help you hold on to the promises in Psalm 34:17, 18; James 1:12; and Joshua 1:9 and to give you victory over your discouraging and anxious thoughts.

A HEALTHFUL
SHABBAT

Richard M. Davidson

If you keep your feet from breaking the Sabbath and from doing as you please on my holy day, if you call the Sabbath a delight and the Lord's holy day honorable, . . . then you will find your joy in the Lord. Isa. 58:13, 14, NIV.

The Sabbath has always been a delight to me, but it was during the six months my family spent studying in Israel that we really discovered *oneg Shabbat* (Sabbath delight) and what it can mean to family health and happiness.

Come with me for a few moments and visit a Jewish home in Israel as the family members welcome the Sabbath.

A white cloth covers the table, and it is set for the Sabbath meal. On it rest two loaves of braided (challah) bread, a bottle of wine (we would use sparkling grape juice), and a goblet, silver candlesticks, candles, and flowers. The family members have dressed in their best clothes. All are ready to receive royalty—"Queen Sabbath."

Long before the sun actually sets, the family in their eager expectation begins its Sabbath celebration. The mother has the honor of officially receiving the Sabbath by kindling the Sabbath lights. The children watch her light the candles. Then we hear her offering a prayer of blessing upon the family: "Grant me and all my loved ones a chance to truly rest on this Sabbath day."

The father tenderly takes his children in his arms or places his hands on their bowed heads and recites a blessing for each.

Then for all comes the priestly dedication: "May the Lord bless you and keep you; may the Lord cause His face to shine upon you and be gracious unto you; may the Lord lift up His countenance toward you and give you peace."

The woman's place of honor on the Sabbath and her exalted position in the home are then again emphasized as the husband sings to his wife from Proverbs 31, extolling her virtues: "Many women have done virtuously, but thou excellest them all!"

Next comes the Sabbath meal, with the special blessing over the challah bread and the special Sabbath courses. On Sabbath the family eats the choicest food of all the week. During the meal the family heartily sings joyous table hymns reflecting the feeling and mood of the Sabbath. In the singing, eating, and fellowship the family can forget their weekday burdens, worries, and sorrows.

What could you do to make the Sabbath a
greater delight for your family?

THE TREE
LINE

June 3

Larry Richardson

Before his downfall a man's heart is proud, but humility comes before honor. Prov. 18:12, NIV.

'**ve** discovered in my years of exercising that a battle rages within my body—a contest between strength and flexibility, two goals that almost seem opposed to each other. I want to be strong, so I usually concentrate on strengthening activities (lifting weights, jogging, push-ups, etc.), which leave my muscles tight and rigid. But I know that I need to stay limber as well. If I neglect my stretching routine, I could easily pull a tight muscle at the wrong time.

As I hike the majestic peaks of the Sierra Nevadas, I'm reminded of the importance of flexibility. As the elevation of the mountain increases, trees begin to disappear, until at about 10,000 feet they cease to grow at all. This transition point is called the tree line. Near the tree line you often see a few twisted and misshapen trees, permanently bent by the relentless winds. Above the tree line even the mighty oak cannot survive the punishing winds and poor soil. At high altitude the barren and rocky terrain seems almost devoid of life. Almost—but not quite.

Look down low, and you will see the soft and supple willow clinging to the rocks, flourishing to a height of no more than six inches. While the mighty winds will crack and break the beefy oak at the craggy peaks, the lowly willow bends, and the wind passes on through.

It is as if God has placed before us a great visual lesson to remind us that the lofty heights of human existence are no place for the proud and haughty. Here only the lowly and humble will survive. God certainly does not discourage ambition and aspiration. Joseph and Daniel both showed great wisdom in the high-pressure, high-profile arena of world politics. But we dare not walk those heights alone, or like the mighty oak, we will be swept off the mountain.

So in my training routine I aim to be as strong as an oak but as supple as a willow. In this way I may also learn to stand for principle against the raging winds of temptation, but yield to my heavenly Father's will in modesty and humility.

Lord, may I stand for principle and be modest and humble as
I scale the heights of possibility within Your will. Amen.

DEVELOPING
A SUSTAINING
SPIRIT

A man's spirit sustains him in sickness, but a crushed spirit who can bear? Prov. 18:14, NIV.

Why is it that some people are so strong when pain, disease, and disability rob them of what we might call the good life? I've observed this many times in my ministry. For example, I've seen the indomitable spirit of my wife, Ruth, as she has suffered excruciating pain for the past 10 years. What gives a person the strength to endure that which the rest of us are quite sure we wouldn't be able to survive?

Proverbs 18:14 indicates that it is possible for people to develop a living connection or faith in God that brings them the spiritual strength necessary to sustain them when everything seems to be falling apart. It's a special quality of life nurtured only by a saving relationship with Jesus.

The Holy Spirit's "plus factor"—that extra Holy Spirit "horsepower"—is available to all during tough times. Without it the pain, disease, or disability would quite likely crush one's spirit.

I visited a Christian woman in the hospital several times. She had terminal cancer. One morning I asked her if she had a favorite Bible chapter that I could read for her, and she requested the twenty-third psalm. When I read the verse that says, "Even though I walk through the valley of the shadow of death, I will fear no evil, *for you are with me*" (verse 4, NIV), she stopped me and said, "Chaplain, this is where I am right now." She looked up at me from her bed of suffering with incredible confidence and assurance in the Great Shepherd. God *was* with her. All was well with her soul. Her sustaining spirit ministered to my weak one. I was in the presence of a woman who was at peace with her God as she traveled down that one-way path. I am certain that the relationship she had with the Saviour and her testimony did more for me than what I had to offer her that morning.

Yes, "a man's spirit sustains him in sickness."

Remember in times of adversity, when accidents or diseases come your way, God will give Holy Spirit power to sustain you.

CHRIST: THE SOURCE OF PERSONAL VALUE

Kay Kuzma

> For God so loved the world that He gave His only begotten Son, that whoever believes in Him should not perish but have everlasting life. John 3:16, NKJV.

When it comes to feeling really valuable, Christians have a big advantage. The world may tell you you're valuable, but that doesn't mean you'll feel that way. If you doubt your worth, humanistic theory says you must simply pull yourself up by your own bootstraps. For emotional and other support it offers encounter groups, therapy sessions, weekend serendipity workshops, and all types of human-made gimmicks to help you believe in yourself.

But what do you do when no matter how you try to pull yourself up by your own bootstraps, you just keep tripping? You've gone to a color analyst, lost 15 pounds, built muscle, and restyled your hair—and you still don't look like Miss or Mr. America. Although you avoid critical and sarcastic comments in order to keep your self-esteem high, still at times you feel rejected anyway. No matter how many skills you develop, you quake when asked to do something new. And as hard as you try, you still yield to temptations and feel bad about doing what you know you shouldn't.

True self-worth is where Christianity parts company with humanistic theories. It has to do with a person's *real* value, not *perceived* value!

The fact is, you *can* feel valuable even though everything in your life seems to be in shambles if you will only believe that God made you. He created you, and not one other person in the entire universe is exactly like you. You are special—known by God from the moment of your conception.

In addition, God said no when Satan condemned you to die because you sinned. Instead, God's Son died in your place so you could live. And do you realize that Jesus would have died for you even if you were the only one who had ever sinned?

God has a plan for your life: a work for you to do that no one else can do, and a plan for you to be with Him forever.

Having Christ is a big advantage when it comes to feeling good about yourself. Don't ever forget who you *really* are!

Think about this statement by Ellen White: "The price paid for our redemption, the infinite sacrifice of our heavenly Father in giving His Son to die for us, should give us exalted conceptions of what we may become through Christ" (Steps to Christ, p. 15).

188

AN ATTITUDE
OF CHRIST

June 6

Jim Cox

Your attitude should be the same as that of Christ Jesus. Phil. 2:5, NIV.

As a police chaplain I encounter a lot of people who have attitude problems. Criminals with a bad attitude are dangerous. Police officers with a bad attitude can cause a lot of trouble for themselves and for others. The word "attitude" is defined, in part, as a frame of mind, or a condition of mind. Our frame of mind determines how we let the things of life affect us. Negatively this can lead to ill health either emotionally and/or physically. But we can, to a large degree, control our attitude and in turn determine our health.

In *Counsels on Health* Ellen White wrote: "That which brings sickness of body and mind to nearly all is dissatisfied feelings and discontented repinings" (pp. 631, 632). What Ellen White is talking about is an attitude problem that needs to be dealt with.

Attitude has an incredible impact on life. It's more important than facts, the past, education, money, circumstances, failures, successes, appearance, giftedness, skill, what other people think, or what they say or do. Chuck Swindoll once made the comment that attitude will make or break a company, a church, or a home. The remarkable thing is that we have a choice every day regarding the attitude we will embrace for that day. We cannot change our past or the fact that people will act in a certain way. Nor can we change the inevitable. The only thing we can do is play on the one string we have, and that is our attitude. I am convinced that life is 10 percent what happens to me and 90 percent how I react to it. And so it is with you—we are in charge of our attitude.

The apostle Paul wrote in Philippians 4:8, 9 that we should fill our minds with things that are true, honest, and just. He said to think on things that are noble, pure, and lovely. We are to dwell on the good things and follow right principles. When we do this, Paul says, "the God of peace will be with [us]" (NIV). This makes for good emotional, physical, and spiritual health.

What rough edges of your attitude do you need to polish to
have an attitude like that of Christ Jesus?

KEEPING TRACK OF THE ENEMY

June 7

Fred Hardinge

Take heed, watch and pray; for you do not know when the time is. . . .
And what I say to you, I say to all: Watch! Mark 13:33-37, NKJV.

Have you ever wondered how Elijah could have become so disheartened and discouraged after the tremendous victory God gave him on Mount Carmel (1 Kings 18, 19)? After all, it was the same man ravens had already sustained miraculously in the wilderness! Yet in his fatigued, worn-out state Elijah's faith and confidence in God failed him. Suddenly terribly afraid, he ran for his life.

We, like Elijah, find ourselves in a contest between good and evil. It is a struggle just as fierce as the one on Mount Carmel, but it plays out in our lives daily.

Let's take a moment to look at the impact fatigue has on modern-day soldiers serving in artillery fire direction centers. Part of their job is to plot the location of artillery targets as requested by forward observers, and to update their situation maps continually.

Studies indicate that when a team has rested, it performs very well. However, when tired, it ceases to keep up the situation map. As a result, its members lose grasp of their position in relationship to friendly and enemy units, and consequently often do not know what they are firing at!

We are like those soldiers too! When we are tired, our vigilance wanes. Our ability to set priorities and focus attention on the tasks at hand vanishes. The events and crises of life drive us, instead of the other way around. Yet we are unaware that anything has affected our performance!

Our Christian life suffers in exactly the same way. Fatigue lessens our spiritual vigilance. We're more likely to have lapses of attention, and it is at these weak moments that the enemy chooses to make his moves. During this state we also easily lose sight of the enemy, thus totally missing him and his maneuvers against us.

Do you consider fatigue a normal part of your life? Remember, fatigue profoundly affects your performance at home, at work, and for the Lord. It was not until Elijah had rested that his faith and confidence in God returned.

Lord, help me to choose to get seven or eight hours of sleep each night so that I can remain a vigilant, watchful soldier for You!

DIET AND
THE DENTIST

> Train up a child in the way he should go: and when he is old, he will
> not depart from it. Prov. 22:6.

The most prevalent disease in the world is dental caries. Ninety-five per-cent of the world's adult population, more than 5 billion people, have cavities. Fortunately, this epidemic is coming to an end. The good news is that we can now control the disease in both children and adults. Today most school-age children in developed countries are caries-free, reflecting a more than 50 percent reduction in caries among the young. A study of Swedish mothers and their children showed that if we could control the dis-ease in a mother, her children might never develop it. Early behaviors can have a lifelong influence!

It is not natural for humans to have cavities. Contrary to popular be-lief, caries is an infectious disease, caused by a specific type of bacteria, the *mutans* group of *Streptococci*. Your dentist can now test to see if you are highly infected, and if so, he or she can prescribe a mouth rinse that can re-duce those bacteria to acceptable levels.

Frequent sucrose (table sugar) consumption tends to encourage the growth of this type of bacteria. Limiting sugar intake between meals can greatly reduce the risk of caries. Teaching children good eating practices will enhance their oral health as well as their overall health throughout their whole lives.

The body fights cavities. Your saliva has everything needed to heal early cavities and, when provided with very small amounts of fluoride, such as through daily brushing with a fluoridated toothpaste, will remineralize the cavities as they initially form.

Body fluids containing antibodies to fight disease cleanse your teeth from the inside out. The quality of your diet affects this natural cleansing action.

God created the mouth to be healthy. Harmful bacteria can enter the mouth only from other people, and the only other persons sufficiently inti-mate to infect extremely young children are their parents. Reducing bacte-rial infection in the mother and father protects the infant from early infection and allows natural protective mechanisms to develop to save the child from the threat of disease.

> *Are you helping or hindering your body in its natural fight*
> *against the infectious disease of dental caries?*

GOD'S BONDING DELIGHT FOR MARRIAGE

Now Adam knew Eve his wife; and she conceived, and bare Cain. Gen. 4:1.

While some more modern translations of the Bible may be more technically accurate, the King James Version portrays the story of Eve and Adam's marital union most sensitively and poetically. It takes sexual union out of the purely physical realm and gives it a dimension of wholeness.

When we say we "know" someone, as we use the term in daily speech, we mean that the person is more than an acquaintance. We feel that we have a relationship that includes respect, understanding, good feelings about, favorable regard for, and an interest in the other's activities and his or her thinking. Knowing someone well takes time, interest, and motivation.

When the King James translators used the word "know" to refer to the sexual experience of the first pair, they were saying something extremely profound. In order for sex to be the bonding delight God intended it to be, marital partners really need to "know" each other in much more than a physical sense. They must try to understand each other's emotional needs and strive to meet them. The couple will be interested in each other's values, goals, and ideas and will share spiritual insights. Only then can they truly "know" each other sufficiently to join their bodies in a complete knowing. And since the years will change their feelings, ideas, and perhaps even their interests, such knowing each other must be a continuous process of communicating and sharing.

Being increasingly able to participate in this type of openness can lead to a higher sense of intimacy. A couple who have only physical proximity of bodies without the other components of togetherness cannot be considered truly intimate. Intimacy denotes a closeness of the whole person.

This type of experience reflects the meaning of the word "within." When married lovers are "within" each other's life boundaries, they are sharing at a level unique to the marital relationship, a space not open to others.

The beautiful part is that when God is central in our lives, He can revive flagging or even troubled marriages. Through God's abiding love we receive the power to love each other as He has loved us.

Dear Father, we know that we can't manufacture love on our own. But we praise You for the promise that You can love through us. Amen.

IS IT TIME
TO OPEN
THE DOOR?

Behold, I stand at the door, and knock: if any man hear my voice, and open the door,
I will come in to him, and will sup with him, and he with me. Rev. 3:20.

Whatever am I doing here? I thought to myself as I prepared to spend my eight-week summer vacation at Uchee Pines Institute. My life had spun out of balance—stressed to the max by working two jobs, eating on the run (empty calories, of course), impulsive snacking, working late at night, and taking no time for my Lord. My blood sugar, triglycerides, and cholesterol were elevated, and to top those off, I was anemic! "I know, Lord, You led me here because You have something in store for my life. But what?"

What was in store for me during that next eight weeks was anything but a vacation! I found myself on a schedule—a balanced schedule. I was up at 6:00 for a personal devotional time. Then after a healthy breakfast I worked out on the farm, sweating in the hot summer sun, bush hogging, disking, picking, and selling produce until 1:00, when I went in to eat.

In the afternoon I'd study and listen to tapes about stress and what I needed to do to live a healthier lifestyle. At night I'd read my Bible. All day Sabbath and on several evenings the institute held meetings that allowed the guests to share a testimony of what God was doing for them. Those testimonies meant a lot to me!

And through it all something began to happen. After seven weeks my second blood test showed everything in the normal range. In addition, I had lost 13 pounds by eating all I wanted of the low-fat, high-fiber vegetarian food, and I felt good.

I had learned I was a workaholic, and the answer was to schedule balance into my life: a time for God, for work, and for study. A time to fellowship with others and to sleep. Plus two regular daily "vacation" times to eat.

Most of all, I rediscovered my heavenly Father and found that He had been knocking on my door all the time, but I had been too busy to open it! My door is open now, and it feels so good to sit down and enjoy His presence.

Your heavenly Father is knocking on your door. Isn't it time
you let Him in?

THE VINE, MY SOURCE OF LIFE

John DeVincenzo

> I am the true vine and my Father is the gardener. He cuts off every branch in me that bears no fruit, while every branch that does bear fruit he prunes so that it will be even more fruitful. John 15:1, 2, NIV.

What does it take to be spiritually healthy? I believe we can find the answer in the object lesson of the vine and branches in John 15. Jesus said, "If a man remains in me and I in him, he will bear much fruit; apart from me you can do nothing. . . . If you remain in me and my words remain in you, ask whatever you wish, and it will be given you. This is to my Father's glory, that you bear much fruit, showing yourselves to be my disciples" (John 15:5-8, NIV).

My avocation is experimental horticulture, and to me these words of our Lord are among the most powerful He spoke. To a society today largely removed from agriculture they may not carry the same impact they had 2,000 years ago.

A cut-off branch (scion) is first completely severed from its parent vine, then grafted into the new vine. When the cell layers (cambium) match, the graft unites with the vine. Then begins a beautiful symbiosis, with the branch supplying photosynthates (sugars) to the vine, while the vine supplies minerals and other soil nutrients (such as nitrogen, phosphorus, etc.) to the branch.

The fruit is unique to the branch. The vine has only minimal influence over the character of the fruit. The genetics within the branch itself determine the type of fruit.

Fruit production begins when the branch is bent. Branches growing straight up do not produce fruit. They are pruned out (trimmed clean) so that the bent branches can receive direct sunlight and produce higher-quality fruit.

As I'm pruning, grafting, and then picking the fruit produced, I realize that the source of life for all of us is the same, but because of our different characteristics, we bear different fruit to meet better the wide variety of needs, purposes, and plans God has for His people.

God needs me to bend to His will so He can have fruit from His vineyard—that unique fruit that each of us is capable of giving.

Lord, I pray that You will graft, bend, and prune me
so I will produce unique fruit for You to use for Your purposes.

HOLDING
ON FOR A
BLESSING

Roger D. Woodruff

Jacob replied, "I will not let you go unless you bless me." Gen. 32:26, NIV.

This text flashed into my mind during a long, pain-filled night following a freak tractor accident. A lengthy recovery loomed ahead of me because of the multiple injuries I had sustained, including a fractured hip socket that had been grafted, plated, and pinned. Nights were toughest to deal with and allowed plenty of time for reflection, wondering, and prayer. My life had been miraculously spared, but what now? I vacillated between hope and discouragement.

As the story of Jacob's all-night struggle against an unknown and unseen foe opened to my thoughts, I identified with the futility of his fight. Switching on the bedside lamp, I turned to Genesis 32 and read again how Jacob had sent his household across the stream and stayed behind to pray, fearing what would happen when he would meet his brother, Esau, whom he had wronged so long ago.

In the middle of the night the Lord came to him, but Jacob apparently thought someone sought to harm him, so he began to fight. "When the man [the Lord] saw that he could not overpower him [Jacob], he touched the socket of Jacob's hip so that his hip was wrenched as he wrestled with the man" (verse 25, NIV). At this point Jacob realized he had been struggling with the Lord, and replied, "I will not let you go unless you bless me" (verse 26, NIV). In spite of pain and discouragement, Jacob held on. Could I?

I desperately longed for something tangible, an anchor point for this crisis in my life. The story of Jacob drew me on as I recalled that he had not left the struggle unrewarded. "Then he blessed him there" (verse 29, NIV).

A blessing! Yes, that was my longing: meaning out of pain and long nights. What more important meaning could there be than a blessing from God? As though a light shone into my troubled mind, I experienced God's blessing as peace and acceptance enveloped my soul!

This anchor point of blessing has become a milestone of encouragement in my life. Jacob's all-night struggle; my dark experience; your blackest hour—God has a blessing waiting!

O God of Jacob, I will not let You go unless You bless me, too!
Though nights are long and struggles fierce, in my weakness I will cling
to You in great anticipation of Your mighty blessing. Amen.

BELSHAZZAR'S
TAMPERINGS

TEKEL: Thou art weighed in the balances, and art found wanting. Dan. 5:27.

Our heavenly Father is a loving and forgiving God, but by our own neglect and indifference we can lose our eternal heritage. King Belshazzar had known of the great God of heaven. His predecessor, King Nebuchadnezzar, had shared with his people the wonderful and powerful workings of Daniel's God, describing how the God of the heavens had intervened in his own life. Belshazzar's mother and grandmother had tried to guide him. But he chose a lifestyle that ignored the God of heaven.

During his drunken revelry Belshazzar had the sacred things of God's holy Temple brought to the feast, and mocked God by using them. Belshazzar tampered with the sacred things of God, and in the words of the eternal God Himself, Belshazzar was found wanting. His kingdom would be taken from him that very night (verse 30).

The Word of God makes it clear that we are not to tamper with sacred things. The sons of Aaron died because they offered profane fire before the Lord (Num. 3:4); Uzzah perished because he ventured to touch the ark of the covenant (2 Sam. 6:6, 7); even 70 men of Beth-shemesh were struck dead for looking into the ark (1 Sam. 6:19). If we, like Belshazzar, Nadab, and Uzzah, tamper with the holy things of God, we will also be found wanting.

A lifestyle that increases the risk of disease and death is a lifestyle that mocks the Creator-God because it tampers with the holy. Therefore, eating rich, fatty foods, drinking caffeine-laced beverages, getting no exercise, and burning the candle at both ends is tampering with the holy! Holding on to such harmful practices shows little respect for that which God considers holy (1 Cor. 3:16). To give honor and glory to God, we must treat with respect the holy things of God. We do this with what we eat, drink, or whatever we do (1 Cor. 10:31).

Is there anything in your lifestyle that might be tipping the scales in the direction of sinful things, rather than toward holy things?

CHRISTIANS IN A VIOLENT SOCIETY

Noah was a righteous man, blameless among the people of his time, and he walked with God. . . . Now the earth was corrupt in God's sight and was full of violence. Gen. 6:9-11, NIV. As it was in the days of Noah, so it will be at the coming of the Son of Man. Matt. 24:37, NIV.

I was called to the emergency department to see a little girl who needed my services. About 5 years old, she was unconscious, bruised, and bleeding from every orifice, a victim of rape and beating.

Nor is this example unique. Every day around our world thousands of innocent victims suffer at the hands of a violent society. It has become our way of life. As I write, the cover story of *USA Today* tells of violence in the workplace. It is everywhere! As a disease, violence has grown to become the number one killer of youth and young adults, accounting for more lost days of productive life than any other malady, including heart attacks and cancer.

Neither are Christians exempt from the effects of the epidemic. Our spouses, our children and parents, our families and friends often fall victim to the plague. Like Abraham's nephew, Lot, living in ancient Sodom (2 Peter 2:7, 8), our hearts often ache from the pain and frustration of our own dysfunctional families and broken homes and the violence that accompanies them.

How are we to live in such a world?

We may run and hide or become so involved in activities that we don't have time to think of our pain and problems. Perhaps we may make-believe that nothing is wrong. Some of us may let alcohol or drugs, sex or sports, computer games or videos, or even our work or religion divert our attentions and fill our time.

Or we, like David of old, may find our peace and comfort in the sanctuary. Ours is the privilege of resting our case with Jesus and trusting Him to carry us through this time of judgment, when everything around us is in frustration, confusion, and turmoil. We can rest in the assurance that He will take care of His own, and one day soon we will celebrate the end of violence and sin.

*Lord, give me the spirit of love and not fear as I live
in this end-time violent society.*

WITHOUT
THOUGHT OF
SPECIAL NOTICE

Let us not become weary in doing good, for at the proper time we will reap
a harvest if we do not give up. Gal. 6:9, NIV.

Henry M. Porter, once a Pony Express rider, later a banker from
Denver, Colorado, was visiting his daughter in Pasadena, California,
when a serious cold suddenly struck him down. At his daughter's sug-
gestion, Porter went to the nearby Glendale Sanitarium for hydrotherapy
treatment. After the treatment, Porter offered the boy who gave it a dollar
tip. The boy declined, saying that it would not be right to accept further
payment in addition to his sanitarium earnings.

Years later, while spending the winter near San Diego, Porter again
contracted a serious cold. Remembering his experience in the Glendale
Sanitarium, he asked whether a similar institution existed nearby. He
learned of Paradise Valley Sanitarium.

While a patient there, every day he opened his door a crack so that he
could watch the unfailing kindness of a student nurse feeding an old man
who had Parkinson's disease. She never knew that anyone was observing her.

Porter soon recovered and returned home. In a few days he was surprised to receive a letter of apology and explanation from the sanitarium
business office and a check for 45 cents. It seemed that the books had not
balanced at the end of the week (bookkeeping was done by hand in the
1920s), and the error, traced to Porter's account, showed that the sanitarium had overcharged him 45 cents.

These small examples of integrity made a lasting impression, and
Porter wrote a letter of gratitude. "I feel I have underpaid you for all your
kind and careful treatment and attention, and I owe you all a debt of gratitude for the kind consideration while with you."

In 1928 he wrote again, asking for the address of the general manager
of these institutions, since he wanted to establish a similar institution in
Denver. This led to a gift of $330,000 (the first of many gifts) for the es-
tablishment of Porter Sanitarium and Hospital in south Denver.

Porter Memorial Hospital, as it has been renamed, is a tribute to the
Porter family, but also to the acts of kindness and compassion quietly done
without thought of special notice or reward.

*Look around you. What kind act can you do for someone
in your family, your church, or your community?*

THE WAY TO A MAN'S HEART

For as in the those days before the flood they were eating and drinking, marrying and giving in marriage, until the day when Noah entered the ark, and they did not know until the flood came and swept them all away, so will be the coming of the Son of man. Matt. 24:38, 39, RSV.

We have all heard the saying "The way to a man's heart is through his stomach." Its truth in a physical sense is readily apparent with even a cursory review of health statistics today. Coronary heart disease reigns as the number one killer. Science has well established the relationship of diet to blocked arteries.

But the saying really isn't talking about a pathway to the physical heart. It's referring to an influence on the emotions—the mind and will. And this doesn't just affect men. How often we use food to alter another's attitude toward us! We employ food and occasions of eating to try to change the mind and make it more susceptible to another's way of thinking. It has been so since the beginning of time.

Think of the many decisions made at tables bedecked with food and drink. Consider the many times we eat, not because we're hungry, but just because we want to. Think of Adam. He wasn't even hungry when he ate with such disastrous results what Eve offered him (see Ellen G. White, in *Signs of the Times*, Apr. 4, 1900).

Think of those who were "eating and drinking" and "did not know until the flood came." The text suggests that how we eat and drink can influence our ability to perceive important issues.

Consider the case of Esau. The more he imagined his favorite food, the more he wanted it, until it became more important than his sacred birthright (Gen. 25:29-34).

And think of the many dinners, receptions, and parties designed to sway others.

Are you ever tempted to eat when you aren't hungry? Or to consume food that isn't really good for you? Can it be that the devil himself knows the way to our hearts? Can it be that he realizes the eternal consequences better than we do?

Follow Christ's example. When Satan tried to tempt Him to turn the stones into bread and satisfy His appetite, Jesus answered, "It is written: 'Man does not live on bread alone, but on every word that comes from the mouth of God'" (Matt. 4:4, NIV).

Lord, help me to resist Satan's strongest temptation by letting Your Word influence my thoughts, not the indulgence of my physical appetite.

AN EMPTINESS THAT WILL NEVER BE FILLED

Why are you downcast, O my soul? Why so disturbed within me? Put your hope in God, for I will yet praise him, my Savior and my God. Ps.m 42:5, NIV.

Make her breathe, Peter! Make her breathe!"

My mind screamed the words to our obstetrician friend, but the delivery room was deadly silent. The child who moments before had been kicking in my womb was now cradled in his hands. So tiny; so fragile. He handed our daughter to me and my husband, and we held her as her heart slowed and finally stopped. Her lungs were too premature to take even one small breath.

I stared at the perfect features of my little girl, etching them forever in my mind. Although I felt the warmth go out of the doll-like body, I still could not give her up. I asked for a basin of water, and with the help of a friend washed her and wrapped her in a soft, white blanket. Then I rocked her gently.

We brought our other children in to see the sister who would never grow up to be their friend. When they had gone, my husband tenderly lifted her from my arms. "They're here for her. You have to let her go."

Of course I did, but it broke my heart.

I thought the tears would never stop. Then to add to the pain, an infection kept me in the hospital through the maze of following days and nights and the funeral. My homecoming, when it finally arrived, was not one of victory, but of desperation. Healing resulted from my physician husband's skilled hands and my sister-in-law's loving arms.

My mind cleared slowly, as if a fog were being burned off by the scent of the lilacs and the laughter of my children. Life returned to what would now be normal. But even after all these years, not a day passes that I don't think of my baby. There is an emptiness deep inside that will never be filled. Oh, how I long for her resurrection!

I wonder, as I think of my pain, how God's heart must break over the eternal loss of even one of His children. I have the feeling an emptiness deep inside Him will never be filled either!

What event in your life makes you long for heaven?

MEASURING LIFE BY DONATION, NOT DURATION

Therefore I tell you, do not worry about your life, what you will eat or drink; or about your body, what you will wear. Is not life more important than food, and the body more important than clothes? . . . Who of you by worrying can add a single hour to his life? Matt. 6:25-27, NIV.

The phone was ringing incessantly. I ran into the room and picked it up. It was my hypochondriac friend, Tina. She sounded distracted and distant. My "Hi, how are you?" let loose a dam of woes.

"Oh terrible!" she responded weakly. "I guess my days are numbered. I have had no appetite for weeks. My stomach feels bloated, and I burp frequently. I have also been losing weight. I'm quite certain I have cancer of the stomach."

"Don't worry, Tina. I think there is nothing wrong with you."

"Sure there is," she insisted. "I even feel nauseated at times. I'm pretty sure I have cancer of the stomach. In fact, I have made an appointment with a specialist to have a gastroscopy on Monday, and I dread what the results will show."

Tina went for the tests, but as I expected, the tests found nothing wrong with her stomach. With this new assurance of her well-being, she regained her appetite and weight.

Then a couple months later Tina was again experiencing the same symptoms—effects of her anxiety over her suspicion that she had another form of cancer. So went the catalog of suspected ailments for as long as I could remember: cancer of the lungs, breast, brain, etc. Each required an X-ray to prove to herself that she had nothing wrong with her before she could take control of herself.

How well the Lord knows our problems when He admonishes us not to be anxious about our life, for ironically, worrying will cut rather than lengthen our life span.

When tempted to be anxious about our life, it will do us well to adopt the attitude of the renowned minister Peter Marshall, who said: "When the clock strikes for me, I shall go, not one minute early, and not one minute late. Until then, there is nothing to fear. I know that the promises of God are true. . . . The measure of a life, after all, is not its duration, but its donation" *(The Best of Peter Marshall,* p. xiii).

How are you measuring your life? Is it by duration, or donation?
Try giving a little more to the needs of others and worrying a little
less about your own, and see what it will do for your health.

JESUS IS
THE WAY
TO LIFE

> Jesus answered, "I am the way and the truth and the life. No one comes to
> the Father except through me." John 14:6, NIV.

It is hard to imagine living without putting food in our mouth or breathing air into our lungs. Yet a healthy, developing baby can grow just fine in its water-filled home within the uterus without ever eating or breathing. God has prepared a very special way for nutrients and oxygen to come into the baby's body and for wastes to be removed. He designed a unique and intricate organ we call the placenta, which is attached to the baby by the umbilical cord.

The placenta takes over many important body functions for the baby, allowing its organs to grow and mature as long as it is in the uterus. It acts as the baby's lungs, providing oxygen to the entire body, and serves as the baby's stomach and intestines, supplying vitamins and nutrients to keep the infant healthy. Also, it behaves as the baby's kidneys, removing wastes from its blood. Immediately after birth the umbilical cord is painlessly cut. Since neither the baby nor the mother needs the placenta anymore, it leaves the mother's body.

Imagine a single organ doing all these special things for the baby when it is unable to do them for itself!

It reminds me of how dependent we are on God. God gave us a placenta to sustain our life while in utero, and then after we were born, each breath and heartbeat is His gift of life to us. But in addition, God has designed a way for us to escape from sin and have eternal life. His way of life, His "placenta" for the condition we are in, is Christ.

"It is impossible for us, of ourselves, to escape from the pit of sin in which we are sunken. . . . Education, culture, the exercise of the will, human effort, all have their proper sphere, but here they are powerless. . . . There must be a power working from within. . . . That power is Christ. His grace alone can quicken the lifeless faculties of the soul, and attract it to God, to holiness" *(Steps to Christ,* p. 18).

Truly God is our life-giver!

Are you trying to be good by yourself? Christ has a better way.
Depend on Him, for His power and grace are the only way for
you to have life eternal!

GET ENERGY
THE NATURAL
WAY

Jan W. Kuzma

> You have plowed wickedness; you have reaped iniquity. You have eaten the fruit of lies, because you trusted in your own way. Hosea 10:13, NKJV.

Most of us work hard to complete certain projects on time. However, with unplanned interruptions and looming deadlines, we realize we need extra energy. Many succumb to society's artificial energy boosters: coffee, tea, or cola. Some wish that they could find a text that would endorse their caffeine habit. They wish that Jesus had indulged in a cup of coffee to give Him that extra boost of energy when facing Gethsemane, but He relied on friends and prayer instead. Probably He knew what artificial stimulants such as caffeine do to the body.

Here's what research has found: caffeine elevates blood sugar; aggravates hypoglycemia; can cause irregular heartbeat; increases urinary calcium and magnesium losses; dilutes and constricts blood vessels, thus increasing blood pressure; increases stomach acid secretion and aggravates a stomach ulcer; can cause tremors, irritability, and nervousness; disrupts sleep and produces insomnia; increases anxiety and depression; heightens symptoms of premenstrual syndrome; lowers tolerance to physical and emotional stress; interferes with higher brain function; and is associated with colon, bladder, and ovarian cancer.

More than 100 years ago God revealed to Ellen White that tea and coffee are "stimulating, and contain poisons" *(Counsels on Diet and Foods,* pp. 419, 420). "Tea has an influence to excite the nerves, and coffee benumbs the brain; both are highly injurious" *(Testimonies,* vol. 4, p. 365). "Tea and coffee do not nourish the system. The relief obtained from them is sudden, before the stomach has time to digest them. This shows that what the users of these stimulants call strength is only received by exciting the nerves of the stomach, which convey the irritation to the brain, and this in turn is aroused to impart increased action to the heart, and short-lived energy to the entire system. All this is false strength, that we are the worse for having. They do not give a particle of natural strength" *(ibid.,* vol. 2, p. 65).

Get energy the natural way. Take walks several times a day, drink plenty of water, get more sleep, spend time with your friends, and ask God to provide you with wisdom to work smart and lead a balanced life.

How long has it been since you read Ellen White's book Counsels on Diet and Foods? *I challenge you to pick up a copy and read it from cover to cover. You'll be amazed at the wisdom and insight of this godly woman with only a limited formal education.*

WHAT
MY DAD
GAVE ME

If you, then, though you are evil, know how to give good gifts to your children, how much more will your Father in heaven give good gifts to those who ask him! Matt. 7:11, NIV.

My dad gave me three gifts that prepared me for a happy, wholesome life. They didn't cost him any money—but today they're priceless treasures. The first: Dad gave me the feeling of being special. Second: He loved my mom. And third: He gave me the gift of optimism!

Three simple gifts, but they have made me what I am.

Dad always thought I was special. I could tell by the way he winked at me from across the room or put his arm around me and gave me a squeeze in church. When I was a teen I worked in his manufacturing plant after school. He loved to say to the businesspeople who visited, "I'd like to have you meet my daughter."

And the last few days before he died he read my first book, *Understanding Children,* not because of his interest in the topic, but because of his interest in me!

The second gift Dad gave me was really loving my mom. When I close my eyes and think of Mom and Dad, I see her standing by the kitchen sink and Dad coming up behind her and putting his arms around her and hugging her. I love that picture.

And as far as optimism is concerned—perhaps that was his greatest gift of all. I don't remember Dad ever being discouraged, even though he struggled for 10 years to keep a manufacturing business alive, and finally, penniless, had to give up. He lost the company, but not hope, and went on to climb new mountains. Before long, Dad's real estate business became so successful he became known as "Humpal—The Mountain Man."

Dad was a dreamer. He always had a million projects tucked away in his head. "Now, someday I'm going to . . . ," he'd begin and would tell us a tiny piece of his dream. Sure enough, before long things would start to take shape.

Yes, Dad gave me three wonderful gifts that were the foundation of a good life, but none of them can compare with the gift my heavenly Father has given me: eternal life!

> *Your earthly father gave you the gift of life, but what else
> did he give? Why not thank him? And while you're at it,
> thank your heavenly Father for Jesus, the best gift of all, for
> without Jesus there would be no eternal life!*

KEEPING OUR IMMUNE SYSTEMS HEALTHY

Remember, your Father knows exactly what you need even before you ask him! Matt. 6:8, TLB.

The human body has a coordinated defense system more sophisticated than any nation's. Unlike military weapons that quickly become obsolete, the body's system never gets outdated. It continually has trillions of "fighter cells" ready for action. One out of every 100 body cells is a defender cell. This fighting force of the immune system is so complicated that scientists are just beginning to appreciate its intricacy and adaptability.

God has designed it to protect the body without human thought or command. Before birth the body gears up its defensive system to fight battles that will rage throughout life. Immediately after birth the immune system receives a big boost in its "firepower" from mother's milk packed with antibodies ready to fight microbial invaders. When you are 10 years of age the human immune system is at its strongest.

Imagine for a moment that disease-causing pathogens slip past the natural defenses of the skin and stomach acids and invade the body. Within 20 minutes these invaders can double in number. An infection starting with just one bacterium can multiply to 1 billion after nine hours and 2 billion after nine hours and 20 minutes! The human system doesn't wait until it's invaded to prepare, however. It has already readied fighter cells, each cell having a specific job to do. They recognize specific enemies and coordinate their battle through their chemical communication "language." Unlike any other defense system, they can reproduce by the millions in a matter of hours.

With age the immune system weakens, so we must be vigilant to keep it active and healthy. Lifestyle choices and environment have a major impact on how effectively the immune system functions.

"God's healing power runs all through nature. If a tree is cut, if a human being is wounded or breaks a bone, nature begins at once to repair the injury. Even before the need exists, the healing agencies are in readiness. . . . So it is in the spiritual realm. Before sin created the need, God had provided the remedy" (*Education*, p. 113).

*What are you doing to keep your immune systems healthy—
your body's immune system to fight disease, and your
spiritual immune system to combat sin?*

THE MOST EFFECTIVE WITNESS

Joyce W. Hopp

But you will receive power when the Holy Spirit comes on you; and you will be my witnesses in Jerusalem, and in all Judea and Samaria, and to the ends of the earth. Acts 1:8, NIV.

C hrist has promised the gift of the Holy Spirit to His church, and the promise belongs to us as much as to the first disciples" (Ellen G. White, in *Review and Herald,* Nov. 19, 1908).

Witnessing by living healthfully poses a special challenge. If we appear to be bragging about our accomplishments, we can turn people off. Instead of wanting to emulate our example, they wish we would shut up.

On the other hand, if we fail to practice what we preach, or to live up to the information we have on healthful living, we are poor witnesses to the power of the gospel to transform our daily lives.

We don't have to be marathon runners, cross-country bikers, or skiers to witness to the powerful effect of living healthfully. Our neighbors will observe the regular walks we take. Friends will notice the low-fat food we consistently choose. And family members will know when we get enough hours of sleep. But how will this make a difference in another person's life?

Jean organized a walking group, "The Happy Wanderers." Every morning they invited neighbors to join. "We talked about everything," she said.

When they first started walking, Lucille could scarcely hold up her end of the conversation because she was so out of breath. Gradually she improved to where she could both talk and walk. She began to ask questions such as Why had God allowed her to have emphysema? Where was God when her daughter died in an accident? Several members of the group provided answers they had found through their study of the Scriptures. No polished presentation, not even a Bible, but Lucille's spiritual steps began to match her physical ones.

"Not by eloquence or logic are men's hearts reached, but by the sweet influences of the Holy Spirit, which operate quietly yet surely in transforming and developing character. It is the still small voice of the Spirit of God that has power to change the heart" *(Prophets and Kings,* p. 169).

We don't use the Holy Spirit—we allow Him to use us.

Lord, I dedicate my daily healthful way of life to You, for the Holy Spirit to use it as a witness to others.

JESUS, THE BREAD OF LIFE

June 24

Bert Connell

> Jesus answered, "I tell you the truth, you are looking for me, not because you saw miraculous signs but because you ate the loaves and had your fill. Do not work for food that spoils, but for food that endures to eternal life, which the Son of Man will give you." John 6:26, 27, NIV.

The Passover approached. Family units made their pilgrimage to Jerusalem through Galilee. Jesus and His disciples hoped to find some rest, but the pilgrims, hearing that Jesus was near, sought Him out. In His compassion Jesus responded to their requests for healing and taught them the way of salvation.

All day long the multitude was so focused upon Jesus' message and activities that they forgot their own physical need for food. Jesus too suffered fatigue and hunger as evening approached. The disciples worried about obtaining enough food to feed the thousands of people.

Jesus, in His wisdom, had a plan to meet their needs. Using a boy's lunch consisting of five barley loaves and two fish, He provided enough food to feed the 5,000 there. His miracle graphically illustrates His loving concern for our welfare and His desire to save us.

Many of His listeners there had warped appetites, just as many of us have today. Jesus leads us to an understanding of a simpler way of eating, as illustrated in the meal served that evening. "Selfishness and the indulgence of unnatural taste have brought sin and misery into the world, from excess on the one hand, and from want on the other" *(The Desire of Ages,* p. 367).

Could you be suffering from the food selections you make to gratify a distorted appetite? Overweight and disease often result from them.

If you would eat more simply, and then, instead of spending hours in the kitchen preparing a large variety of fancy, rich, high-calorie gourmet dishes, spend that time with Jesus, the true Bread of Life, I wonder what a difference it would make in your spiritual, as well as your physical, well-being.

Jesus Christ shows us a way. By feeding the 5,000 there on the side of the mountain, He taught us to turn our thoughts away from what we will eat next, and toward Him as the source of our daily sustenance and the way to salvation.

Lord, may my thoughts be on obtaining my daily bread of life from You, and not on satisfying my perverted physical appetite.

HEALING
WOUNDS

I will restore health unto thee, and I will heal thee of thy wounds, saith the Lord. Jer. 30:17.

A wound is a disruption of the skin, usually because of an injury or surgical procedure. But if properly treated, we expect our wounds to heal. However, at times something will block the natural healing process. Maybe you've gotten a splinter or a piece of glass embedded in your skin. At first it didn't feel that uncomfortable. But instead of healing in a day or so, your wound festered, turned red, and became sore. The problem was the infection caused by a foreign body implanted in your skin.

Cancer, the destruction of the autoimmune system by AIDS, or a poor blood supply can also prevent healing.

Sometimes it takes radical measures to deal with these barriers to the healing process. Unless we eradicate them, the skin will never function as it should so that healing can occur. It will never be able to act as the first line of defense against infection.

As our skin needs to be undamaged to function, so must we if we are to reach our full Christian potential. Unfortunately, underlying and often unnoticed festerings affect our spiritual lives. We become infected with destructive habits, embedded with idols that we value above all else, filled with malignant hurt feelings, or suffer from either low self-esteem or self-sufficiency—all of which prevent us from being healthy Christians. Only under the Holy Spirit's spiritual guidance can we identify and treat these problem areas.

Even when healing occurs, it can leave scars behind as reminders. Some are barely noticeable; others are ugly and glaring. The scars themselves can become symbols for either thankfulness or guilt. Since we'll have these scars until Jesus comes and makes us completely new, we need the Holy Spirit's help for us to keep them in proper perspective. We must allow the Master Physician to direct our healing process.

Interestingly, in heaven only Jesus will have scars—your scars and mine, from Calvary!

When you look at a certain scar on your body, what do
you remember? What will you remember throughout eternity
as you look at Jesus' scars? Why not thank Him
today for those scars?

TAKING THE TRIP OF YOUR LIFE

Christine Neish

> Those who know your name will trust in you, for you, Lord, have never forsaken those who seek you. Ps. 9:10, NIV.

We were prepared for our 10-mile trek in Utah's canyon country. In just a few minutes our Navajo guide and 10 horses would arrive, and we would begin the trip of a lifetime to Rainbow Bridge.

Let the faint of heart arrive by boat, take a short walk, and view that glorious sandstone arch. We were going to follow the land route—riding horses and camping, doing it the right way. Only after we saw three out of the 10 horses we had requested and met our 81-year-old guide did we begin to worry just a bit. Unfortunately, our trip coincided with the first weekend of hunting season. Somebody else had snapped up all trailworthy horses and our original guide. The ride/walk began.

As we descended from Piaute Mesa to the canyons we marveled at the beauty of the red rock, the narrow and winding canyons, and the feeling of aloneness. It was a great experience. Occasionally we would ask about our progress but would not receive an answer from our guide. Fortunately, one of our members spoke some Navajo. Our guide, it seems, did not speak English. No matter, he was nearly deaf, and besides, he had never been to Rainbow Bridge before. Yes, this was going to be a good trip.

By the time we dragged ourselves home we had walked 50 miles, been rained and snowed upon, had our food stolen by those friendly dogs who began the trip with us, and had eaten a meager ration of sandy scrambled eggs. What a trip!

When I remember our trek, I think of today's children of God. We know our destination—but what lies ahead? What will we do for clothing, shelter, food? We have our Guide, but can we trust Him to get us there? How long will it take? How are we doing?

Jesus tells us to trust Him. We can. He hears us, has been there before, and will care for us.

When you don't know where life is leading you, "trust in the Lord and do good; dwell in the land and enjoy safe pasture. Delight yourself in the Lord and he will give you the desires of your heart" (Ps. 37:3, 4, NIV).

TRAPPED

David Beardsley

> And she shall bring forth a son, and thou shalt call his name Jesus:
> for he shall save his people *from* their sins. Matt. 1:21.

Many years ago, during the summer, my brothers and I were building a house for our parents, I dug a deep hole for a septic tank. Unfortunately, it caved in and buried me up to my shoulders. There was absolutely nothing I could do to free myself. It was a helpless feeling. I was totally dependent on aid from my brothers to get out of my trapped condition. After some discussion and joking, they started to work and freed me.

Spiritually we are all trapped by the sin that is so much a part of our natures. Equally helpless to do anything to free ourselves from our predicament, we need outside assistance—a Saviour.

If we all have a Saviour, why do we so often remain trapped by our sin? Could it be because we don't really believe that anything can rescue us from it? Could it be because we believe that our Saviour will save us *in* our sins instead of *from* our sins?

While I was buried up to my shoulders, how satisfying would it have been to me to have my brothers tell me that they were sorry about my condition, but they could not get me out? How would I have felt if they had told me they would bring me food and drink and make me as comfortable as they could, but I would have to stay trapped by the sand?

That's how absurd it would be to believe that our Saviour would leave us trapped in our sins and still save us. He is a powerful deliverer. "God's ideal for His children is higher than the highest human thought can reach. 'Be ye therefore perfect, even as your Father which is in heaven is perfect.' The command is a promise. The plan of redemption contemplates our complete recovery from the power of Satan" *(The Desire of Ages*, p. 311).

How big is your God today? Can He overcome sin in your life?

Dear Lord, thank You for not leaving me trapped in my sins,
and for providing a way for me to live a more vibrant life. Amen.

FOOD AND EXERCISE FOR THE SOUL

Kay Kuzma

When I consider your heavens, the work of your fingers, the moon and the stars, which you have set in place, what is man that you are mindful of him, the son of man that you care for him? Ps. 8:3, 4, NIV.

Ralph Waldo Emerson once said, "The sky is the daily bread of the eyes." Just as food feeds our body and gives us strength and health, so it is that what we see nourishes our soul. And here is where we have a choice. We can become anemic and stressed out by bingeing on the empty calories of visual junk food: crowded streets, concrete cities, and pollution; the messy house, paper-strewn desk, and dirty laundry; or television and videos produced to titillate our passions and imprison our creativity. Or we can look up and feed on something beyond humanity that can lower stress and heighten spirituality, something that has always been there and always will be: *the sky.*

The sky is "God's original diet" for the human soul, to take us from mundane, minuscule human thoughts to ones centering on God. Human beings have desecrated the earth in many places, but the sky belongs to God. It was the very first thing He created. "In the beginning God created the heavens" (Gen. 1:1, NIV). And throughout the ages the sky has been the major link between God's created creatures and the Creator. When we doubt, when we are tempted to lose faith and stumble into discouragement, all we have to do is look up.

Viewing the sky can be good soul exercise, too. "Wherever I am," says poet David Accord, "the night is full of familiar stars, and every day—unless rain or snow or illness has interfered—there is at least one uncrowded moment of renewed adventure through the cumulus mountains, down the black canyons of storm, across the mackerel Sahara, up the cirro-vapor trails or under the drifting cotton of a summer afternoon."

Pause now and listen to the words of the music of the sky: "The heavens declare the glory of God; the skies proclaim the work of his hands. Day after day they pour forth speech; night after night they display knowledge. There is no speech or language where their voice is not heard" (Ps. 19:1-3, NIV).

For soul health, look up.

When you're discouraged and your soul is hungry, feast on the sky. It's always there. Its immensity can turn heaviness and hate into hope; its blazing beauty can turn discouragement into delight; its blue haze can quiet and calm your stormy spirit.

A BRAND
PLUCKED OUT
OF THE FIRE

And the Lord said unto Satan, the Lord rebuke thee, O Satan; even the Lord that hath chosen Jerusalem rebuke thee; is not this a brand plucked out of the fire? Zech. 3:2.

I was definitely "a brand plucked out of the fire." Although I was born of very religious parents, I became involved with drugs during my early 20s. Heroin, cocaine, and marijuana were my gods. The police arrested me more than 40 times in the Denver area between 1966 and 1984 on a variety of drug-related charges, and I ended up in prison. I lost my family, my home, and my employment as the result of my 20-year drug habit.

And then in 1985 I realized I needed help. God says, "Ask, and it will be given to you; seek, and you will find; knock, and it will be opened to you" (Matt. 7:7, NKJV). When I turned my life over to Him, I found even more than I had ever hoped or dreamed of finding.

I met Freddie one Sabbath in church, I proposed the next day, and three months later we were married. Next to the Lord, she has been my inspiration, my constant companion, and my soul mate.

During my 20-year struggle I had no one to help me get off drugs. Every time I'd try to keep clean for a couple days, something would happen, someone would tempt me, and I was right back where I started—or even worse!

I was a bricklayer by trade. But once I became converted, Freddie and I began to dream of providing more than just brick walls for people. We wanted to give others the support they needed to break their addictions, and to prevent as many young people as possible from experimenting with fire. And so, shortly after our marriage, we moved from Denver to Grand Terrace, California, and through a series of miracles started DAP—the Drug Alternative Program. Together we have given our lives to helping pull other "brands" from the fire of drug dependency. We've made a lifetime commitment. No retirement.

I tell my story to give you hope. Whatever your addiction, God is the answer. He can pluck you from the fire, for He is "able to do exceeding abundantly above all that we ask or think" (Eph. 3:20).

Look to Jesus. He is the answer to life . . . and the source of all liberty!

TWENTY-ONE DAYS TO A HABIT

Obey me, and I will be your God and you will be my people. Walk in all the ways
I command you, that it may go well with you. Jer. 7:23, NIV.

All true obedience comes from the heart. . . . And if we consent, He will
so identify Himself with our thoughts and aims, so blend our hearts
and minds into conformity to His will, that when obeying Him we
shall be but carrying out our own impulses. The will, refined and sanctified,
will find its highest delight in doing His service. When we know God as it
is our privilege to know Him, our life will be a life of continual obedience.
Through an appreciation of the character of Christ, through communion
with God, sin will become hateful to us" *(The Desire of Ages,* p. 668).

That's quite a statement. I often wondered how it could be true. Then
I began to study the brain and how it functions. Repetition causes a small
bouton to form at the end of the sending fiber of the brain nerve cell. It enlarges and multiples by more repetition, and thus a habit gets established.

Dr. William Sadler, a psychiatrist, says that our established habits
make literal pathways through the nervous system. Frequent repetition of
the same thought, feeling, or action creates a stronger and more permanent
pathway, just as repeated walking over the same place on a lawn will wear
a deep path in the sod.

Since the frequent repetition of thoughts, feelings, and acts patterns or
wires our brain, if our choices are based on Scripture and by beholding
Jesus, and if they are strengthened by the power of the Holy Spirit, then
there is going to be a long-term effect!

It doesn't make any difference whether you are trying to form a good
health habit, such as flossing your teeth, eating nutritiously, or exercising
daily, or a good heart habit, such as spending time with Jesus or cultivat-
ing loving relationships with your family—*you can do it in 21 days!* The
boutons that you form by repetition will be large and numerous enough in
just three weeks to establish the habit.

So take courage! You can be obedient, and His will can become your
own as His will unites with yours to transform you.

*Thank You, God, for creating my brain with the capacity
to form thought, feeling, and action pathways that
conform to Your will and purpose for my life.*

THE RUNNER'S HIGH

July 1

Larry Richardson

A cheerful heart does good like medicine, but a broken spirit makes one sick. Prov. 17:22, TLB.

Feeling happy is certainly something we all strive for and deserve to enjoy. Unfortunately, some people rely on dangerous drugs to induce euphoria. Long ago I found that a good half-hour run produces the same results with much less risk.

The phenomenon is commonly referred to as the "runner's high," and most joggers feel it after about 30-40 minutes on the track. For some it takes longer, while others encounter it sooner. The sensation results from a natural narcotic produced by the body, called beta-endorphins. After a period of extended aerobic activity the body releases the chemical into your system, which acts as a painkiller and mood elevator. For the runner, the sense of exhilaration makes you feel that you could go on running forever. Some runners call it "catching your second wind."

I often bring on this "runner's high" while jogging, and it is physically and mentally energizing. In fact, it is often my most creative time. I find that my most inspired thoughts and insightful times occur while I am exercising. Whenever I'm confused, discouraged, or just in need of rejuvenation, I simply go for a run. Ideas pop into my head so fast I need a secretary bicycling beside me to write them all down. Why am I so creative while jogging and not while sitting behind a desk? I believe it is because of the energizing qualities of human motion and those wonderful beta-endorphins.

I actually know a psychiatrist who uses the jogging track rather than his office couch to counsel patients. Instead of letting them lie down while pouring out their woes, he takes them for a run while they talk.

"You'd be amazed how many patients feel great after our sessions," he told me. "The truth is, most problems could be solved with a good run."

Solomon tells us that a merry heart is like a medicine. What physiologists are now discovering is that the body already comes equipped with the medicine that produces a cheerful heart—endorphins. So when someone invites you to "get high," tell them, "That sounds great," and take them for a five-mile run.

What can you do to experience God's natural "high" when you feel low?

FIREWORKS

Isak Wessels

Then Samson prayed to the Lord, "O Sovereign Lord, remember me. O God, please strengthen me just once more, and let me with one blow get revenge on the Philistines for my two eyes." Judges 16:28, NIV.

The tragic story of this phenomenally powerful yet incredibly weak young man is well known. The pitiful final result of Samson's foolish infatuation with a bewitchingly beautiful woman was the loss first of his hair, then of divine power, followed by freedom, and ultimately by both of his eyes, which motivated his suicidal act. His anguished petition screams out feelings many people will suffer this month, as their eyes are also brutally injured while enjoying enchanting visions.

According to the Centers for Disease Control, hospital emergency rooms treat approximately 12,000 fireworks injuries every year. The estimated cost is more than $24 million. One in five injuries involves the eyes, with half of them resulting in blindness or removal of the eyes. Three types of fireworks were most responsible for injuries: firecrackers; bottle rockets (which caused 72 percent of hospitalizations); and sparklers (producing severe burns by reaching temperatures as high as 1,800° F, which can melt gold). In 1991 fireworks started an estimated 25,500 fires, causing more than $33 million in property damage.

Fewer than a dozen states ban all private fireworks; some have no laws whatsoever, and unregulated mail-order sales or bootlegging disseminates these explosive devices. Many of the injuries occur from misuse (intentionally aiming a rocket at people, or throwing it after lighting it) or from malfunction such as erratic flight, premature explosions, or ricocheting off a hard surface. Almost 80 percent of injuries occur around the Fourth of July, and more than half affect children and teenagers.

Fireworks have a captivating excitement and seductive beauty that Samson would recognize. Only too late did he realize that the seductive Delilah would be one of the very last things he would ever see. How high the cost and how brief the thrill! It reminds me of the proverb "Can a man scoop fire into his lap without his clothes being burned?" (Prov. 6:27, NIV).

Lord, let me not play with fire!

215

WHAT SABBATH DOES TO GOD'S PEOPLE

Niels-Erik Andreasen

Here there is no Greek or Jew, . . . but Christ is all, and is in all. Therefore, as God's chosen people, holy and dearly loved, clothe yourselves with compassion, kindness, humility, gentleness and patience. . . . And over all these virtues put on love, which binds them all together in perfect unity." Col. 3:11-14, NIV.

Father was a small farmer, eking out a modest income working the soil, planting vegetables and flowers, and taking them to market. As a young man he had nurtured great ambitions to study medicine and become a missionary. But the war had interfered, and he had ended up farming, never quite comfortable in the overalls and wooden shoes farmers used in those days.

Thus I remember well the dramatic contrast in his appearance Friday evening at the beginning of Sabbath. He came down slowly from the upstairs bedroom just as the sun was setting. The steep staircase did not reveal his full height at once. First I saw the black wingtip shoes, polished to a brilliant shine. Then the black socks, the well-creased trousers, the bottom of his waistcoat, the white shirt with tie, open jacket, hair groomed to perfection.

"Are we going somewhere?" we would ask with excitement upon seeing him dressed up.

"No," he replied, "we are not going anywhere, but Someone is coming tonight, and we must be ready to meet Him."

Years later Father entered business and eventually became a pastor. During those difficult war years he may have appeared to be a common laborer struggling with serious physical ailments, but deep inside he remained a man of great dignity, extraordinary personal and mental health, and stubborn faith, who never lost sight of his calling. And once a week, on Sabbath, at God's invitation, he became the pastor he always wanted to be. There never was a common laborer like him in our village, with such inner balance, such spiritual health, such dignity for all to see on one day each week: God's day.

On the Sabbath day we are equal before God. No one gives the other an order or demands a service. On this day janitor, university president, student, and faculty member share the same pew and study the Bible on an equal basis. That makes a healthy community. What is more, we do not achieve such equality by putting everyone down to the same level, but by lifting everyone up to the same level, namely, that of a son and daughter of God.

How can you make the Sabbath day special and on this day be the person God created you to be?

216

SIN AND
THE SUN

July 4

Kay Kuzma

For God cannot be tempted by evil, nor does he tempt anyone; but each one is tempted when, by his own evil desire, he is dragged away and enticed. Then, after desire has conceived, it gives birth to sin; and sin, when it is full-grown, gives birth to death. James 1:13-15, NIV.

It was July 4, and I was 12. Our family went to the mountains for a picnic by a stream. I decided a good tan would make me beautiful, so I spent most of the day in the sun. By evening I could feel the tenderness. Coated with lotion, I walked with my family to the University of Colorado stadium for the fireworks display and became increasingly miserable. By the time it was over I was violently sick, shaking with chills. Crying in agony, I thought I was going to die. And then a week later my "beautiful" skin peeled off! I learned a painful lesson that day. Too much of a good thing can be bad.

The same beneficial ultraviolet rays that destroy bacteria and help our bodies manufacture vitamin D are the major cause of skin cancer and premature aging of the skin. But you can enjoy the warmth and delight of the sun if you take some simple precautions.

First, a little sun goes a long way. In fact, you can get enough sun to reap all the benefits even in bed, if you will just open a window and let the sun shine on part of your face for five minutes!

Second, apply sunscreen 30 minutes before going out, even if it's overcast, because ultraviolet rays penetrate the clouds. And if you're in and out of the water or perspiring heavily, be sure the sunscreen is waterproof, or reapply it often.

Third, wear a hat or loose protective clothing if not swimming, and sunglasses for eye protection.

Fourth, don't get burned. There's less danger in the early-morning hours before 10:00 or 11:00, and again in the late afternoon.

Fifth, eat a low-fat diet, because fat increases the production of defective skin cells, allowing ultraviolet rays to do more damage.

Sin is something like a sunburn. It can sneak up on you before you realize what's happening. At the moment it seems pleasurable. But afterward the consequences can be agonizing. Apply generously the sunscreen of God's Word, ask for Holy Spirit protection, and avoid temptation.

What is the sunscreen of protection against sin?
What can I do to apply it each day?

THE CLEANSING POWER

If we confess our sins, He is faithful and just to forgive us our sins and to cleanse us from all unrighteousness. 1 John 1:9, NKJV.

The summer heat was already intensifying as I stood and stretched my aching muscles. Even at 9:00 a.m. the July sun was potent. I had learned that the never-ending work of maintaining a yard was best done early in the day. Wiping the sweat from my face, I smiled at the results of this morning's work. The flower bed was again rid of those noxious, prickly thistles. It looked pretty good, though I couldn't take credit for the rainbow array of perennial flowers that brightened our landscape. The previous owner had shown a real talent for arranging and planning flower beds that would complement the uneven terrain. My job was to try to keep the weeds removed.

Returning the gardening tools to the garage, I gratefully headed for the shower. The dust and dirt of the garden mixed with sweat might be a sign of honest labor, but it was hardly a thing to cherish longer than necessary. As the warm water and soap removed the unpleasant aroma of my morning's toil, I thanked the Lord again for the convenience of abundant hot water and modern plumbing. Not only did the soap and water remove the dirt, but they also brought relief to muscles unaccustomed to such agricultural pursuits.

When God created the skin to cover the human body, He could have made it as tough as that of the turtle's shell. Instead our skin is supple, strong, and so sensitive that, according to Paul Brand and Philip Yancey in *Fearfully and Wonderfully Made,* we can discern a thousandth of an ounce of pressure on the tip of a half inch of hair. No wonder the warm spray of a shower is so delightfully refreshing!

Rejuvenated, I stepped from the shower ready to tackle the rest of the day's tasks. The psalmist had recognized the restorative power of water when he prayed, "Wash away all my iniquity and cleanse me from my sin. . . . Cleanse me with hyssop, and I will be clean; wash me, and I will be whiter than snow" (Ps. 51:2-7, NIV).

Thank You, Lord, that Your cleansing water of life is even more available than the warm water in my shower.
Please wash me every day.

ONE
LITTLE
LIFE

July 6
Leonard L. Bailey

> It is not the will of your Father who is in heaven that one of these
> little ones should perish. Matt. 18:14, NKJV.

How old is she?" we asked as deep inside another youngster's heart the surgeon placed the final stitches around a cloth patch used to close a large hole between the two main pumping chambers. "And can you keep her going until we get this one finished?"

A cold, ashen-gray, air-hungry, and now nearly limp 3-year-old girl had been brought urgently into the bustling six-bed intensive-care ward of the Tribhuven University Teaching Hospital of Kathmandu, Nepal. Dr. Glenn Van Arsdell and I and our Nepalese associates were rushing to finish the second of three scheduled children of the day while our principal anesthesiologist, Dr. Stanley Brauer, assisted the ICU team in their desperate effort to keep the 3-year-old from perishing.

Members of the Loma Linda University overseas heart surgery team exhibited this day the best that God had given each participant, for the nearly dead child got her chance for the urgent operation she needed to restore life and hope for a future. In less than 30 minutes we had the congenitally sealed valve leading out of her heart to her lungs opened wide and circulation through her lungs and body restored. She left the operating room another 30 minutes later somewhat stunned, but with a warm, pink glow that promised new life.

The girl recovered completely. Perhaps more than any of the other 30 infants, children, and young adults who had their malformed hearts repaired during our brief mission tour to Nepal, she exemplified the Creator's love for us all.

This one little life became a metaphor of God's day-by-day promise of life anew, a promise we seek to exemplify as individuals and as a team in our work at home and abroad. This one little life reaches out to each of us with God's message of hope. "Even though I walk through the darkest valley, I fear no evil; for you are with me" (Ps. 23:4, NRSV).

Do you sometimes feel insignificant? Hold on to the reality
that God doesn't want even one of His children to perish.
Like the shepherd searching for his one lost sheep,
Jesus seeks for you and provides a way for you to be saved.

PARABLE OF AN HEIR

I have come that men may have life, and may have it in all its fullness. John 10:10, NEB.

Once upon a time there lived a girl named Juliana. Born "with a silver spoon in her mouth," she possessed a wealth of assets for a long and enjoyable life. Her parents raised her carefully, conserving her fortune until she was old enough to handle her own wealth wisely and responsibly.

When Juliana came of age, she began to manage her inheritance herself. Soon she noticed that many people sought her company, hoping she would invest her time and wealth in their enterprises. At first all the choices she could make intrigued her. But after a while she began to notice that her friends seemed to fall into three categories.

Some were very attractive, fun to be around, and flattering. They assured her that their projects would be a "sure bonanza." But every time she gave them money, it vanished. Worse, often she had to spend more money to pay off the legal fees and other costs resulting from their projects. Investing in them appeared to be a consistently losing proposition in spite of the enthusiastic promises. She wondered, *Could these really be my friends?*

Another group also sought for her attention, but not in flashy ways. She noticed the money she lent them didn't seem to make large profits, but her investments were always repaid. She considered them reliable and steady friends, though not very glamorous nor paying high returns.

The members of the third group were reserved, almost difficult to develop friendship with. However, she found they not only repaid whatever she invested in them, but also yielded a high rate of financial return. Such friends were highly profitable people to know.

The key to the parable? "Health is wealth."

Like Juliana, we must choose how to use our health capital. Some so-called friends—alcohol, tobacco, caffeine, and other drugs—seem fun to be around, but always deplete our health balance. Other friends, such as sleep, eating nourishing foods, drinking pure water, and playfulness, maintain our wealth. And a few consistent winners require effort to make our friends: exercise, eating prudently, meditation, serving others, praising God.

Lord, thank You for the treasure of health. Help me to invest it wisely.

GOD HAS
A PLAN
FOR YOU

Nancy Rockey

For I know the thoughts that I think toward you, says the Lord, thoughts of peace and not of evil, to give you a future and a hope. Jer. 29:11, NKJV.

Muscles tensed and body rigid, she stood beside her little rollaway bed. She had done this many times before when frightening but familiar sounds penetrated her world. How does a child of 6 or 7 cope with a violent, drunken father whose rage is out of control?

Paralyzed by fear, she focused on Mother's safety and Father's rage, stiffening every muscle. Her father was beating her mother again. Previous episodes had caused Mother to isolate herself in her bedroom for several days. Beth would be alone. Would this be one of those nights that Father would approach her, drunk, violent, and naked?

Desperately she tried to hold her world together in a family whose behavior was irrational and out of control. Beth was everybody's victim. The youngest girl of 10 children, she was tortured and sexually abused by her father as well as siblings whose pain was equal to her own. Feeling totally alone, abandoned by family, she insulated herself from people and lived in a world of her own, trusting no one. The torture of her home life was a secret to be left at home.

In her late teens Beth met Bert. He was the gentle stability she needed and longed for. They married immediately after her high school graduation. While Bert was not without problems in his life, his were different than her own. He was an Adventist, and since Beth's only place of safety had been an open-door neighborhood church, she rapidly embraced Bert's religion. Weekly they attended services, but their interaction with other members was minimal.

Finally after 15 years of silent remembering and sadness, Beth opened up to her pastor's wife because they had built a trusting relationship. Beth chose to recover by learning about the emotional damage that cripples our emotional development. Given the proper knowledge and tools, and relying on God's power, she chose to grow up (see Eph. 4:14).

Today Beth is active in ministry to others damaged in similar ways. Bert has chosen to walk the road of recovery beside her, and as a result, their marriage has blossomed and become a benefit to others.

Praise God! No matter how desperate our circumstances or how damaged our beginnings, God has a plan for us to be whole.

MOTIVATED

July 9

Kenneth I. Burke

And yet I show you a more excellent way. 1 Cor. 12:31, NKJV.

I once knew a woman who suffered from anxiety. Added to all her other anxieties was a big one called "healthful living." She had to do everything right, to be *religiously* healthful, if you will. She thought God said so!

Another time I knew a man who said he was going to practice "health reform" if it killed him. It almost did.

What's wrong with this approach to health?

A friend of mine uses the expression "health by faith" to denote a healthful lifestyle. Perhaps Jesus went to the root of health by faith when He observed that it isn't what goes into a person, but what comes from his or her heart, that defiles.

What did He mean, anyway? Was He endorsing a diet of all chocolate bars, pizza, and sodas? Are cockroaches suitable for food—if you give thanks for them?

Hardly. I understand Jesus' words to mean something like this: You and I are more, much more, than what we put into our mouths.

Ellen White wrote that "many of the diseases from which men suffer are the result of mental depression. Grief, anxiety, discontent, remorse, guilt, distrust, all tend to break down the life forces and to invite decay and death" *(The Ministry of Healing,* p. 241). Long before that King Solomon said much the same thing: "The spirit of a man will sustain him in sickness, but who can bear a broken spirit?" (Prov. 18:14, NKJV).

Because a broken spirit produces illness, Jesus treats the soul needs of His patients. For a closer look at His compassion, read the Gospels. Notice how tenderly Jesus cares for those who live right—and even those who don't. And how, in the encouragement of His love, some who have squandered health in one way or another find themselves motivated to go and do so no more.

We hear a great deal about fitness. People urge us to get fit to feel better, live longer, look sharper, think clearer—all legitimate motivations.

And all second-rate.

Let me suggest (with apologies to the apostle Paul) that a more excellent way is love.

Imagine that Jesus comes up to you and heals you. Can you think of anything He might tell you to go and do no more?

222

STANDING FOR INTEGRITY

Because the Sovereign Lord helps me, I will not be disgraced. Therefore have I set my face like flint, and I know I will not be put to shame. Isa. 50:7, NIV.

Thomas More is well known as one of the great moral and ethical heroes of the Western world, and each of us lives his story in microcosm in the daily decisions we face.

The great question of his life was how to respond to the divorce and remarriage of King Henry VIII. Frustrated by her inability to produce a male heir, Henry divorced Catherine of Aragon and married Anne Boleyn. The church opposed the divorce and delayed approving the new marriage. Henry put pressure on Parliament to pass the act of succession to transfer the royal lineage from the children of Catherine to the children of Anne.

The members of Parliament, with various degrees of enthusiasm, ultimately went along, with one exception—Thomas More.

More paid a high price for his faithfulness to principle.

His reputation for integrity was well known. More's approval would have helped to silence the king's conscience, but his refusal to go along pricked the king's comfort and disturbed his peace.

The king had More confined in a filthy dungeon and his income cut off. His wife and daughter were reduced to poverty. England watched and the king waited for More's signature approving the act of succession.

More held out for two years, but his wife lost all patience with his unyieldingly principled life.

Tradition says that someone entered his filthy cell and found More surrounded by vagabonds, brigands, thieves, and killers. The gentle scholar sat emaciated, clad in rags, shivering from the cold. The visitor had brought the list of parliamentary signatures, signatures of friends and companions from law and life. He begged More to sign and save his life: "But Thomas, look at these names. You know these men. Can't you do what I did, and come with us, for fellowship?"

More responded: "And when we stand before God, and you are sent to heaven for doing according to your conscience and I am sent to hell for not doing according to mine, will you come with me for fellowship?"

Are you living according to God's principles, or do you find yourself compromising when tempted? Think about More's response.

WHAT'S PRAYER GOT TO DO WITH HEALING?

Delbert W. Baker

He will call upon me, and I will answer him; I will be with him in trouble, I will deliver him and honor him. Ps. 91:15, NIV.

People are receiving the best medical care money can buy. It is a good thing, because they are seriously ill. They used to believe in prayer—before they got sick. But now, what does prayer have to do with the possibility of restoration to health? Many reason, in light of medical technology and the breakthroughs in health care, why pray?

We may group people's attitudes toward prayer and healing in at least four broad categories. First are *prayer resisters*. This group rejects the idea of prayer and spirituality in general. They may not deny God's existence, but they don't see the connection between the spiritual and secular. To them prayer is a placebo, a spiritual opiate that has little real value except as a feel-good.

Second are *prayer enlisters*. Here the attitude is "if prayer works or might work, use it—in my condition, I'll try anything." Individuals in this category don't necessarily believe in the power of prayer, but they will seize any opportunity to achieve healing.

The third group can be called *prayer insisters*. They must pray because "there is no other way." People with this attitude reject any medical advice or treatment. They hold the opinion that to do anything else but pray would show a lack of faith.

The fourth group we can call *prayer persisters*. They persist in prayer not as an end in itself, but as a means to recognize, invite, and free God to do what He desires—the accomplishment of His will. Prayer is not a crutch, a quick fix, or a cure-all. They believe that God is able, willing, and dependable to heal, and see prayer as a means by which God can bless, heal, and accomplish His sovereign will.

Your beliefs about prayer and healing make a difference in your whole outlook on life—and death. What you believe will affect what you do and think. Which category do you fall in? A *prayer resister*, a *prayer enlister*, a *prayer insister*, or a *prayer persister*?

Thank You, God, for answered prayer. Like the father of the boy who was convulsing and foaming at the mouth, my prayer for healing is "Lord, I believe; help my unbelief!" (Mark 9:24, NKJV). Amen.

SPECIAL
DELIVERY

In love he predestined us to be adopted as his sons through Jesus Christ, in accordance with his pleasure and will. Eph. 1:4, 5, NIV.

During a period of about six years our son begged for a baby sister, even though he knew it would be dangerous for his mother to have any more children. We had mentioned this fact to our cousin, who worked in the labor and delivery unit of a hospital, in case a baby became available for adoption.

Four years passed. We had long forgotten the conversation with the cousin when the phone rang one rainy Sunday afternoon. Our cousin asked if we were still interested in adopting. After we prayed and all agreed, we arranged to meet with the social worker and doctor within the hour.

Within three hours we had decided on a name and were looking at our little pink bundle. Twenty-three hours after the call we had our baby home, while our family and the church family arranged for bottles, blankets, clothing, a car seat, a bassinet, formula, diapers, and even a pediatrician.

Question marks ran through our minds, however: would we love Traci as we did Matthew? Would she respond to us? Would we make it through the adoption process? What if her parents changed their minds? What about Traci's genetic background?

Soon Traci's new daddy knew he couldn't possibly love his little girl more. Her mommy adored her energy and personality, and her brother delighted in holding her and tickling her tummy. Nothing else mattered.

As we've watched Traci respond to our love, we've become more aware of what God has offered us as His adopted children and how deeply hurt He must be when we deny Him.

The God of the universe has said to us: "I will make you my sons and daughters; . . . you shall become members of the royal family and children of the heavenly King" *(Testimonies,* vol. 2, p. 592).

If only we would respond as does little Traci—with utmost love and confidence—and accept the incredible honor of being part of His family. If we choose to be "specially delivered" by Jesus, we can all be adopted heirs of the King, and what heavenly rejoicing that will bring!

What does it take to be adopted into God's family? "Come out from among them, and be separate, saith the Lord, and I will receive you, and ye shall be sons and daughters of the Lord Almighty. What a promise!" (ibid.).

BEING A TRUSTWORTHY ENVOY

Jan W. Kuzma

A wicked messenger falls into trouble, but a trustworthy envoy brings healing. He who ignores discipline comes to poverty and shame, but whoever heeds correction is honored. Prov. 13:17, 18, NIV.

Being overweight is a major health hazard. You may or may not fall into this category. But all of us have family and friends who do, and their good health is important to us. That's why we must do everything possible to be supportive and encouraging.

Few of us realize that obese people face three times the risk of heart disease, and are four times more likely to have high blood pressure. They also have five times greater risk of developing diabetes, and five times the likelihood of having elevated blood cholesterol.

Furthermore, overweight individuals face six times the chance of developing gallbladder disease, and they will also experience more cancer of the colon, rectum, breast, cervix, uterus, ovaries, and prostate than average-weight people.

But the list of hazards doesn't stop there. Health experts estimate that only 60 percent of obese people reach the age of 60, compared with 90 percent of those who aren't overweight.

A recent survey of Adventists showed that 24 percent considered themselves moderately or considerably overweight. And if you meet one who does, perhaps you can get better acquainted and possibly learn the reason for their condition. Is it their inactive job, their cultural habit of snacking, their lack of moderation, a missing exercise program such as walking, their anxiety or depression that makes them want to eat more than they should? Is it a hereditary problem? Or is it the lack of information and no supportive friends?

Once you get to know them and are a trusted friend, it's easier to provide helpful information or to work together on a weight reduction plan. You must be sympathetic and supportive, not judgmental. The same survey indicates that 76 percent of those overweight *are* interested in changing their condition, and you may be just the person who will make the critical difference in their lives.

You might not be the good Samaritan who picks up the bloody man on the side of the road, but you can lift up the hope and expectation of someone wanting to get control of their weight problem. Having good support and encouragement is one of the keys for success.

If you fall into the overweight category, seek out supportive friends who can help you keep your commitment to adopt a healthier lifestyle.

THE JOY
OF CREATING

Lois Rittenhouse Pecce

Thou art worthy, O Lord, to receive glory and honour and power: for thou hast created all things, and for thy pleasure they are and were created. Rev. 4:11.

My husband says he's never going to get old. You might chuckle as you note that the "salt and pepper" of his once dark hair has blended into silver. "Laugh," he'll say, flexing a set of muscles that in his fifty-ninth year threaten to rival those of the Incredible Hulk. (I exaggerate a little!)

"I've been watching people," he'll say, "and when they hit their 50s, they must let their bodies go to mush. By the time they retire, they're old and flabby and have no strength for anything."

So he works out, faithfully, diligently—exercise, weight-lifting, watching his diet. But where he works sometimes the hardest, where he feels the most intense pains of disappointment and the keenest pleasures of achievement, is not with his weight machine but with his wood-turning lathe. There is where he takes dull, rough wood and with care and patience creates from it a thing of beauty.

Though our living room may seem cluttered with varied vessels of his creating, I see him eager to tell anyone who enters there the story of each piece. And each piece does have a story: a new tool, a different wood, a reluctant finish. I watch his animation as he talks. There is something wonderful and pleasing and powerful and health-enhancing in the act of creating with one's hands and mind.

Knowing our simple human pleasures in creative ventures, how they quicken the mind and energize the spirit, I can only imagine how God delights in His creations. Indeed, each has a story.

Health is more than working the body, proper nutrition, and living long. Ultimately, health is quality of life. God created us for His pleasure, and it's using that God-given gift of creativity that can bring the crowning glow of joyful health to one's face.

"Lord, make me creative. Help me not to look at life as all duty and drudgery, but teach me to catch a glimpse of the Divine and to see in each person's life the potential there. Whether working in the media of art or with human 'clay,' may I see the pattern that will glorify You."

When did you last give yourself the time and
pleasure to create something?

HOPE
FOR THE
TROUBLED HEART

The fruit of righteousness will be peace; the effect of righteousness will be quietness and confidence forever. My people will live in peaceful dwelling places, in secure homes, in undisturbed places of rest. Isa. 32:17, 18, NIV.

Hannah wanted a son almost more than life itself. No longer could she take the jealousy and taunting of Peninnah, the wife that Elkanah took so he could have children. So in agony she silently pleaded with the Lord.

When Eli the priest saw her lips move in silent prayer, he drew the hasty conclusion that she was drunk and reprimanded her. "How long will you keep on getting drunk? Get rid of your wine" (1 Sam. 1:14, NIV). His reaction must have added insult to injury to Hannah's troubled heart. "'Not so, my lord,' Hannah replied, 'I am a woman who is deeply troubled. . . . Do not take your servant for a wicked woman; I have been praying here out of my great anguish and grief'" (verses 15, 16, NIV).

Chagrined, Eli said, "Go in peace, and may the God of Israel grant you what you have asked of him" (verse 17, NIV).

Immediately Hannah felt better. Hope changes things. She felt hungry, then ate something, and her face no longer mirrored despair.

Unwanted mental distress comes, in one form or another and at various times of life, to practically everyone. It can be triggered by thwarted hopes, severe disappointment, grief, remorse, unfulfilled ambitions, or as in Hannah's case, a problem that has no obvious solution.

The best way for God-fearing persons to respond to distress is to do as Hannah did—pour out your soul to the Lord.

Mental distress is an unnatural, unhealthy state of mind. When allowed to persist, it upsets the balance by which the brain unconsciously regulates the actions of the body's various organs. Thus any one of the so-called functional diseases may develop, such as stomach ulcer, colitis, some kinds of arthritis, heart difficulties, some forms of diabetes, persistent headache, and sexual aberrations. Science has proved Ellen White right when she said, "The sympathy which exists between the mind and the body is very great. When one is affected, the other responds. The condition of the mind has much to do with the health of the physical system" *(Testimonies,* vol. 4, p. 60).

When distressed, remember: "When we beseech the Lord to pity us in our distress, and to guide us by His Holy Spirit, He will never turn away our prayer" (Thoughts From the Mount of Blessing, *p. 132).*

Never despise one of these little ones; I tell you, they have their guardian angels in heaven, who look continually on the face of my heavenly Father. Matt. 18:10, NEB.

We have all seen it happen: frantic mother speed-racing her shopping cart through rush-hour traffic at the supermarket while a tired and bored little boy stops whining only long enough to grab boxes of extra-sweet cereal off the shelves. She makes endless threats about the pain she is about to inflict if he doesn't behave—without breaking eye contact with the soup can label.

Finally his energy level outlasts hers, and she explodes. As his howl reverberates to the frozen foods section, she calls him every demeaning name she can recall. She delivers wounding blows to his self-esteem as well as to his behind. And only after he is whimpering and submissive on the lower rack of the shopping cart does quiet return to the marketplace.

We remember paintings from our childhood in which a white-winged angel in robes hovers over a little child as he is about to cross a narrow bridge over a raging stream. The artist's comforting intentions are that God assures the safety of children. But a careful observer realizes that children are far more likely to carry lifelong scars in their souls than on their knees. The wounds that do the most damage are the shame-based ones that cause a growing child to say, "I am a nuisance; I am not loved; I really am rotten to the core, because my mother and my father told me so."

Jesus desired to plant a very specific image in the minds of His hearers. Before they spoke to their children, He wanted them to remember that other beings were watching those same children. And these were beings who had just been in the presence of the Divine. Fresh from the throne room of heaven, they were honored to behold young, promising reflections of that divinity. Such an awareness will always elevate how we talk to our children.

To do so will raise our children's estimation both of their parents and of God. They'll be as happy to be our children as to be God's children.

The next time you're tempted to raise your voice or hand in such a way as to cause pain, picture the child's guardian angel next to the child, and see what a difference it might make.

TIME—GOD'S GREAT GIFT

For in six days the Lord made the heavens and the earth, the sea, and all that is in them, and rested the seventh day. Therefore the Lord blessed the Sabbath day and hallowed it. Ex. 20:11, NKJV.

Knowing that His human children would need time to refresh mind and body after a week of work, at the end of Creation week God prescribed the Sabbath. His prescription still works. Weekly He provides His children time to enjoy His companionship and handiwork.

Our family loves the outdoors, and on Sabbath we take time to bask in God's natural beauty.

Our Sabbath refreshment has included a summer of Sabbath mornings when we watched four baby foxes grow up in the field behind our house. Then one Sabbath afternoon we followed a mother deer and her speckled fawn as they strolled down Lehigh Street, the mother walking protectively between the cars and her baby. Another Sabbath at sunset we watched a beaver eating supper at Rocky Mountain National Park. And one Sabbath a herd of more than 100 elks milled around our jeep, eating and bugling, close enough that we watched without binoculars.

My very favorite Sabbath refreshment took place on the peaceful Moose River in Maine. We took our motored canoe out to a narrow passage and dropped anchor. Sudden movement to our right caught our attention. A family of beavers slid silently into the water and began nibbling twigs and leaves from overhanging branches. A mosquito landed on my nose, and I swatted. A slap of a beaver's tail sent the whole family underwater. We sat motionless, waiting. Then the beavers surfaced and continued with their meal.

Downriver two otters swam toward us, their humped backs rising and falling above the water as they played. As a climax, a deer with a large rack of antlers walked into the water and stood facing us, silhouetted in the sunset colors. Darkness would soon descend, and knowing we had to thread our way through some rocks on the way back to the dock, we reluctantly started the motor. The animals disappeared into the forest. No one can erase from our memories the refreshment that God's gift of time gave us.

And best of all, God's prescription for rest comes every week, not once a year like Christmas. What a wise God!

Take time on the Sabbath to refresh yourself with peaceful scenes of God's creation, and you too will be revitalized.

FINDING GOD'S LOVE IN YOUR WORLD

Walter Thompson

> Lift your eyes and look to the heavens: Who created all these? He who brings out the
> starry host one by one, and calls them each by name. Because of his great power
> and mighty strength, not one of them is missing. Isa. 40:26, NIV.

had just left a trying day in the Los Angeles area and decided to drive out across the high desert on my way to Redlands, California. Although I thought that it would be relaxing and quiet, I discovered just the opposite. I was hot, tired, and stressed out, the scenery was disappointing, and the road was much longer than I had remembered. In the depths of my despair I noticed a cloud forming in the east. Shortly I was driving through a most refreshing cloudburst, and then I spotted a rainbow. Contrasted against the black cloud, it could not have been brighter or more beautiful. And just then I knew that it was all OK. That rainbow told me all that I needed to know. God was at the wheel and would guide me through.

Since then I have developed a game that I play nearly everywhere I go. I look for rainbows. I watch to see where they may be hiding and what the elements are that lend to their creation. Sometimes there are rainbows in the spider webs wet with dew on a late summer morn. At other times rainbows form on the ice that crusts over patches of melted snow. Even the snow crystals glittering in the late February sun aid my search for this evidence of God's love.

But I have learned that it is not only in the rainbow that we can find evidence of God's love. When I look up into the sky at night, I remember the creative power of love as contrasted with the destructive nature of selfish lust, and I know that it is love that put and holds the stars in place. Even along the concrete streets of the city I see bright yellow, white, and cobalt blue flowers defying the restrictions of modern civilization, and I know who placed them there, and why.

Recognizing God's love in all of these places and things not only tells me about His goodness but also reveals something about my value to Him. There is so much good health in being wanted!

Why not practice looking for the evidence of love in the world around you? When you find it, you'll find God, because God is love.

HOW TO WIN THE RACE

Do you not know that those who run in a race all run, but one receives the prize?
Run in such a way that you may obtain it. 1 Cor. 9:24, NKJV.

We've got an enemy that's always trying to trip us up on our race through life. Satan wants us to become weary and tired, so he has filled life with all kinds of stressors, many of our own doing. Such stresses become trials that sometimes lead to sickness and death. What makes the difference between living victoriously or losing in defeat may be simply how much exercise we engage in each week.

Two researchers, David Holmes and Beth McGilley, chose 34 high-fit and 34 low-fit people to determine how their heart rate would respond to stress. Half of each group went on an intensive 13-week aerobic training program. The other half served as controls. The low-fitness half who did not undergo any training (who served as controls) showed no change in heart rates between pre- and post-test. The low-fit subjects who exercised had a similar starting heart rate, but they were able to lower their resting heart rate significantly as a result of the training. The low-fit individuals who did not have any training had an 11.8 beats per minute (bpm) increase in response to the psychological stressor. When it combined with their already high resting heart rate, the low-fit individuals exhibited a 29 bpm higher rate change than their trained and untrained high-fit counterparts and their trained low-fit teammates.

Why is this important? We know from animal studies that rapid rises in heart rate and blood pressure greatly increase the risk of damage to the lining of the arteries and therefore aggravate the process of atherogenesis in damaged arteries. In a nutshell, unfit individuals who experience stress respond with higher heartbeats, which increase their risk of developing atherosclerosis of the arteries and early death from heart attack or stroke.

The bottom line is that if we wish to win this race called life, we must be physically fit as well as spiritually fit. The Creator-God designed our bodies to function best when exercised.

How can you run the race of life to obtain the prize of good health?

THE DAY
NICKY FELL

July 20
Nicole Sydenham

Yet there is one ray of hope: his compassion never ends. It is only the Lord's mercies that have kept us from complete destruction. Great is his faithfulness; his lovingkindness begins afresh each day. . . . The Lord is wonderfully good to those who wait for him, to those who seek for him. Lam. 3:21-25, TLB.

It was a hot July 20 at Camp White Sand in Saskatchewan when I heard, "A child's fallen from a horse." I rushed to the scene. "It's Nicky," someone screamed. Suddenly my knees weakened. Nicky was my 10-year-old daughter.

"Nicky, Nicky, it's Mommy," I said as I bent over her. When I saw her eyes and vomiting, I knew her head injury was serious.

At the hospital the doctor said, "Madam, it is *very serious*. You will need a lot of prayer. In six months to a year she might regain 90 percent of her brain capacity, or it could be worse."

Around the world people prayed for her.

For 10 days the doctors kept Nicky in an induced coma and under as many as 15 medications at one time to attempt to reduce the pressure on her brain and keep her alive. She had 19 tubes and wires hooked up to her.

When she was transferred to a children's ward, she almost died twice. We could tell she couldn't breathe, but no one would believe us, so we prayed, "Please bring the right nurse or doctor." Ron, my husband, felt he had to do something, so he put Nicky in a wheelchair and pushed her out into the hall. A doctor "happened" by and yelled, "This child can't breathe. Rush her to surgery. I'll go scrub," and he put a tracheostomy in.

One day Ron was standing by Nicky's bed, crying, "Lord, please save my little girl." Her body was burning with fever, but the hand he held was limp and ice-cold. And in response, he heard, "Yes, Ron, I do want to save your daughter from her fall, just as I want to save all My children from the Fall, and restore them to My original design."

I held on to Lamentations 3:21-26 and Jeremiah 29:11-14. *The Living Bible* translates verse 14: "I will . . . restore your fortunes." I would substitute Nicky's name for the word "fortunes."

After 46 days in the hospital, Nicky was released, still with a tracheostomy, but miraculously with 100 percent brain capacity! God had restored our "fortunes."

Thank You, my Saviour, for giving Your life to save me from the Fall!

ARE YOU A TEN-TALENT COOK?

July 21

Ellen G. White

She gets up while it is still dark; she provides food for her family. . . . Give her the reward she has earned, and let her works bring her praise at the city gate. Prov. 31:15-31, NIV.

Often health reform is made health deform by unpalatable preparation of food. The lack of knowledge regarding healthful cookery must be remedied before health reform is a success.

"Good cooks are few. Many, many mothers need to take lessons in cooking, that they may set before the family well-prepared, neatly served food.

"Before children take lessons on the organ or the piano they should be given lessons in cooking. The work of learning to cook need not exclude music, but to learn music is of less importance than to learn how to prepare food that is wholesome and appetizing. . . .

"It is a sin to place poorly prepared food on the table, because the matter of eating concerns the well-being of the entire system. The Lord desires His people to appreciate the necessity of having food prepared in such a way that it will not make sour stomachs and in consequence sour tempers. Let us remember that there is practical religion in a loaf of good bread.

"Let not the work of cooking be looked upon as a sort of slavery. What would become of those in our world if all who are engaged in cooking should give up their work with the flimsy excuse that it is not sufficiently dignified? Cooking may be regarded as less desirable than some other lines of work, but in reality it is a science above all other sciences. Thus God regards the preparation of healthful food. He places a high estimate on those who do faithful service in preparing wholesome, palatable food.

"The one who understands the art of properly preparing food, and who uses this knowledge, is worthy of higher commendation than those engaged in any other line of work. This talent should be regarded as equal in value to ten talents; for its right use has much to do with keeping the human organism in health. Because so inseparably connected with life and health, it is the most valuable of all gifts" *(Medical Ministry,* pp. 270, 271).

"The foundation of that which keeps people in health is the medical missionary work of good cooking" *(ibid.,* p. 270).

What could you do to enhance your cooking skills?

THIS IS
THE DAY . . .

This is the day the Lord has made; let us rejoice and be glad in it. Ps. 118:24, NIV.

God's in His heaven—all's right with the world!" I exclaimed, drawing open the blinds of our condo.

"But all is not right with the world," my sister replied. "There is murder, rape, famine, floods. . . . This world is a mess!"

My sister was right, if that's the way you choose to look at the world. But from my vantage point that day, I was overwhelmed with God's goodness to bring us five sisters and my two daughters from four states for a week together in Colorado. We could view Mount Baldy from our balcony, take early-morning walks along the picturesque river flowing through the little mountain town, hike in the woods, ride mountain bikes, white-water raft, and just bask in one another's company.

It's easy to get burdened down with the world's cares and miss the little things that can lift a person's thoughts. That's why when walking in the early mornings near my Georgia home I try to look up at the heavens instead of down at my feet. It helps brighten my spirits and bring positive thoughts to mind. The exercise makes the healing endorphins flow to strengthen my immune system. It's even great walking in the rain or frosty weather.

I praise the Lord for the privilege of getting out in His nature, viewing the fluffy clouds against a blue sky, listening to the birds, watching the squirrels, enjoying my neighbors' lovely yards, and having a release from my day-to-day stresses.

I try desperately to be an "up" person, not darkening the paths of those around me by speaking of depressing things. And I believe that laughter is good for the soul. It, too, makes those healing endorphins flow.

My sister was right. Perhaps I shouldn't say, "All's right with the world." But God is still in His heaven, so now as I open the blinds in Colorado, or look up at the lovely Georgia sky, I say, "This is the day the Lord has made; let us rejoice and be glad in it!" We can praise Him for that.

Praise God as you open the blinds of your day.

LOOK FOR
LITTLE GIFTS
FROM GOD

He who forms the mountains, creates the wind, and reveals his thoughts to man, he who turns dawn to darkness, and treads the high places of the earth—the Lord God Almighty is his name. Amos 4:13, NIV.

As soon as I got out of my car and started across the large parking lot, I felt it. A warm, gentle morning breeze. A breeze that played with my hair and fluttered my shirtsleeves. It had been so hot and still lately, and I accepted the breeze as one of those little gifts from God.

Closing my eyes and breathing the air in deeply, I tried to imagine how God does it. *Is the wind God's breath blowing from the heavens? Did He start the wind sailing across the earth with a wave of His mighty hand? Or is it caused by angels swinging from the trees?* It was one of the really perfect winds—not too hard or too soft—and for a moment I imagined that paved parking lot was Paradise. When the wind blows, I can't help thinking of His awesome glory—the Creator of the air we breathe, everything it brings life to, and the entire universe.

God created our amazing, life-giving atmosphere that we take for granted. By itself it's invisible and silent, but with a little force behind it, it can be a gentle breeze or a powerful blast. It's a wonderful gift that brings us life-sustaining qualities and also serves to rejuvenate the mind and body, relaxing us and serving as a great de-stressor. Also, it reminds us of God's power and gentleness.

Occasionally I seek release from the large office building where I spend much of my day by hiking down three flights of stairs and out the back door—into the fresh air. Almost instantly God's marvelous creation does its job. It clears my mind and allows me to reorganize my thoughts and put Jesus Christ back as top priority.

Try to get a little extra fresh air today, especially at times when you need a break. Step outside, take a deep breath, relax, and meditate on Christ. And the next time you feel a warm, gentle breeze, don't worry about your hair—think of it as a refreshing gift from your Creator.

Thank You, God, for the gentle breeze that reminds us that You are the Creator of the air we breathe. Indeed, You are the breath of life to regenerate our sagging souls.

IS YOUR
JOB KILLING
YOU?

July 24

Jan W. Kuzma

About the eleventh hour he went out and found still others standing around. He asked them, "Why have you been standing here all day long doing nothing?" Matt. 20:6, NIV.

Working persons, especially middle-aged ones, may face a health hazard at work. No, we're not talking about dangerous jobs such as walking on scaffolding or driving race cars! We're speaking about ordinary office jobs that require you to sit for long periods of time.

A study conducted by the National Institutes of Health showed that physical exercise decreases the risk of developing cancer. Inactive men were more likely to develop lung, colon, or rectal cancer, and inactive women were at an increased risk of developing cervical and breast cancer. Other studies have indicated that those who get very little physical exercise are more likely to suffer a hip fracture later in life and have a greater chance of becoming obese.

This study's results reminded me of a statement Ellen White once made: "Perfect health depends upon perfect circulation" *(Testimonies,* vol. 2, p. 531).

It is interesting to observe in the analysis of the Adventist Mortality Study that for men the factor that made the largest difference with respect to longevity wasn't smoking, weight, or vegetarianism, but exercise. Those who exercised lived five years longer, a difference twice as much as for any of the other three comparison groups.

If your job is an inactive one, get involved in a regular exercise program: use the stairs, walk briskly during break times, or work out during lunch. Turn "idleness" at your desk into some type of movement. Every hour take a few minutes to stretch, run in place, or do jumping jacks, or as you sit, exercise your muscles. Don't let your job be a hazard to your health. You want to go home with a paycheck and the health to enjoy it. The paycheck alone is just not worth it.

God designed your body for movement. Your muscles, joints, and bones need motion to be able to function optimally, or they atrophy. Even if it's the "eleventh hour," Jesus invites you to work to keep His "machinery" in good operating order. And remember to exercise your faith to keep your spiritual life in order as well.

Are you working for a paycheck, or for your health? What can you do to make sure your workplace is a healthy place?

237

THE EARTH
PANTS FOR
WATER

George M. Lessard

As the deer pants for streams of water, so my soul pants for you, O God. Ps. 42:1, NIV.

I just recently completed a trip across the U.S. by light airplane. Hour after hour I flew over green fields, green forests, green valleys. Green, green, green! Near Tucumcari, New Mexico, the color began to change to more and more brown. By Albuquerque the only green I noticed was on the mountains or in the river valleys where human habitation occurred. Why the difference? Water, life-giving water!

It is not surprising that the Bible, written as it was in the arid country now known as Israel, uses the vision of water to symbolize life-giving power. More than 70 percent of our body mass consists of water. While we can live weeks without food, we can survive only hours without water. Water is the basis of life. It provides the environment in which life processes occur. The medium for the biochemical reactions essential for life, it also carries away the wastes generated by all living cells.

But do we really know about water? Most people take it for granted. The small molecule H_2O, having only two hydrogen atoms and one oxygen atom, has a mass of 18. Other molecules this size exist at room temperature as gases. Water is unusual in that it remains a liquid at room temperature because of differences between parts of the molecule. Oxygen nuclei attract electrons more than do hydrogen nuclei. Because of this, one end of the molecule is more positively charged than the other. The resulting positive and negative ends form what we call a dipole. The dipolar nature of water molecules causes them to be attracted to each other by what we call hydrogen bonds. These hydrogen bonds link every water molecule to other water molecules, creating a cohesive fluid with all the properties needed to make life possible.

What if God had not designed this molecule to function as it does? What if the differences within each molecule had not led to unity of the whole? Can we ask this question of other unique creations of God? Can differences between us lead to unity among us? I certainly hope so!

I praise You, Lord, for Your divine wisdom that created this world—and its water. And may I daily drink deeply from the "living water" of Your Word.

BACON OR BANANAS?

Samuel DeShay

Let the wise listen and add to their learning, and let the discerning get guidance. Prov. 1:5, NIV.

Three statements by Ellen White have intrigued me:

• "Whatever disturbs the circulation of the electric currents in the nervous system lessens the strength of the vital powers, and the result is a deadening of the sensibilities of the mind" *(Testimonies,* vol. 2, p. 347).

• "If Adam, at his creation, had not been endowed with twenty times as much vital force as men now have, the race, with their present habits of living in violation of natural law, would have become extinct" *(ibid.,* vol. 3, p. 138).

• "The system is vitalized by electrical force of the brain to resist disease" *(ibid.,* p. 157).

Where does this vital force, or electrical current, come from?

Each cell has the potential of generating electricity, if the voltage from the activity of the sodium-potassium pump that transfers the sodium out of the cell and potassium into the cell keeps the cell's battery charged. If a diet is too high in sodium chloride and too low in potassium, the sodium-potassium pump tends to slow, allowing the battery to run down not only in the cells of blood vessels but also in cells throughout the body. When the battery runs down, your electricity goes down, depleting your energy or vital force and making you hypertensive and susceptible to other diseases.

Dr. Norman Kaplan, one of the chief researchers in hypertension, says that hypertension problems are more closely related to low potassium levels than to high sodium.

Now contrast God's diet for His incredible human machine with humankind's diet in terms of the salt and potassium content. Bacon and ham are cured meats with three times as much sodium as potassium. Potato chips and processed foods all contain salt. But fruits (especially bananas and figs), vegetables, grains, seeds, and nuts contain hundreds of times more potassium than sodium. Exactly what your cells need to keep electrically charged!

If you want to feel young again, with vital energy surging through your veins, you've got to keep your cells' sodium-potassium pumps in good working order. You do that by avoiding humankind's sodium-filled foods and enjoying God's potassium-filled ones.

Bacon or bananas? I'll take a banana, thank you!

Think about what you regularly eat. How much potassium is your body getting to keep your sodium-potassium pumps working effectively to charge the sodium "batteries" in your cells?

I CAN
CHOOSE

So God created man in his own image, . . . male and female he created them. Gen. 1:27, NIV.

reated in the image of God, we are uniquely gifted with the ability to think, to reason, to create, and to choose. What a risk God took, and what a responsibility is ours by our life choices to reflect the image of the loving God who created us. Revelation and research both agree that the positive exercise of the power of choice contributes to health and prolongs life.

I can choose . . .

- To eat healthfully of the nutritious bounty of God's garden.
- To exercise—walk, run, bike, swim, move with freedom and joy.
- To rest, relax, enjoy a siesta, take a holiday, vacation with friends.
- To sleep, refreshing the body, recharging the nerves, restoring the spirit.

I can choose . . .

- To laugh freely and often, with others and at myself.
- To hope in the face of fear and failure, disappointment and despair.
- To learn about my world and the people who inhabit it, about myself.
- To grow, as did Jesus, in strength and wisdom and favor with God and human beings.
- To think, to ask questions and search for answers.
- To work with my hands and with my mind, with energy and purpose.
- To play, just for the fun of it!

I can choose . . .

- To nurture relationships, talking and touching, giving and taking.
- To participate in life, speaking up, taking a stand, being counted.
- To volunteer in the hospital, the school, or the homeless shelter.
- To be a neighbor to a single mom or an aging couple with Alzheimer's.
- To keep my promises and honor my commitments.
- To affirm the good, the noble, the giftedness of others.

I can choose . . .

- To believe in a divine purpose for my life.
- To worship the God who made me for joyful relationship with Him.
- To pray, living in communion with my Creator-Friend.
- To forgive those who hurt me, releasing my bitterness.
- To forget . . . yes, it is possible!
- To act with integrity, honesty, and purity.
- To love . . . for God is love.

What will you choose today?

MIGHTY MORPHING CELLS

Trust in the Lord with all thine heart; and lean not unto thine own understanding. In all thy ways acknowledge him, and he shall direct thy paths. Be not wise in thine own eyes: fear the Lord, and depart from evil. It shall be health to thy navel, and marrow to thy bones. Prov. 3:5-8.

On television sensational "morphing" effects look like visual magic as one image changes into another. Fantasy-based movies frequently use this computerized technique. For example, a cat's face becomes a human face, or a person transforms into a super metallic being or even into a vehicle. In movies, morphing distorts reality.

In reality, the body has a Creator-programmed mighty morphing system of its own. This fantastic feat takes place in the red marrow of bones. The bone marrow produces precursor cells. As they mature they morph into red or white blood cells. The white cells then morph into a virtual army of specialized cells trained to recognize, destroy, and remove the body's invaders. Every day this efficient system pours forth billions of cells to replace worn-out red and white blood cells.

Through morphed images, movie viewers are thrilled, chilled, and enthralled by fictitious stories and unreal superwarriors. But their exploits pale in comparison to the complex battles fought each day by the immune system and the workload carried by red blood cells transporting their gaseous loads to and from trillions of body cells.

All of God's natural health laws affect the blood-producing work of the bones. It is impossible to produce the best-quality blood with poor-quality food, lack of rest, and intemperance. Guilt, depression, and negative attitudes affect the production of the bone marrow.

David understood this when he decried his weakness and condition of the marrow of his bones because of the guilt of his iniquity. "Be merciful to me, O Lord, for I am in distress; my eyes grow weak with sorrow, my soul and my body with grief. My life is consumed by anguish and my years by groaning; my strength fails because of my affliction, and my bones grow weak" (Ps. 31:9, 10, NIV).

Ellen White put it this way: "A contented mind, a cheerful spirit, is health to the body and strength to the soul. Nothing is so fruitful a cause of disease as depression, gloominess, and sadness" *(Testimonies,* vol. 1, p. 702).

When you're tempted to be discouraged, remember how David ends Psalm 31: "Be strong and take heart, all you who hope in the Lord" (verse 24, NIV). Holding on to this philosophy should strengthen your immune system.

ONE-FLESH
MARRIAGE

> For this reason a man will leave his father and mother and be united
> to his wife, and they will become one flesh. Gen. 2:24, NIV.

Writing one's own marriage vows is not a new idea. Adam spoke his own words during that first ceremony. We wish we knew more about this memorable event. No bride was ever surrounded by more beauty. Flowers, vines, shrubs, all in their pristine beauty, formed a background.

Was there music? How could there not be? Celestial music always accompanied important events: Creation, when the morning stars sang together (Job 38:7); Moses' song of deliverance from Egypt (Ex. 15:1-19); at Jesus' birth, the sound of "Glory to God in the highest!" (Luke 2:13, 14); and the greatest of all events—the song of Moses and the Lamb when Christ returns (Rev. 15:3, 4). Why, of course there was wedding music!

Without doubt the refreshments were the best that any caterers could ever boast of, and most trouble-free! Picking the delicious fruits right off the trees and feeding them to each other must have been a great delight for the bride and groom.

What about the homily? Ellen White says: "God celebrated the first marriage" *(Patriarchs and Prophets,* p. 46). He may have told them that marriage was one of His first gifts to the human race. We can be sure that He gave them some instructions as to their responsibilities in their new relationship. After all, they had no other experience to model, no library resources to check out. All their instruction came from Him, so there was never any doubt about its absolute trustworthiness.

God was also their instructor in reference to their sexuality. In the area of being fruitful and multiplying they had absolutely no knowledge. In beautiful simplicity He explained to them His plan for their one-fleshness. They would never wonder if their loving embrace was proper, dignified, or blessed. He assured them that in offering their bodies to each other they were exactly fulfilling God's purpose for them in the marriage act.

No wonder Eve and Adam were able to enjoy their sexuality for hundreds of years! And still God's desire for every marriage is that sexuality will continue to be an expression of joy and commitment.

God, our Creator, help us to realize our part in emphasizing
the good news about sexuality in our marriages,
and in our homes, schools, and churches.

BURY THE
BITTERNESS

July 30

Mary Wong

> One who is slow to anger is better than the mighty, and one whose temper is controlled than one who captures a city. Prov. 16:32, NRSV.

Hurrying between classes at the university one Friday, I stopped at the telex office to collect a fax someone had sent to me. Because it was a letter from my home country, I read it with eager anticipation. Then all of a sudden I felt anger like a thunderbolt exploding in my brain. My blood pressure soared and my heart pounded against my rib cage. Classes the rest of the day passed in a blur as I burned and seethed with anger at the recollection of the insulting words in the letter: anger at the unjust accusations; anger at the injustice done to my reputation.

At vespers that night and church service the next morning, while the servants of God were busy expounding biblical truth from the pulpit, I, in my pew, was busy composing a searing response to the writer of the letter—one that I hoped would scorch him worse than he had burned me. The obsession to get back at him continued to hold me in its grip during the following days. I was totally unable to function during the day because sleep eluded me at night. My appetite was also gone, for my stomach was in knots, and I suffered terrible ulcer pains. Needless to say, being spiritually and physically drained, I had found the fastest, surest, and most unhealthy way of losing weight.

My health deteriorated under the tremendous emotional strain until one day I awoke to the fact that the one being hurt most—physically, mentally, and spiritually—by my angry feelings was none other than I myself. For me then, Ecclesiastes 7:9, "Do not be quick to anger, for anger lodges in the bosom of fools" (NIV), took on new significance, and I was ready to take the Lord's advice to forgive others for having wronged me, even as God has forgiven my sins (Matt. 6:14, 15). Only then was I able to experience a sense of physical and spiritual well-being.

Is there someone in your life who has said or done
something to you that made you angry? Maybe it's
time to forgive and to bury the bitterness.

BICYCLE BOB AND HIS WIFE THERESA

Then He who sat on the throne said, "Behold, I make all things new." And He said to me, "Write, for these words are true and faithful." Rev. 21:5, NKJV.

When Bob Anderson was 66 he retired as a building contractor because of debilitating arthritis in his lower back. "I could hardly make it out to the mailbox," Bob said, "so I started driving my old car the 200 feet to get the mail. I had no energy. I was 60 pounds overweight, smoked three packs of cigarettes a day, and was always short of breath."

His wife's health wasn't much better. Theresa suffered from high blood pressure and diabetes and was overweight and extremely depressed.

Then Dr. Hans Diehl came to their town of Creston, British Columbia, with a Live With All Your Heart Seminar. Its message was simple: "Our diets are killing us. Our excesses in meat, rich dairy products, sugar, alcohol, salt, and tobacco must go, or we'll eat and drink ourselves into early graves."

The results of their HeartScreen health evaluation jolted the Andersons into action. Their blood pressure, cholesterol, and blood sugar were all too high. When they realized their rich diet and sedentary lifestyle were contributing to their heart disease, diabetes, hypertension, and osteoarthritis, they dumped their vodka down the sink and filled three garbage bags with the "junk" food they cleaned out of their refrigerator. They burned Bob's cigarettes (a 35-year-long habit) in their fireplace, and started walking. First just one block, then two, three, five—and more.

They say God can make crooked things straight, and that happened to Bob. By the sixth month his back pain disappeared; he stood straight and walked without a limp. Their blood pressure, cholesterol, and blood sugar levels returned to normal. Both took up bicycling and shed 50 pounds, and three years later, at age 69, Bob cycled 3,210 miles from Creston to Ottawa, Ontario, in 60 days.

Theresa says, "No more are we simply enduring retirement. We are living our lives to the hilt! We both have bicycles and love life on the road. And as our physical health improves, we are growing spiritually. We've been born again and are active in our church. Now we have a purpose and sense of direction in our lives."

If you don't want to just endure retirement, the time to do something about your lifestyle is now. Determine what must change in your life, and make a commitment to God that you will start your new life today.

EXERCISE
YOUR MIND

> Every athlete in training submits to strict discipline, in order to be crowned with a wreath that will not last; but we do it for one that will last forever. That is why I run straight for the finish line. 1 Cor. 9:25, 26, TEV.

Stan had been sick for several months, confined to bed with a painful infection. The inevitable vicious cycle of weakness ensued as he lost both physical and emotional strength. One day as he complained to me that he despaired of ever working in his beloved garden again, I suggested, "Stan, the Creator has put into our bodies tremendous healing powers. Start walking just a few minutes twice a day and you'll be amazed at what happens."

About a month later Stan came to me all excited. He'd been working in the garden and could once again stoop to pull weeds! When I wondered at the dramatic transformation, he explained, "I walked a quarter of a mile twice a day for a while, then increased gradually, and now I'm back to normal!"

The dictum "use it or lose it" obviously applies to physical strength, but what about mental or spiritual strength? Recent research at the University of California at Los Angeles substantiates what many have felt applies to the mind: regular exercise strengthens brainpower. When examined at autopsy the brain cells of bridge players appeared much more healthy than those of people whose pastime was playing bingo. A kindergartner can play bingo, but bridge requires constant analysis and decision-making.

Paul uses the example of an athlete to describe his spiritual life. If you want to win a race you must discipline yourself. Paul said, "I am like a boxer who does not beat the air; I bruise my own body and make it know its master, for fear that after preaching to others I should find myself rejected" (1 Cor. 9:26, 27, NEB).

You may exert your body when you're preparing for a sporting event, but do you exercise your mind when it comes to Bible study?

If you read through Scripture in a perfunctory manner, it avoids exercising your brain and may be like playing bingo—the words pass through your mind without leaving any real impact. However, if you get out several versions of the Bible, read the context, look up some background material, and then discuss your findings, you've exercised your mind. You're running "straight for the finish line"!

Have you exercised your brain with some in-depth
Bible study today? What else could you do to make sure
you are running "straight for the finish line"?

STAYING FIT

Larry Richardson

I am the vine; you are the branches. If a man remains in me and I in him, he will bear much fruit; apart from me you can do nothing. John 15:5, NIV.

When it comes to our bodies, nothing lasts forever. First we are young, then we grow old. After eating a meal, we get hungry again. We drink to our fill, but need more water later. And no matter how much we exercise to stay in shape, that effect wears off if we do not repeat it regularly.

Experts in exercise physiology tell us that the body starts to decondition after 48 hours of nonactivity. That means if you rest too long between exercise sessions, your body will begin to lose its tone. If you neglect exercise long enough, you will eventually lose most of the benefits of your previous efforts.

I learned that lesson myself with great frustration one year when a knee injury forced me to suspend my jogging routine for several months. Prior to this injury, I was averaging 20 miles a week. After my recuperation I returned to the track and could barely run a mile without feeling winded. It was a discouraging setback and a painful reminder to me that exercise must be continual for the benefits to linger. I cannot take this year off and expect last year's efforts to carry me on indefinitely.

When it comes to my relationship with God, the rules are very much the same. A healthy Christian experience requires a regular routine of prayer, study, and connection with our heavenly Father. Like eating, sleeping, and exercising, it demands daily attention. And like our physical bodies, our spiritual vitality quickly atrophies with indolence.

God could have designed us to draw all our nutrition by simply breathing the required nutrients from the air around us. Then we wouldn't have to deal with the daily necessity of eating. He could have engineered our physiology so that a one-mile jog would yield Olympic results for a lifetime. But He didn't, and I suspect He had a reason, with a lesson to teach us.

Human physical and spiritual requirements are similar. Ignore your body's needs, and you pay a price in weakness and debilitation. Neglect your relationship with God, and your spiritual health will wither like a branch cut off from the vine.

So, get fit—but don't forget to *stay* fit.

It's time to get organized. What in your physical or spiritual life should you schedule into your day, to make sure you stay fit?

For God did not call us to be impure, but to live a holy life. Therefore, he who rejects this instruction does not reject man but God, who gives you his Holy Spirit. 1 Thess. 4:7, 8, NIV.

God cares about our everyday lives and calls us from impurity and unhealthful practices. But is willpower alone enough to keep us from temptation and enable us to accomplish a needed change of health behavior?

Jean had a cabin cruiser on the river. She often spent her weekends there, inviting others to join her and enjoy the escape from the hot summers in the city. Her guests frequently brought food for the weekend meals.

"What did they leave this time?" Jean asked herself after the last batch of guests left. "A whole box of chocolates!"

Although Jean was well aware of her health problem that could be triggered by eating concentrated sweets, she thought, *Just one won't hurt!* But a chocolate binge was in the offing. Before she knew it, she had eaten the whole box. The penalty followed quickly, as she fell into the bunk, unconscious and alone for many hours. Only the timely visit by the dockman, who knew the potential of her ailing pancreas, brought her the needed emergency help.

"I should have known better," she said later. "But my willpower is challenged by a box of chocolates!"

What is it that challenges your willpower? It's easy for those who are not tempted by harmful substances such as smoking, drugs, alcohol, or chocolates to criticize the binge behavior of others. But what about overeating? You know you shouldn't, and yet you do it. Even the apostle Paul had the problem of doing things he knew he shouldn't (see Rom. 7:15, 16). Let's face it—we're all tempted by something!

But the good news is "The Lord knoweth how to deliver the godly out of temptations" (2 Peter 2:9).

God cares about our everyday lives, and summons us from impurity. Because willpower alone is not enough, "Christ has given His Spirit as a divine power to overcome all hereditary and cultivated tendencies to evil" (Ellen G. White, in *Review and Herald*, Nov. 19, 1908). The Holy Spirit is the most powerful agent of behavior change and will bolster the weakness of our willpower.

Lord, I admit I'm tempted to do things I shouldn't.
Give me Holy Spirit power today to resist the devil.
And may this be my prayer every day!

"Whoever drinks the water I give him will never thirst. Indeed, the water I give him will become in him a spring of water welling up to eternal life." John 4:14, NIV.

Jesus is the fountain of living water, and if we drink from that fountain daily, He will supply our spiritual needs. Not long ago, however, I had an experience that demonstrated the importance of drinking often and deeply from a literal water fountain as well!

I woke up one morning with a severe pain in my lower abdomen that persisted for more than an hour. When the pain became unbearable I went to the hospital's emergency department. The doctor examined me and then left without comment. After a while I called one of the nurses to find out what was happening. The nurse told me that the doctor was trying to get the surgeon from the operating room to examine me and explain why I might need surgery.

The thought of surgery frightened me. When the doctor came back, I told him I was not prepared to have surgery, and asked to be discharged, since I was feeling better. Although concerned, he wrote up my discharge papers and gave me a prescription for painkilling tablets. He said if I continued to have pain I should return for a thorough examination and be prepared for possible surgery.

The following day I went to see a specialist in natural remedies who suggested that my problem could be with my bowels, because I had not been drinking very much water.

I started drinking six glasses of water daily. Shortly thereafter my pain gradually disappeared. I continued to drink six glasses of water every day since and have not had any more problems with pain in my abdomen. I was fortunate that the cure for my problem was so simple, since I realize that persistent abdominal pain can indicate serious problems that might indeed need surgery.

This incident has been an important object lesson to me. Just as we need to drink daily enough water to preserve our physical health, so we must continue to drink daily from the spiritual fountain to preserve our spiritual health. If the supply is insufficient, we will not experience the full spiritual benefits that we need.

Lord, help me to remember to drink six to eight glasses of water each day to keep my body healthy, and give me constant drinks of Your water of life so I won't be spiritually thirsty either.

LIKE PLANTS
AND PILLARS

August 5
Betty M. Hoehn

Then our sons in their youth will be like well-nurtured plants, and our daughters will be like pillars carved to adorn a palace. Ps. 144:12, NIV.

Saturday night we were seated around the table as Uncle John led in the scriptural reading of the marriage ceremony and had the blessing. In the library hung a 25-year-old wedding dress with a man's tuxedo next to it.

Two teenage sons had planned the surprise event and arranged the menu. One son and his cousin had blindfolded the couple and brought them to my house. But dinner with the extended family was only the beginning of what their sons intended for the twenty-fifth wedding anniversary celebration.

The boys told their parents what they should pack for their extended weekend. They put their father's golf bag, shoes, and other items into the car without the father or mother knowing it. Then the boys arranged for their parents to spend a night in their honeymoon cabin on the lake, and then made reservations for a hotel and evening entertainment for the next.

As three generations gathered in the room around that large dinner table, I was thankful my grandsons had such a positive example of what a stable Christian home should be. There was no shouting, yelling, or confrontational episodes. The example of the grandparents had been exemplified in the parents and was being passed on now to the third generation. Solomon said it best: "Children's children are the crown of old men; and the glory of children is their father" (Prov. 17:6, NKJV).

After much perusing of the wedding pictures from 25 years before, the boys chauffeured their parents to the cabin on the lake.

The next morning my daughter was surprised to see that her sons had stocked the refrigerator and even set the table for two. Not until then did they see the computer printout of the plans their teens had made for their parents' trip to the Smokies.

What fun these young people had surprising their parents. And what fun it was for me to see the rewards of positive family relationships. Certainly when children are loved into maturity, boys become like "well-nurtured plants," and daughters like "pillars carved to adorn a palace." I love that word picture of a healthy family!

Thank You, Lord, for family.

THINK HAPPY, FEEL BETTER

Jan W. and Kay Kuzma

Whatever is true, whatever is noble, whatever is right, whatever is pure, whatever is lovely, whatever is admirable—if anything is excellent or praiseworthy—think about such things. Phil. 4:8, NIV.

Did you know that . . .

● Socially active married people tend to live longer than less active separated, divorced, or single people? And happily married women have the strongest immune systems of all?

● Men who participate in social activities at least once a week outlive men who don't?

● Confiding in someone else can result in a significant improvement in immune-system function?

● Those men who were most pessimistic at age 25 had more severe illness during their 40s, 50s, and 60s?

● There is a relationship between psychological factors and susceptibility to colds—i.e., pessimists are more likely to get colds?

● Even thinking about love can raise the levels of salivary immunoglobulin A in some individuals?

● When patients were trained to focus on the positive aspects of their postsurgery hospital stay, they used only half as many painkillers and stayed in the hospital an average of two days less than others?

The brain and the immune system have a strong linkage. For example, Donald Robinson tells of a long-term study reported in the prestigious British medical journal *The Lancet* on 57 breast cancer victims that had undergone mastectomies. Seventy percent of the women who had a "fighting spirit" were alive 10 years later compared to only 20 percent of the women who "felt hopeless." Three fourths of those who merely accepted their diagnosis also died.

In 1987 Candace Pert, while at the National Institute of Mental Health, suggested a molecular equivalent of telephone lines between the brain and the immune system by which white blood cells receive messages directly from the brain to fight off disease invaders.

What message is your brain sending to your immune system? Is it any wonder that God inspired the apostle Paul to instruct us to think about things that were true, noble, right, pure, lovely, admirable, excellent, and praiseworthy?

Dear Lord, help me to focus on the positive and
spend time with my friends and family.

GIVING UP
CONTROL

Linda B.

Blessed are all they that put their trust in him. Ps. 2:12.

Pain, arguing, and loneliness often overshadowed the fun times of growing up. As the years went by I began to question, *If God could not help
my caring Christian parents to be happy and peaceful, how can He
possibly help me?*

For a time I believed "Mr. Right" would be the solution to my problems. But when my boyfriend and I broke up, I was through trying to live
God's way. It was time for me to be in control. And thus began a 20-year
battle, a secret nightmare.

On the outside my life seemed perfect. But the truth of my controlling
ways, driven by fear and resentment, surfaced in binge eating and then
throwing up.

Bulimia is now well recognized as a life-threatening eating disorder.
But at that time it was not even in the medical textbooks. I feared I was
demon-possessed because no amount of prayer, determination, or off-campus witnessing seemed able to keep me from this destructive practice. By
my junior year it was so bad I was suicidal.

My husband and son have been through much emotional pain, not
knowing what to expect from me, or if life would ever be normal and
happy. Hospitalization and Overeaters Anonymous (OA) helped me to see
I was living just to serve myself and to make myself feel and look good.

OA is based on the 12-step recovery program of Alcoholics
Anonymous and teaches that we are powerless over food (or sin, or whatever our problem is). Only a Power greater than ourselves can help us live
to be of service to God and our fellow human beings. Making amends to
those I had hurt was very painful, humbling, and slow. I started to let God
be more and more in control of my life. Giving rather than taking is becoming more a part of my way of living. A previously unknown joy and
contentment is growing inside me. I'm learning that God's way is good and
that every victory is a gift, not something I can take credit for.

For me, bulimia has been a life-and-death struggle. Maybe all addictions
are. But then, don't we all have to choose between life or death in the long run?

*Who is in control of your life? Pray each morning, "Lord, I choose life.
Take control of my thoughts and my actions. May I unselfishly live
today for You and others, instead of for myself. Amen."*

251

A MODERN-DAY
MIRACLE

This is the assurance we have in approaching God: that if we ask anything according to his will, he hears us. And if we know that he hears us—whatever we ask— we know that we have what we asked of him. 1 John 5:14, 15, NIV.

In the early 1970s I was working on the morning shift as a nurse at the orthopedic surgery unit at Loma Linda University Medical Center.

Many of the patients there were older women who had broken their hips. After menopause a woman's bones demineralize and weaken. Since the hip is a major weight-bearing joint, often their hips would break and they would fall, rather than falling first and breaking their hips from the blow. The treatment, then, rather than months in a plaster cast, was surgery in which a metal nail would be used to stabilize the fracture.

This story is about one such woman. The relationship she had with her grown sons caught everyone's attention. They were loving and kind. One or both would come every day to sit with her while she ate and to help her.

Her wound, however, instead of healing, became infected. Despite our best efforts, she got worse and worse.

My heart ached for her. I wanted to help her, so I turned to God. I felt so unworthy to ask for a miracle healing. While I had no doubt in my mind that God *could* heal her, *would* He? I knew it had to be her faith, as well as mine, so I went to her bedside and asked her if she believed in God. "Oh, yes," she said, so I asked God to heal her, if it was His will, and then we thanked Him for answering our prayer.

The next day I hesitantly went into her room. She looked up at me and smiled one of the most beautiful smiles I had ever seen. I noticed her cheeks were rosy! Trembling, I removed the dressing from her hip wound. I could not believe my eyes. It looked as if two full weeks of healing had taken place overnight. We praised God. She fully recovered and went home to her family.

I believe God healed her to help her, but also so that this story could be told to strengthen my faith and that of others.

God is a God of miracles. Approach Him with the words of Psalm 150: "Praise the Lord! Praise God in His sanctuary; praise Him in His mighty firmament! Praise Him for His mighty acts; praise Him according to His excellent greatness!" (NKJV).

THE TRUE MEASURE OF SUCCESS

August 9

Steven L. Haley

For you make me glad by your deeds, O Lord; I sing for joy at the works of your hands. How great are your works, O Lord, how profound your thoughts! The senseless man does not know, fools do not understand. Ps. 92:4-6, NIV.

I was invited to give a devotional talk to a group of professional businesspersons of various faiths. My appeal to them that day was to consider measuring their success by a very different standard than one they were normally accustomed to. Instead of bottom lines, positive cash flow, net assets, hours spent in the office, why not evaluate the health of their business and their personal lives by how much time they gave to themselves personally, to their families, and most important, to their God? As I shared my thoughts, I could see in their faces a polite agreement to hear me out, but a silent message that said all too clearly that no matter what, time will always mean money.

For centuries Western civilization has lived the philosophy that we are a self-made people. We work hard, play by the rules, minimize our mistakes, and maximize our opportunities, always living by a tenuous promise that we're certain someday to have it all.

Psalm 92, David's psalm for the Sabbath, refocuses and reprioritizes our lives from the horizontal to the vertical plane; to the spiritual dimension where great are His works, not ours, and profound are His thoughts, not ours. Every seven days the Sabbath challenges us to a self-examination of time and priorities and life direction.

Before you this week are six 24-hour "windows" of opportunity. For those six days you will work, study, play, achieve, and probably accumulate a little—if nothing more than debt! At the end of those six days God has set a seventh day that calls you to a higher place. A place of refuge and communion where He alone, not we ourselves, is Lord. A place in time where we recognize that we are not the owners of ourselves, or our time, or our fortunes. They all are His.

"Fools" do not understand how this works, but through the experience of Sabbath, we understand and know that all we have is His, and all we have—including how we spend our time—must glorify Him!

What can you do this Sabbath to live on the higher plane of measuring success in how much time you give to yourself, your family, and your God?

PERFECT
PEACE

August 10

Mary Paulson Lauda

You will keep him in perfect peace, whose mind is stayed on You,
because he trusts in You. Isa. 26:3, NKJV.

've always loved Isaiah's promise that if we keep our minds on God and trust Him, He'll give us perfect peace. But I never thought I would have to see this promise fulfilled in one of my children. During a four-year period I watched Doreen struggle to live with a glioblastoma, an extremely fast-growing type of cancer in the right frontal lobe of her brain.

After her first surgery the physicians estimated that she would have six to 18 months to live. She was only 47 and had a 9-year-old daughter and a husband to live for, so she chose to go to the Livingston Clinic in San Diego, where they treat cancer by building up the immune system. She followed their program religiously, which included a diet of natural, unrefined, organically grown foods, vitamins, and a multitude of herbs.

Soon after her first surgery she followed the biblical instruction of anointing and prayer for healing. She searched her soul and made sure all things were right with God and fellow human beings before the anointing, and the result was that an incredible peace spread over her face. Her comment was "I may not be cured or made well, but I am healed."

For two years she enjoyed a good life, until the growth caused a condition similar to a stroke. Following a second surgery she came back remarkably, and another year was hers. Then the third surgery and radiation. But time was running out. After the fourth surgery she was partially paralyzed and needed full-time nursing care. Four months later she died.

But throughout it all she was such a patient, quiet, long-suffering person and continued her careful diet until she could no longer take nourishment. She continually witnessed to all she met, and more than one doctor shook his head in disbelief that she could still be alive. Then she would point them to God and say, "It's called divine intervention!"

As I think about it, God intervenes in many ways, sometimes with miraculous healing. But perhaps the greatest intervention of all is that of perfect peace in the face of death.

*If you are troubled and facing an unsure future, or even if
you aren't, ask for God's divine intervention of perfect peace.
He has promised it to all, if we have faith and will
keep our minds focused on Him.*

CONTENDING WITH HORSES

If you have run with the footmen, and they have wearied you, then how can you contend with horses? And if in the land of peace, in which you trusted, they wearied you, then how will you do in the floodplain of the Jordan? Jer. 12:5, NKJV.

A few years ago I was playing softball and doing my impression of a weekend athlete. Giving all "for the sake of the team" and in denial of my real age, I slid into second base in an attempt to break up the double play, only to tear the cartilage and several ligaments in my right knee. It didn't take long to realize that I should have settled for being called out and avoided the major league heroics. As a physical therapist I knew the importance of exercises and rehabilitation, so I began physical therapy as soon as possible. I returned to work a few days after the injury, exercised with weights, swam, walked, and resumed my routine activities of daily living.

An interesting thing happened about eight months after the injury. I tried to jump on one foot and hop from side to side to test my maneuvering ability, but I couldn't do it. Although I said to myself, "Jump," I remained there, flat-footed. My muscles could not produce adequate strength, tension, and force quickly enough to jump. I realized I had not fully rehabilitated my knee. My exercises had prepared me for walking and swimming, but not for more complex and challenging activities such as jumping or hopping.

That experience raised other thoughts. Our spiritual exercises of church attendance, returning a faithful tithe, and being vegetarians can enable us to be respectable Christians. But alone they are not enough to prepare us for the more challenging and complex spiritual activities such as keeping silent when we are being insulted; speaking words of kindness and encouragement instead of censorship and hatred; loving unconditionally; accepting someone who may believe differently than we do; or reflecting Christ's character. If our spiritual exercises and rehabilitation do not prepare us for more complex spiritual activities, how can we contend with spiritual "horses" and a Jordan overflowing its banks?

Today, why not consider more industrious physical and spiritual exercises that will prepare you for whatever "horses" and/or Jordan experiences may come your way.

*Lord, show me where I am weak, and show me
the way to become strong for You.*

HOW HEALTHY IS YOUR INHIBITORY SYSTEM?

Kay Kuzma

Jesus answered, "If you want to be perfect, go, sell your possessions and give to the poor, and you will have treasure in heaven. Then come, follow me." Matt. 19:21, NIV.

You know the story. The rich young ruler asked Jesus, "What do I need to do for eternal life?" Jesus said to obey the commandments. "I've done that since I was a kid," the young man replied. Jesus' response has made people ponder through the ages. What did He mean by "If you want to be perfect, go, sell your possessions and give to the poor"?

Should every Christian sell everything and donate the money to the poor? If they did that, who would there be to support missions, build churches, and finance Christian radio?

Rather than take this literally, I believe the principle is self-denial. The first thing Jesus said when He called His disciples was "If anyone desires to come after Me, let him deny himself, and take up his cross, and follow Me" (Matt. 16:24, NKJV).

In a day when many psychologists are saying, "Be good to yourself. Don't deprive yourself; that's legalism," Christ urges that we crucify self and follow Him.

After numerous postmortem studies on the brains of criminals, Dr. Richard Restak, a neurologist in Washington, D.C., said, "These studies and many others have convinced me that the hallmark of a healthy mind is a healthy inhibitory system."

What's an inhibitory system? It's the system in our brain that puts the brakes on. It says no to tempting desires and allows us to practice self-denial.

Dr. Elden Chalmers, a psychologist specializing in brain development, says, "It is a good practice to deny yourself at least one pleasurable thing each day, just to exercise the inhibitory system and keep it working at peak performance." You never know when you'll need it in an emergency to control your emotions and behavior, to keep yourself out of trouble, or to keep from hurting others.

For your own good, Jesus might want you to sell everything, or He might ask you to say no to a second helping at fellowship dinner or that snack between meals. Or maybe to deny yourself some tempting not-so-good-for-you food.

The secret to good mental health *and eternal life* is a healthy inhibitory system.

What simple pleasure could you deny yourself today, just to maintain your inhibitory system in good condition?

PARTS OF
THE WHOLE

August 13

John DeVincenzo

> But God has combined the various parts of the body, giving special honour to the humbler parts, so that there might be no sense of division in the body, but that all its organs might feel the same concern for one another. 1 Cor. 12:24, 25, NEB.

All too often I find myself wondering why God doesn't use me in some great and noble work for Him—to preach to the masses, to make an important scientific discovery, to produce a secular movie with a Christian message, to possess great wealth so it can be given to His work. And then I pause and look around me and see all the beautiful children of God, both past and present, who were/are the seemingly unimportant parts of the body of Christ.

Think of our body for a moment. It requires millions of endothelial and connective tissue cells to make one tiny blood vessel running from the heart to the brain. How important the brain and unassuming the vessel, but should this tiny vessel rupture . . .

Every person is vital and important to God—each His own gift and each needed by God for that perfectly functioning body, the church, ultimately Christ's bride.

Jonathan Goforth, that great early missionary to China, would take long trips away from his mission post. On one of those to Manchuria he had one of the most memorable three-day missionary campaigns of his life. Hundreds came to the Lord and were baptized. Years later he was speaking in England and mentioned the incident. A woman happened to hear of it and showed him her diary. During the exact three days that he was having such a remarkable evangelistic campaign, God mysteriously led her to fervently pray for His work.

Never should you feel discouraged or insignificant because your life seems so unimportant. God needs your talent. He needs you to share your testimony with others to encourage and uplift them. You are a significant part of His universe and can play a vital and needed role in His plan for His church.

May each of us seek God's direction so He can fit us into His body where He wants us. May we serve Him with gladness, and may joy fill us as He uses us to do just what He needs for His church.

Ask God what He wants you to do today. Stay on your knees
long enough for the Holy Spirit to tell you at least
two things you could do for God.

HEART
ATTACK
AT 27!

August 14

Vivian Raitz

Let the morning bring me word of Your unfailing love, for I have put my trust in You. Show me the way I should go, for to You I will lift up my soul. Ps. 143:8, NIV.

"It can't be a heart attack. My husband is only 27 years old!" Patty was in a state of shock. It was Christmas Day 1994. Her husband, Jim, and her father had had a couple mixed drinks, had done some target practicing, and then enjoyed the big family Christmas dinner. After the meal Jim took a nap. Upon awaking, he stepped outside to smoke a cigarette. Feeling some indigestion, he took some medicine. His symptoms increased: nausea and clammy sweat. He felt hot, but lying down with a fan blowing on him didn't help. Finally he consented to be taken to the hospital emergency room. The physician diagnosed a heart attack.

Jim was a tall, muscular supervisor in a carpet plant. But his job was a stressful one, and although his main summer sport was waterskiing, during the winter he didn't do much of anything except sit and watch TV.

After the scare of the heart attack, Patty said to Jim, "Honey, we must change our lifestyles." The couple had heard that one could reverse heart disease by following a healthy diet and by exercising regularly. They knew that Americans eat too much fat and rich foods, which cause plaque to build up in the arteries.

So searching for answers, they went with a vanload of people attending a satellite downlinked vegetarian cooking class in Chattanooga, and then they participated in the follow-up sessions at the Dalton Seventh-day Adventist Church. They joined the local health club and began exercising regularly. Jim has now quit smoking and has become much more physically active. Careful about their diet, emphasizing fruits, vegetables, whole grains, and beans, they avoid adding margarine, mayonnaise, and other visible fats to their food. But most important, they have rededicated their lives to Christ.

Nearly a year after his heart attack Jim is enjoying a normal life, and continues to follow a healthy lifestyle program.

One can understand why one of Jim and Patty's favorite texts is: "Show me the way I should go, for to You I will lift up my soul."

Challenge: Make Psalm 143:8 your philosophy of life.

LOVE IN ACTION

> Now there was at Joppa a disciple named Tabitha, which means Dorcas. She was full of good works and acts of charity. Acts 9:36, RSV.

What if you were in charge of miracles? What if, at your whim and desire, you could decide who would be miraculously healed and who would die from a painful disease? What if you could choose what lost child suddenly gets found, what miraculous scientific breakthrough would create a wonder drug?

Even though this is the kind of thing Hollywood movies are made about, the idea is intriguing, because to have a handle on such power tells us something about our values. And that's why this amazingly brief reference from Acts 9 is so intriguing. It just may tell us something about God's values.

Imagine the setting: The young church is growing, mostly (we think) because courageous individuals such as Peter and Paul are standing in public places and preaching to large crowds who stand in rapt attention. Should one of those great early preachers become ill, we would convene a large prayer meeting. We might even urge an all-night prayer marathon, reminding God how vital and necessary the person is to His cause.

But in this barely mentioned event we see a woman whose credentials don't list sermons or degrees. In that community she has the reputation as the one who mends worn overalls for the poor carpenters and delivers casseroles to the harried young mothers. She stays up late and gets up early because she's so good at what people really need—tender listening and skilled touching. And when she dies, she leaves a love-shaped vacuum so large and deep that God says, "This is a real loss."

So He has two men send for Peter from a nearby town, and the disciple receives permission to bring Dorcas back to life. When Peter died, he did not receive the same favor. Sure, God always has lots of things to take into account when working miracles. But the case of Dorcas emphasizes His esteem for love in action.

In what ways can you be a Dorcas to your family, church,
or community, and put love into action?

HUMBLING
ME FOR
HIS GOOD

Mary McDonald

> Remember how the Lord your God led you all the way in the desert these forty years, to humble you and to test you in order to know what was in your heart, whether or not you would keep his commands. Deut. 8:2, NIV.

After graduating from Stanford University, I married my college sweetheart. While he attended medical school and did residencies, I obtained a Ph.D. in developmental psychology and completed a postdoctoral fellowship. By the time I was 31 we had four beautiful children, two boys and two girls. I had more than 20 publications, and my scientific career was booming. We had a nice house, even a new minivan. Life was *good*.

At church, when friends asked me how I did it all, I'd think to myself, *I really am amazing.* When I needed help, which wasn't often, I'd ask God and plunge on. I perceived myself to be in control.

Then unexpectedly the diagnosis came—multiple sclerosis, a crippling, progressive disease.

No! Please, God. Let me keep doing great things. What about the kids? my career?

I fought back, but the condition didn't go away. Why, God? Why?

But always, through it all, then and now, I feel the love of God. And slowly I have learned and am learning that "God causes all things to work together for *good* to those who love God, to those who are called according to His purpose" (Rom. 8:28, NASB). And God's meaning of *good* is wonderful beyond human definition. In His all-knowing wisdom *good* is knowing Him, loving Him, becoming more like Him. For these things, through God's grace, I now strive.

I am realizing the glory and goodness of the Lord, who loves me so much that He didn't want me to suffer spiritually in my state of health but allowed health to be taken from me for a greater purpose. So He permits the disease that I might leave worldly accomplishments and be brought into His joy.

All things, including our well-being, are in the hands of our omniscient Lord.

I still have much to learn. My disease seems to have stabilized for the past few years. While I experience visual problems and weakness, I am comforted in knowing that God is in control. He sees the big picture, because He made it. God is so *good*.

Perhaps you are going through a humbling time right now. Remember, God is in control. Just as He brought the Israelites through 40 years in the desert so they would be ready to inherit Canaan, He is working in your life for good.

260

GET THE CHARGE OF YOUR LIFE

Draw near to God and He will draw near to you. James 4:8, NKJV.

S unlight electrically charges air molecules and makes them negative. But the problem for most of us is that we end up breathing too much positively charged air from heating and air-conditioning. This can result in headache, nasal obstruction, fatigue, and dizziness. In addition, it's been shown to depress the adrenal glands and diminish secretion of hormones essential in dealing with stress. That's why, for your well-being, it's so important to exercise in the sunshine and take deep breaths of that negative-ion-charged fresh air.

Isn't it interesting that before scientists discovered this information about some of the harmful effects of breathing stale air, Ellen White wrote, "Air is the free blessing of heaven, calculated to electrify the whole system. . . . The effects produced by living in close, ill-ventilated rooms are these: The system becomes weak and unhealthy, the circulation is depressed, the blood moves sluggishly through the system because it is not purified and vitalized by the pure, invigorating air of heaven. The mind becomes depressed and gloomy, while the whole system is enervated; and fevers and other acute diseases are liable to be generated" *(Testimonies,* vol. 1, pp. 701-703).

A similar thing applies to our spiritual lives. Ellen White says: "The influence of every man's thoughts and actions surrounds him like an invisible atmosphere, which is unconsciously breathed in by all who come in contact with him" *(ibid.,* vol. 5, p. 111). That's scary, since we don't want our negative attitudes affecting others. But there is a remedy. "When the Lord sees the determined effort made to retain only pure thoughts, He will attract the mind, like the magnet, and purify the thoughts, and enable them to cleanse themselves from every secret sin" *(A Solemn Appeal,* p. 76).

So let God's Holy Spirit magnet draw you, and you will get the charge that can change your life!

God is the greatest source of spiritual power in the world.
What are you doing to get plugged in to His infinite supply?

WHEN YOU FEEL
A WORRY
COMING ON

Caroline Watkins

You will keep in perfect peace him whose mind is steadfast, because he trusts in you. Isa. 26:3, NIV.

Lyndon B. Johnson, former president of the United States, once told an audience in Stonewall, Texas, that he was feeling fine because he had followed the advice of an old woman who once said, "When I walks, I walks slowly. When I sits, I sits loosely. And when I feels worry comin' on, I just goes to sleep." That old woman was not a psychologist, but she gave great advice to those who live in a high-tech, high-stress world plagued with depression, worry, and anxiety.

First, "When I walks, I walks slowly." In other words, don't rush through life. Slow down enough to enjoy the scenery and stop to smell the flowers along the way.

Second, "When I sits, I sits loosely." Don't get too comfortable with what you have, who you are, or what you do. Life is difficult, and sometimes circumstances beyond your control can rip your security away and force change upon you. It's best to be flexible in times like this. As those in the West Indies say, "Hang loose, mon"!

And third, "When I feels worry comin' on, I just goes to sleep." Sleep is a great battery charger. As life falls apart and you don't think you can cope, one of the best things you can do is get some sleep. Things always look brighter in the morning!

God has some great advice too. Read again Jesus' words in Matthew 6:27-35. Why do you worry, since if God takes care of little things such as birds and flowers, He can take care of you even more? All He asks you to do is live one day at a time.

Peter underscores this same message in 1 Peter 5:7, in which he says we should give our cares to God. Letting go and allowing Christ to take care of you and your problems isn't as easy as it sounds if you're used to fixing things yourself. But God says if you'll just trust in Him, He'll give you perfect peace. Why not give it a try?

*Give all your worries to the Lord and trust that He will
answer your prayers, and He will give you perfect peace.*

LAZY HANDS

Therese L. Allen

Lazy hands make a man poor, but diligent hands bring wealth. Prov. 10:4, NIV.

After an automobile accident in 1972, I missed my freshman year of high school. But I loved the physical therapy I had to take, and during that year I worked so hard that my therapist told me *he* needed a rest! You see, I knew the harder I worked, the sooner I'd walk out of there and back to school.

Nobody told me I had a badly damaged spinal cord. It probably wouldn't have mattered anyway, because I was very stubborn. I remember thinking that a broken neck is like a broken arm or leg. They heal, and everything gets back to normal. Sometimes ignorance is bliss.

The next year I went back to school—but not walking. I'd regained feeling and a little movement, however, on my left side. I had begun my life right-handed, but now I was an unwilling southpaw. I could sign my name, mark T or F, circle multiple-choice answers, borrow classmates' notes, and take essay exams orally. Did I really need to learn to write?

Yes, according to my English teacher. Mr. Jones told our class we had to write a one-page essay a day. I thought I'd get an extra 10 minutes to read, study, or whatever. Not so. When I said I couldn't write without a table, he said to use his desk. And when I said I couldn't write a page, he told me to compose three or four lines. I couldn't talk my way out of this one. So I wrote and I wrote—and I hated it. If Jones and I hadn't been friends, I don't know how things would have turned out.

With Jones's discipline, the care he had for me, and God's continuing gift of healing, I began writing with my left hand. If God hadn't cared about my writing, and Jones hadn't allowed God to use him, it's highly unlikely I'd be sharing this with you today.

I know that we can all do more than we think we can, *if we don't give up*, and we give God a chance to work out His will for us in our lives.

Have you been putting off learning a skill or doing
something you've never done before because it's hard work?
Why not start today to put in the extra effort needed for
God to work out His will in your life?

JESUS AS
SHEPHERD

He will feed His flock like a shepherd; He will gather the lambs with His arm, and carry them in His bosom. Isa. 40:11, NKJV.

Our son Chuck's tombstone has Revelation 21:4 carved on it: "And God shall wipe away all tears from their eyes." I felt it would be a comforting verse and a witness for others, because it soothed my own breaking heart every time I read it.

For my own stone, though, I would choose Isaiah 40:11. My favorite vision of Jesus is as shepherd, for as shepherd He brings love and comfort. As shepherd He understands when anguish covers us with darkness and pain and we find ourselves lost in a fog of circumstances that leave us numb.

Jesus enfolds us to His heart according to our need. I like to think in particularly agonizing moments that those of us who have immediate needs He holds even closer to His breast. It reminds me of that wonderful verse in John: "Then, leaning back on Jesus' breast . . ." (John 13:25, NKJV). We need to lean back on Jesus' breast every moment, but at certain times we need to yield totally and allow Him to carry both us and our burden.

The following anecdote from *Farm and Fireside* illustrates wonderfully this point: "An aged, weary-looking woman with a heavy basket upon her arm entered a train. Carrying her burden down the aisle, she found a seat and dropped into it, resting her heavy basket on her lap. A friendly workingman sitting across from her watched her for a long time, and then finally leaned across and spoke. 'Madam,' he said, 'if you will put your basket on the floor, the train will carry you and the basket, too.' How much truth there is in that kind remark. How often we do as the woman did, come to Christ for our soul's salvation, and yet steadfastly refuse to let Him bear our burdens and look after our daily lives. We are willing to get on the train, but refuse to lay down the burdens."

How blessed we are to have a Shepherd who clasps our weary heart and body to His own pierced heart!

> *Ask God to lift your burden today. Then hold fast to this thought: "Because the Lord is my shepherd, I have everything I need!" (Ps. 23:1, TLB).*
> *Aren't we blessed that Jesus is our shepherd?*

HEALING IN
THE SUN

Jan W. Kuzma

The Mighty One, God, the Lord, speaks and summons the earth from the rising of the sun to the place where it sets. From Zion, perfect in beauty, God shines forth. Ps. 50:1, 2, NIV.

I love to get up early in the morning and go out on the deck of our house, which looks east over the hills and ridges to the Smoky Mountains. There I stand in awe as the sun's first rays blaze across the horizon, awakening the misty valleys and warming my soul. Stretching my muscles, I breathe deeply and bathe in the beauty. And I think about God.

I've always loved the sun. Perhaps it's a part of my European background to spend some time each day exposing my skin to the sun.

But it wasn't until I read in a recent medical journal about sunlight and colon cancer that I realized the far-reaching benefits of this wonderful fiery orb that lights up the sky and our spirits.

Here's what I've found. Researchers at the University of Washington studied cancer rates in nine regions of the United States. The results were impressive. Men from Southern states had much less colon cancer than Northerners. When Michigan, Connecticut, and Washington men were compared with New Mexico men, the colon cancer rates were 50 to 80 percent higher.

Why might sunshine ward off colon cancer? Vitamin D, known to suppress growth of cancer cells, may be the answer. Our bodies make Vitamin D when we get adequate ultraviolet light from sources such as the sun. This may explain why people living in cities with more air pollution that blocks out ultraviolet rays may have more colon cancer.

While too little sunshine means a likely increase in colon cancer, too much sunshine means possible skin cancer. So, as in all things in God's nature, be moderate. Your body needs about 400 units of vitamin D each day. By exposing your face to sunlight for as short a time as five minutes daily, you can get all the vitamin D you need. What a healthy gift from God! But it's impossible to get it inside!

No wonder Ellen White advises: "Go out into the light and warmth of the glorious sun, you pale and sickly ones, and share with vegetation its life-giving, healing power" (*Health Reformer*, May 1, 1871).

Enjoy the health benefits of the sun. It's a gift from your Creator.

GETTING YOUR PRIORITIES STRAIGHT

Dan Day

> All this is from God, who reconciled us to himself through Christ
> and gave us the ministry of reconciliation. 2 Cor. 5:18, NIV.

We all have certain things we do in life that we value. But how much of a good thing is too much? For example, is there such a thing as being too religious? too concerned with your health? too generous? My first instinct is to respond, "No. These are all good things, and none of us are in any danger of doing too much of them." However, on second thought, what about the person preoccupied with his or her own salvation to the neglect of others? Or what about the person who makes health his or her god, putting physical perfection above all the other important priorities in life? And what about the person whose generosity results in distributing to strangers what the family really needs to survive?

The truly healthy person is one who seeks balance, who recognizes a time and a place for everything. When I come home from work each evening, my 2-year-old, Caitlin, thinks the first hour of the evening is her time. She believes that my job is to play blocks with her. Now, I'll be candid enough to say that some evenings playing with blocks isn't the highest thing on my personal agenda. But I'm also aware that it is very definitely the highest thing on hers. So I spend most evenings playing with blocks. I don't do it because I love blocks, but because I love Caitlin.

Life is like that. We choose the components in our life not just from among the things we enjoy but from among the things that contribute to what we value. God values reconciling us to Himself, and enlisting us in reconciling others to Him through a witness for Him that is open, loving, and accepting. Is that what others sense in us?

"In the life of the true Christian there are no nonessentials. . . . We shall be judged by what we ought to have done, but did not accomplish because we did not use our powers to glorify God" *(Prophets and Kings,* p. 488).

> *List the five most important things in your life. Did the way*
> *you spent your time yesterday reflect those values?*
> *What changes should you make so the values you*
> *live reflect the values you claim to hold?*

GOD'S SPECIAL
GROWING PLACE

You are my hiding place; you will protect me from trouble and surround me with songs of deliverance. Ps. 32:7, NIV.

I've been delivering babies for more than 20 years, and I never cease to marvel how God designed the human body to meet the needs of babies before their birth. Consider the womb or uterus, the special place in a mother's body that God has prepared to protect the baby and to allow it to grow in safety. It is truly an incredible organ!

The uterus is hollow with walls of smooth muscle. Before a woman becomes pregnant the uterus is about the size of a pear, weighing two to three ounces with walls about one-third inch (1 centimeter) thick. The space within the uterus would hold about two tablespoons (30 milliliters) of fluid. As the pregnancy progresses, God has designed that it will continue to enlarge to hold the growing baby regardless of its size. The way this happens is nothing short of amazing.

No other organ in the human body changes in size so rapidly as does the uterus. Soon after conception the smooth muscle cells in the uterine wall start to enlarge gradually. They do this by growing in all dimensions, becoming longer and wider and thicker. By the time the uterus reaches its maximum size prior to the birth process, these smooth muscle cells have enlarged to 20 times their original size. The uterus now fills almost the mother's entire abdominal cavity. The space within the uterus has increased by a hundredfold—capable of holding almost a gallon of fluid!

An even more amazing fact is that after the baby's birth the size of the uterus quickly starts to shrink. The muscle cells of the uterine wall rapidly decrease in size until within four to six weeks they are back to their former dimensions.

The power of God knows no limits in providing a growing place for the developing baby, but He also has a growing place for the developing Christian. King David called it a "hiding place." That special place is in Jesus. He meets all our needs and protects us. And it is through Him that rebirth is possible.

When you're frightened and frustrated, go to Jesus' "hiding place."
You can always feel safe and secure with Christ.

SOWING
WILD OATS

There was once a man who had two sons; and the younger said to his father, "Father, give me my share of the property." So he divided his estate between them. A few days later the younger son . . . left home for a distant country, where he squandered it in reckless living. Luke 15:11-13, NEB.

Foolish choices lead to sorry consequences. Between the fair-weather friends and continual carousing, the prodigal son not only went broke, but probably became addicted to alcohol and sexual pleasure. But when his money ran out, his friends evaporated. He had sown his wild oats and discovered he had no crop at all.

A severe famine came, and he began to feel the pinch, so he took a job feeding pigs. In later Jewish custom, if a person even touched a pig, they became unclean and could be rejected, disowned by their family. This boy knew that taking this job could disqualify him for ever returning to his family and sonship, but he thought that was the only way to survive. Still, even working in that stinking pigpen, he wasn't able to get enough food to fill his stomach. Finally he came to his senses and recognized that he was in a helpless and hopeless condition.

Alcoholics Anonymous (AA) describes this change as the first of the 12 steps of recovery: you admit you are powerless over addiction—that your life has become unmanageable.

In his pit of despair the miserable youth remembers the love and bounty of his father's home. He knows that his father takes good care of his servants. Although he realizes he has no chance that he can return as a son, at least as a servant he would survive. This is the second step of the AA program: to believe that a Power greater than you can restore you to sanity.

So, faint with hunger, in rags, stinking from living with the pigs, the young man surrenders and sets out for the long journey home. He has decided to turn his will and life over to God's care. As he plods along, he has time to reflect on his actions, honestly face his real self, and confess—the next steps of AA.

The route of the prodigal addict coming home is the same today as Jesus outlined so long ago.

Remember, it's never too late to turn from addiction toward home!

THE RUNNING
FATHER

August 25

Pat B. Mutch

> But while he was still a long way off his father saw him, and his heart went out to him. He ran to meet him, flung his arms round him, and kissed him. Luke 15:20, NEB.

Have you ever pictured God running toward you to welcome you to heaven? He is, for He is the Father in the prodigal son story.

Day after day the father had watched for his lost son. Perhaps he had asked passing travelers of news; perhaps he even knew of his disappearance from the social scene and was grieving, wondering if the boy had even survived. But faithfully he watched anyhow. One day a stumbling form appeared on the horizon. Somehow the father recognized that gait and ran to meet him.

Jesus did something here that rejects the culture of His time. People in positions of authority, especially if moral and religious righteousness was the basis of their authority, did not go out to meet and greet anyone. They held audiences in imposing surroundings. If apologies were to be made, the wrongdoer came and confessed to them. Forgiveness had to be earned. But in this wonderful cameo of God the unconditional love and welcome He has for each erring child is the reality He wants etched in our understanding.

Not only did the father run to meet his lost son, but he gave him an exuberant welcome! Ignoring the pig smell and dirt, he threw his arms around his son and kissed him. Immediately the boy began his carefully rehearsed apology and appeal. He admitted his sin and said, "I am no longer fit to be called your son" (verse 19, NEB). But strangely, the father didn't pay any attention. He never responded at all to the confession! You see, what the son had done didn't matter to the father's unconditional love. All that was important was that his lost son had returned. When the helpless, hopeless addict surrenders, Jesus makes it clear that he or she is welcome.

An openmouthed servant went quickly to fetch the household's finest robe to throw around the young man's filthy, gaunt body. The father placed the ring of sonship on the boy's finger and gave directions to prepare a feast. It was time for a party, "for this son of mine was dead and has come back to life; he was lost and is found" (Luke 15:24, NEB).

Thank You, Father, for running toward me, Your wayward child, and offering me the life of a royal child and gifts I don't deserve.

269

PERFECTION
ISN'T ENOUGH

August 26
Pat B. Mutch

Now the elder son was out on the farm; and on his way back, as he approached the house, he heard music and dancing. . . . But he was angry and refused to go in. Luke 15:25-28, NEB.

Did you know that the point of the prodigal son story is not about the prodigal?

The Jewish leaders didn't like the tax gatherers and other bad characters crowding in to listen to Jesus, so they criticized, "This fellow . . . welcomes sinners and eats with them" (Luke 15:2, NEB). Jesus answered by telling three stories: the lost sheep, the lost coin, and the lost son. By portraying the anger and resentment in the elder son's heart toward his prodigal brother, Jesus revealed the thoughts of the critical Jewish leaders.

You remember the story. As the older son nears home at the end of the day, he hears the merriment and laughter. It surprises him—after all, being a good son is serious business! He asks a servant what's going on. When he learns about the return and welcome of his younger brother, the writer Luke says he was angry. Furious might be a better word. He must have made his displeasure plain, because the servant goes to tell the father about the problem.

When his father comes out to plead with him to join the party, all the older brother's jealousy and resentment spills over: "You know how I have slaved for you all these years; I never once disobeyed your orders; and you never gave me so much as a kid, for a feast with my friends. But now that this son of yours turns up, after running through your money with his women, you kill the fatted calf for him" (verses 29, 30, NEB). Notice, it's not "my brother" but "your son" who has returned.

The older son's righteous deeds are the most important thing in his life—more important than his relationship to his brother or his father. He is addicted to his righteousness—an obsession called "religious addiction." He is the victim of compulsions about righteous behavior to earn God's acceptance, of trying to feel good about self, but unable to achieve joy and peacefulness. In the search for perfection the religious addict tries harder, fails, tries even harder, still fails—and inside the polished exterior shell the rage builds. Then a crisis comes, the person lashes out verbally or physically, and the true addiction stands revealed.

In a way all the addictions of these two sons represent all of us.
Some of us cling to unhealthful habits, and others frantically hold
on to righteousness above relationships. Which addict is more
typical of you, and why? How can you avoid becoming an addict?

270

WAITING ON THE BACK PORCH

> "My boy," said the father, "you are always with me, and everything I have is yours. How could we help celebrating this happy day? Your brother here was dead and has come back to life, was lost and is found." Luke 15:31, 32, NEB.

Have you ever felt like the elder son in the story of the prodigal son? Perhaps you have upheld the moral standards of our church; been consistently strict with your diet; abstained from harmful drugs; stayed by while others sowed their wild oats. Isn't that important to God? Isn't He pleased with your righteousness? Shouldn't the prodigals in the world have to prove they have really repented and reformed? Why should there be celebration when they deserve censure?

To the older son it just didn't seem right to celebrate over someone who had wasted his life on wine and women. Jealousy makes a person lash out, or pout. And in this story the older son pouted. He walked away and refused to participate.

But the point of the story is this: God never gives up on any of us. He loves the proud Pharisee and the hopeless publican. Both are His children. God loves both unconditionally—while they are yet sinners. He wants both "inside" the family of God.

So the story tells how the father tried to reason lovingly with his angry older son. "My boy," he began gently. He assured the older brother that "everything I have is yours."

Yes, there are rewards for conscientious religious efforts. Those who stay in the church have the blessings that accompany obedience to God's laws. Living in harmony with the laws governing His universe does bring us positive consequences: health, intact homes, serenity. But it doesn't earn God's love.

The father continued as persuasively as he could: "But how can we help celebrating this happy day? Your brother who was dead has come back to life." And the story ends.

Interestingly enough, this seems to be the only parable that Jesus did not finish. The father is left standing on the back porch, appealing to the proud but empty-hearted "righteous" son to come inside and join the family. He longs for both kinds of sinners to acknowledge their complete dependence on Him and accept His loving lordship. As you stand there, what will your answer be?

Father, forgive me for my self-righteous attitudes.
Help me to see the wayward sinner as my brother,
not my competitor, and rejoice at each homecoming.

THE GARDEN
OF YOUR MIND

A man will always reap just the kind of crop he sows! If he sows to please his own wrong desires,
. . . he will surely reap a harvest of spiritual decay and death; but if he plants the good things of
the Spirit, he will reap the everlasting life which the Holy Spirit gives him. Gal. 6:7, 8, TLB.

A young bride-to-be carefully selected flower seeds in just the right colors for her summer wedding in her family's yard. She drew up a plan and left it with her mother.

Spring sunshine warmed the soil. The rains left it moist and perfect for tilling. Weeds were already thriving, but after considerable nagging from her overworked mom, her dad finally set aside one morning for seed planting. After a night of too much worry and too little sleep he hastily did the job, quickly checked the automatic watering systems, and considered his duty done.

Nature has laws of germination and growth. Seeds bear genetic traits and reproduce after their kind. Garden plants develop and grow silently, continuously, and imperceptibly in an environment with adequate sunshine, water, and nutrients. Weeds do the same. Both yield their flowers, fruits, and seeds. And so it was with the family garden. No one paid much attention as it grew.

Shortly before the wedding the bride returned home. To her distress, she found almost as many weeds as flowers growing. The yard was a hodgepodge of plants and colors, nothing like her plan. Her parents had been too busy to care. She felt disappointed and unloved.

So it is with the garden of the mind. It too follows laws of nature and produces according to the care given. The quality of the yield and resulting harvest is the character we develop by our personal choices.

"By the laws of God in nature, effect follows cause with unvarying certainty. The reaping testifies to the sowing. . . . On the unfaithful husbandman the harvest passes sentence of condemnation. And in the highest sense this is true also in the spiritual realm" *(Education,* p. 108).

Have you looked at the garden of your mind recently? What's growing in it? Weeds of intemperance, thorns of conflict, and briars of immorality? Or are you carefully tending your garden and enjoying a rich harvest of love, joy, peace, patience, kindness, goodness, faithfulness, gentleness, and self-control (see Gal. 5:22, 23)?

Lord, help me to plant the good things of the Spirit,
and weed out harmful tendencies and bad habits that
will destroy the possibility of enjoying
a rich harvest later in life.

> Woe to you, O land whose king was a servant and whose princes feast in the morning.
> Blessed are you, O land . . . whose princes eat at a proper time—for strength
> and not for drunkenness. Eccl. 10:16, 17, NIV.

Early one morning I received an urgent telephone call from my physician telling me to report as quickly as possible to a designated hospital. An electrocardiogram taken a week earlier had shown some form of heart irregularity.

Lying in anxiety in the cardiac-care unit, I observed on the monitor the effect that my slightest body motion had on my pulse rate and blood pressure. The psalmist's declaration that we are fearfully and wonderfully made came instantly to mind.

After two weeks with no clearly defined diagnosis the hospital discharged me. Six months later my doctor advised me that esophagitis, a common condition related to my hiatal hernia, was my problem. Hiatal hernias are known to produce symptoms that mimic certain heart ailments, but are not life-threatening. Undoubtedly my stressful managerial position had exacerbated the hernia, causing an acute reaction.

Thankful for the alert, I resolved to become more actively involved in my personal health. A sedentary lifestyle had increased my weight to 200 pounds. It was time to make some changes.

For me the advice of the wise teacher and king of Israel in Ecclesiastes 10:16, 17 was the best remedy. "Eat at a proper time—for strength." I wondered how many times had I eaten a meal even when I wasn't hungry because food was there? How many times had I, although full, gone back for another helping?

I stopped eating a big breakfast before I was hungry, allowing my body ample time to use up stored calories from the day before. Instead I began spending time working in my vegetable garden during the early-morning hours. Only after engaging in such strenuous activity did I have a desire for food. Then I would break my "fast" and eat a healthy meal.

Within months I lost 20 pounds and stabilized at a normal weight. My hernia became manageable and controllable, with none of the side effects I'd experienced earlier.

For more than 10 years now I've followed this healthy regimen of eating for strength, and I have no need for the stomach remedies my doctor prescribed. I thank God that His remedies provide the best medicine.

Take the 10-day challenge: eat for strength and not for appetite,
and see if it doesn't make a difference in how you feel.

Up, for this is the day in which the Lord hath delivered . . . into your hand: is not the Lord gone out before you? Judges 4:14.

What wonderful words to start this new day. Jesus has already gone before me preparing the way. He knows my travel contacts, problems, cares, joys, and sorrows for this day. And He knows the decisions I must make. I'm not alone, because He's chosen me to be on His team, and I can do all things through Him (Phil. 4:13).

Morning manna is the way to get a healthy start for your day: "Consecrate yourself to God in the morning, make this your very first work. Let your prayer be, 'Take me, O Lord, as wholly Thine. I lay all my plans at Thy feet. Use me today in Thy service. Abide with me, and let all my work be wrought in Thee'" *(Steps to Christ, p. 70)*.

I've made this my prayer every morning for more years than I care to remember, and I know it works. At the beginning of each new day I surrender my life to Jesus and make plans for that day according to what He impresses me to do.

Carefully and prayerfully notice what happens when you make it your policy to talk to God before speaking to human beings. "When you rise in the morning, do you feel your helplessness and your need of strength from God? and do you humbly, heartily make known your wants to your heavenly Father? If so, angels mark your prayers, and if these prayers have not gone forth out of feigned lips, when you are in danger of unconsciously doing wrong, . . . your guardian angel will be by your side, prompting you to a better course, choosing your words for you, and influencing your actions" *(Testimonies, vol. 3, pp. 363, 364)*. Isn't that awesome?

But if you forget your morning manna and try to get through your day on an empty spiritual stomach, notice what happens: "If you offer no prayer for help and strength to resist temptations, you will be sure to go astray; your neglect of duty will be marked in the book of God in heaven, and you will be found wanting in the trying day" *(ibid.)*.

Have you had your morning manna today?

The number one habit of successful Christians is to talk to God before talking to fellow humans.

GOD LOVES
TO BUY LOW
AND SELL HIGH

You made him a little lower than the heavenly beings and crowned him with glory and honor. You made him ruler over the works of your hands; you put everything under his feet. . . . O Lord, our Lord, how majestic is your name in all the earth! Ps. 8:5-9, NIV.

God's investment policy for people is to buy low and sell high. He loves to pick up bargains and turn them into benefits. The Lord delights in rescuing the downhearted and turning them into dynamic testimonies about what He can do for people.

His philosophy is "I want you to trust me in your times of trouble, so I can rescue you, and you can give me glory" (Ps. 50:15, TLB). When you've run out of options and can't help yourself, that's the very time Jesus wants to pick you up. And the result? You have to give all the glory to Him!

Just look at who Jesus invested in. He took fishermen and turned them into successful evangelists. He took a slave and turned him into the second most powerful man in Egypt. He took a condemned murderer and made him the powerful deliverer of the Jewish nation. He took a prostitute and lifted her to the honor of being named in the lineage of Christ.

So if you're discouraged today because you feel like a nothing and nobody seems to care, remember, Christ has purchased you, and He is right now in the process of producing someone of incredible value. He does that with all His investments!

We need to have the same people investment policy ourselves. Too often we ignore the down-and-outer and buy in with our time and attention when a person is riding the crest of success. The very time when people need rescuing, when they're sick, discouraged, and struggling, is often the time we withhold investing.

Andrew Carnegie, who amassed a fortune in business, once had 43 millionaires working for him, but they didn't start out millionaires. When asked how he did it, he replied, "You develop people the same way you mine for gold. When you mine for gold you must literally move tons of dirt to find a single ounce of gold. However, you do not look for dirt—you look for gold." His philosophy was that no one can become rich without enriching others.

If Jesus is willing to buy low and develop His investment into a priceless gem, shouldn't we be willing to make the same investment in our fellow humans, and then mine for gold?

GOD'S IDEAL
FOR MALES
AND FEMALES

Alberta Mazat

> So God created man in his own image, in the image of God he created him;
> male and female he created them. Gen. 1:27, NIV.

Male and female he created them." Have you ever wondered why God chose to introduce into His new, beautiful earth male and female units? True, it was His chosen means of populating our planet. But God could have done that in many different ways. He could have spoken inhabitants into existence until He was satisfied that there were enough.

But how much we would have missed! Father and Son had known the joys of an intimate relationship since the beginning (John 17), and He wanted earthlings to know a similar joy in several areas of their relationships. So since He chose to make us in His image, He provided for a special relationship between the male part of His image and the female part of His image. It was to be the hallmark of His earthly creation—the gift of the power to create.

How carefully He went about this Edenic event. Adam's significant contribution came from his side. Eve was dependent on him for that. He was dependent upon her for the continuance of life from his seed. Complete interdependence.

Adam slept during this first surgical procedure, not because God was not a painless surgeon, but more likely so that the first man could never be tempted to employ the argument "I was there. I witnessed your origin." To do so would not have been fair!

Then God said four significant things to both of them together. He blessed them equally; He told them to be fruitful and multiply, for which both were equally essential; He told them to subdue the earth, involving them both in implementing submission over it; and He enjoined them to have dominion over His nonhuman creation—in effect, to be comanagers. No wonder Ellen White can assure us that Eve and Adam were equal at Creation *(Patriarchs and Prophets,* p. 46).

How thankful we can be to God for His ideal plan, which brought male and female together in a relationship of oneness, side by side and equals in perfect harmony.

O Creator-God, may I show my spouse the respect and admiration
of a side-by-side, egalitarian, Edenic relationship, God's
original purpose for male and female.

NURTURING
RELATIONSHIPS

September 2

Ted Hamilton

A friend loves at all times. Prov. 17:17, NIV.

I was straightening my desk today when I came across a birthday card that I received two months ago. The front of the card pictures a small animal with a quizzical expression on its face, saying, "Happy Birthday. Even with your ageless good looks, brains, and talent, you still manage to be a regular person!" Inside the card, the punch line reads "I guess you eat a lot of fiber."

I enjoyed the experience of reading this card again several weeks after I had initially received it, partly because of the "fiber" line, but more because of the friendship it expressed. The birthday card was from my sister, Becky. She never forgets my birthday. Nor my brother's, nor those of our parents, of our spouses and children, or of countless cousins, aunts and uncles, in-laws, outlaws, casual acquaintances, and total strangers.

Becky loves people, and she lets them know it. She keeps a calendar, regularly updated, that contains vital statistics regarding the significant people in her life. Not just birthdays, but anniversaries, graduations, first tooth, first step, first date . . . she has recorded all the times and circumstances.

And whenever possible, she's there. Weddings, funerals, reunions, holidays, and homecomings, she's part of the action—preparing, organizing, cooking, decorating, photographing, loving.

If she happens to be traveling within 100 miles or so, we can count on a visit. It's like the arrival of the Pony Express. Because she initiates communication, people reciprocate, and Becky has all the news.

My brother sells industrial adhesives. Companies use his products primarily in labeling and packaging to provide a reliable seal for wrappers and containers. Bob's glue ensures product freshness and protects the integrity of packaged goods. Major manufacturers depend upon Bob and his company to provide quality products and service.

Becky is the communal adhesive of our family. Her ongoing commitment to communication and participation in the lives of her family and friends contributes to the freshness of our experience and supports the integrity of our relationships. We depend upon her to help us maintain the quality and richness of our lives together.

Nurturing relationships produce health and happiness.
How can you be like Becky today?

TAP INTO GOD'S WATER SUPPLY

For I will pour water on the thirsty land, and streams on the dry ground; I will pour out my Spirit on your offspring, and my blessing on your descendants. Isa. 44:3, NIV.

It all started when mountaineering teams from several nations sought to be the first to conquer Mount Everest, the tallest mountain in the world. The elite Swiss team, considered by many to be the best, made the first attempt, but failed.

A year later, in 1953, the British decided to try. As they carefully studied the records of the Swiss expedition, they made an interesting discovery. The Swiss team members drank less than two glasses of water each day. Could that be the reason for their failure? Consequently, the British climbers ordered extra snow-melting equipment. The men drank 12 glasses of water a day, and they reached the top!

Most people underestimate the amount of water they lose while active. Some athletes lose up to five quarts. If you don't replace this lost fluid, not only do you feel severe fatigue, but you lose essential salts as well. If you wait until you feel thirsty, that's too late. Your body is already suffering from dehydration and symptoms of exhaustion.

Water is nature's energy source on tap. It can help you get your house painted or your lawn mowed. The vital fluid gives you energy to finish that marathon you never thought you could run, or climb a mountain peak!

But water can do more than that. Have you ever visited Palm Springs? On one lot you'll see nothing but sand and desert brush, and right next to it grow lush green grass, shady palms, and flowers of every variety. What makes the difference? Water.

God's Spirit is a lot like water. When it comes into people the change is dramatic. Energy, motivations, and talents blossom into life. People now have power to say no to habits that have held them captive for years. They have strength to conquer mountains of guilt and confusion that had seemed hopeless. But just as a few days without water turns the garden into a desert, so it is with us. So for best results, drink freely of God's Spirit throughout the day.

Drink eight glasses of water today, even if you don't feel like it. The results will far outweigh your efforts.

TWO SETS OF FEARS

For God has not given us a spirit of fear, but of power and of love and of a sound mind. 2 Tim. 1:7, NKJV.

Seven-year-old Laurie, clinging to her mother's arm, eyed her pediatrician like a scared rabbit. Mother had brought her to see the doctor because she had been vomiting for the past four weeks. It had begun the day after Labor Day. The doctor was quick to discover that the day after Labor Day had been the day Laurie had started school for the first time. Thrust into a new situation that filled her with fear, she had developed an anxiety that had sent nerve impulses that tightened her stomach, causing her to vomit.

Adults also suffer from fear and anxiety, manifested by a variety of feelings. Some of the main ones we can describe by the acronym **FEARS:** Frustration, Envy, Anger, Resentment, and Sadness. These negative feelings cause changes in various organs in our body. They influence the amount of blood that flows to an organ. When we are embarrassed, for example, our face and neck turn red. As too much blood rushes to the head, headache may result.

Stress affects the heart. Repressed hostility has been associated with heart attacks. Also, stress can elevate the level of adrenal hormones—epinephrine and corticosteroid—which can raise the blood pressure as well as suppress the immune system. In addition, stress affects the muscles, causing neck tension and back pain, and the gastrointestinal and nervous systems as well.

To overcome stress we can use the same acronym, **FEARS.** F is for Faith in God—we need to trust God, who knows all our troubles. Exercise, both physical and spiritual, is crucial. We need Acceptance of ourselves and others. "Be kindly affectioned one to another with brotherly love; in honour preferring one another" (Rom. 12:10). R stands for Rest—not only physical rest but also the rest Jesus is so willing to give us (Matt. 11:28). S is for Singing. When your spirit is low, take a short walk and sing a chorus such as "Jesus, loving Jesus, sweetest name I know, fills my ev'ry longing, keeps me singing as I go." We need not fear when we have Jesus.

*What **FEARS** do you have? The first set: Frustration, Envy, Anger, Resentment, and Sadness; or the second set: Faith, Exercise, Acceptance, Rest, and Singing?*

AN UNBEATABLE COMBINATION

Richard A. Schaefer

As for God, his way is perfect; the word of the Lord is flawless. Ps. 18:30, NIV.

On September 5, 1866, the first Seventh-day Adventist health-care facility, the Western Health Reform Institute (later Battle Creek Sanitarium), opened to the public.

On September 5, 1966, the president of the United States, Lyndon B. Johnson, and the president of the American Medical Association, Charles L. Hudson, M.D., met in Battle Creek, Michigan. There they participated in the centennial celebration commemorating 100 years of Seventh-day Adventist medical emphasis. On that day Hudson delivered a speech entitled "Medicine and Religion, an Unbeatable Combination."

Ironically, it had been this same combination of medicine and religion that had nearly prevented the founding of the denominationally operated medical school. The school's leaders had been told that the American Medical Association was not prepared to recognize a church-operated school of medicine. Yet those struggling to establish the school found in Scripture those general counsels, and in the messages given through Ellen White those timely and specific counsels that gave them the faith to overcome every obstacle. George I. Butler, longtime president of the church, attributed the success of the church and its medical program to following these instructions. He wrote: "We have found in a long, varied, and in some instances, sad experience the value of their counsel. When we have heeded them, we have prospered; when we have slighted them, we have suffered a great loss" *(Review and Herald, Aug. 14, 1883).*

Ellen White herself, speaking of the results of following God's counsels, said, "In reviewing our past history, . . . I can say, Praise God! As I see what the Lord has wrought, I am filled with astonishment, and with confidence in Christ as leader. We have nothing to fear for the future, except as we shall forget the way the Lord has led us, and His teaching in our past history" *(Life Sketches, p. 196).*

As we continue the health program we must remember George Butler's words: "When we have heeded [God's instructions], we have prospered. When we have slighted them, we have suffered a great loss."

Lord, help me never to forget the way You have led
me in the past. Thank You.

GROWING CLOSER TO HEAVEN

Teach us to number our days aright, that we may gain a heart of wisdom. Ps. 90:12, NIV.

The summer is waning. Our garden has passed its peak, and I caught the first rustle of fallen brown, crisp leaves blown across the walk the other day. Today on my way to town I got stopped behind a school bus. How quickly seasons come and go.

But God has a time and purpose for everything, and although many fear the aging process, I like the words of Tryon Edwards: "Age does not depend upon years, but upon temperament and health. . . . Some men are born old, and some never grow so."

When I look in the mirror, I'm shocked with the person I'm becoming on the outside: the touch of gray, the sagging chin, a few more age spots, and deepened laugh lines. Inside I'm 25, looking forward to children, raising a family, and pursuing a career; or I'm 35, in the midst of the hustle and bustle of getting kids off to where they need to be and back home again; or maybe I'm 45, with a houseful of teenagers who are eagerly anticipating emancipation as much as I am. But 55 and beyond—is that really me?

So I find myself pondering, as did King Solomon, What is the meaning of life? I know "there is a time for everything, and a season for every activity under heaven: a time to be born and a time to die" (Eccl. 3:1, 2, NIV). But more important, how shall I live my life so that I can have the heart of wisdom that Solomon's father talks about?

Jean-Paul Richter's words bring insight: "Like a morning dream, life becomes more and more bright the longer we live, and the reason of everything appears more clear. As winter strips the leaves from around us, so that we may see the distant regions they formerly concealed, so old age takes away our enjoyments, only to enlarge the prospect of the coming eternity."

And E. H. Chapin's thoughts give hope. "An aged Christian, with the snow of time upon his head, may remind us that those points of earth are whitest which are nearest to heaven."

Look forward to each new day, not as a sign of growing older, but for the incredible potential of growing closer to heaven and the person, Jesus Christ, who makes heaven possible.

CLASS REUNION: LOOKING GOOD AND FEELING GREAT

September 7

Vivian Raitz

After that, we who are still alive and are left will be caught up together with them in the clouds to meet the Lord in the air. And so we will be with the Lord forever. 1 Thess. 4:17, NIV.

My fortieth college class reunion was coming up in two months. "I would love to lose at least 15 pounds, but I can't seem to. My weight set point has gone from 120 up to 130, and I even weigh 134 now. That's the heaviest I've ever been except when I was pregnant," I told my physician-husband.

I'm a health educator, so I'd been going faithfully to a local track and jogging. I thought I was watching what I ate on my semi-vegetarian diet and allowed myself dessert only on Saturdays. But as hard as I tried, my weight would not drop below 130. Then I heard a health lecturer talk about a very low-fat, starch-based total vegetarian diet that included fruits, vegetables, whole grains, beans, peas, and lentils.

"Substantial changes bring substantial results," he said. Well, I was motivated! I prayed for God's help with my sugar addiction and stopped eating desserts entirely, except for fruit. I joined a health club, began walking vigorously two miles three or four times a week, and cut back on dietary fat.

Wonder of wonders! I couldn't believe the bathroom scale. One to three pounds a week started dropping off. I could start wearing clothes on the "too small" pile in the attic. As I lost the 15 pounds, my borderline cholesterol came down 25 percent within a month, my resting heart rate reduced to the 60s, and my energy level was high.

The class reunion was great fun, but best of all, I'm still on the new lifestyle. My weight stays down as long as I continue to eat this way and to exercise. I still have to keep a close eye on my hereditary cholesterol problem, so I can't get lazy about the exercise.

There's nothing like going to a class reunion looking good and feeling great! I'm looking forward to another "class reunion." That's when Jesus calls all His "students" home to live with Him forever. Since He made me what I am, I want to make sure when He sees me that I'm looking good and feeling great!

Are you looking good and feeling great spiritually? There's always room for improvement. Follow God's biblically based program and live abundantly.

RECOVERY
TIME

September 8
Larry Richardson

've read that the true measure of the condition of a runner is not how high his or her pulse gets while running, but rather how long it takes for the pulse to lower once the runner stops. This is called recovery time. In other words, runners should check their pulse immediately at the end of a run, then again after two minutes' rest. If the beats per minute drop 40 beats or more, it indicates that the runner is in excellent cardiovascular shape.

So, for example, if my heart rate measures 180 beats per minute at the end of my run, it should drop to 140 after two minutes' rest. A lengthy recovery time would indicate poor cardiovascular shape. Thus if my heart rate continued to race even after several minutes of rest, I should be concerned that I'm out of shape.

It seems to me that we can measure other qualities in life similarly. Most people will, from time to time, push themselves to their limits in their work, in commitments at church, in hobbies, interests, and activities, just as runners can push their heart rates to the max. At times they may even exceed their limits, overextend themselves, promise more than they can deliver, and disappoint both themselves and others.

But the measure of a person is not necessarily how far they can reach, how hard they can try, or even how often they succeed, but rather how well they recover when they fail. It has been said that in this life almost everyone will stumble and fall on the road to their goals. Occasional setbacks are inevitable. The quitters are the ones who don't get up and try again. Overcome at the first discouragement, they simply don't recover. The real winners in life, like the experienced runner, have a quick "recovery time." They get right up when they meet adversity, assess the cause for their roadblock, formulate a new plan, and press forward.

So learn to overcome those everyday discouragements and develop a healthy recovery time.

In what areas do you need to shorten your recovery time?

THE WONDERS OF WATER

September 9

Dona Daniel

You care for the land and water it; you enrich it abundantly. The streams of God are filled with water to provide the people with grain, for so you have ordained it. Ps. 65:9, NIV.

Thousands of years ago God put into operation the finest water recycling program the world has ever known. I am in awe when I think that the water I drink or use was not long ago in the ocean, then drawn up into the clouds, where it was purified. Winds blow the clouds across the land to deposit their life-giving load in the mountains, where it flows down to the rivers and into the ground for our use. When I have used it, it is carried again into the rivers and back to the ocean to be recycled. What a fantastic imagination God has!

How much enjoyment and usefulness we get from water. Not only does God's water provide us with an abundant harvest, but water provides great opportunities for recreation. From playing in the snow and ice skating, to swimming or watching children play in the puddles left by the last rain; from watching moon jellies in the sea aquarium and birds in a birdbath, to drinking pink lemonade and eating watermelon, water plays an important part in our daily lives.

Plus, there is nothing like the wonderful feeling of a cold shower after hot, sweaty yard work, or relaxing in a warm bubbly bath on a cold evening.

But water is also essential for the inside of me. Not a cell in my body could exist without water. I can't even blink my eye without water! Water helps me digest my food and carries waste products and toxins from my body—especially important when I am sick. It helps to make good blood, which in turn flows to all parts of my body, including my brain.

I am reminded that the work of the Holy Spirit is very much like that of water. He cleanses us from spiritual impurities and fills us with the pure Living Water. My prayer is "Lord, flood me with Your Living Water; wash me inside and out. Make me a pure vessel for You." I hope that's your prayer too!

How should you plan your day in order to drink as much of the Living Water as possible?

STOP AND SMELL THE ROSES

Nancy Hadaway

Which of all these does not know that the hand of the Lord has done this? In his hand is the life of every creature and the breath of all mankind. Job 12:9, 10, NIV.

As a working mother of two young girls, my busiest, most stressful time of the day is not during office hours, but between 6:00 and 8:00 a.m., when I'm trying to bathe, dress, feed, and transport all of us to where we need to be on time.

One day Diana, my eldest, reminded me of one of life's simple lessons. Diana has cerebral palsy and is mentally disabled. Although she was 8 years old at the time, she functioned more as a 3- or 4-year-old.

After dropping my youngest at school, I was already running five minutes late as I whizzed Diana to her baby-sitter. I was hurrying up the sidewalk when Diana stopped and said in her singsong voice, "Mom, do you hear that?" Still trying to prod her along, I said, "What is it? I don't hear anything. Come on, come on, let's go!" She wasn't budging just yet.

"The birdies. Don't you hear the birdies, Mommy? Where are they?"

Realizing I wouldn't get her moving unless I showed her where the birds were singing, I pointed them out to her in a nearby tree. I grabbed her wrist again to hurry her along, but she continued her leisurely stroll. She turned to the array of spring flowers blooming along the baby-sitters' front walk. "Which flower do you like best, Mom?"

With a sigh I gave up trying to make a quick exit. Finally, realizing the innocence with which Diana was enjoying the morning (oblivious to my need for speed), I answered, "I like the purple ones best. Which ones do you like?"

"I like the yellow ones and the pink ones and the white ones and the orange ones . . ." She continued listing colors through the rainbow. Finally we made it up the walk and I got to work about 10 minutes late, but with a much brighter outlook on my day, having been reminded to "stop and smell the roses."

And what more beautiful rose is there than the life of a child?

Have you stopped to smell the roses today?

September 11

David and Carrie Grellmann

In Joppa there was a disciple named Tabitha (. . . Dorcas), who was always doing good and helping the poor. . . . She became sick and died. . . . Peter . . . prayed. Turning toward the dead woman, he said, "Tabitha, get up." She opened her eyes, and . . . sat up. Acts 9:36-40, NIV.

Our daughter Kristi died September 11, 1994. She was only 4½. The battle for her life started two years before when we discovered a firmness in the right side of her abdomen. Kristi had a neuroblastoma, and it was growing fast. Only three out of 100,000 children get this tumor. Highly malignant, it had spread to the bone. She had a one-in-three chance of survival. And for that chance her treatment would have to be severe: six months of chemotherapy, then radiation followed by a bone marrow transplant. The agonizing treatment would leave its marks on her body for life, but we had to try.

We celebrated the one-year posttransplant milestone, then a couple weeks later Kristi's fourth birthday. Life was good again. Kristi was going to make it. Then 17 months out from transplant the tumor was back, and our brave little girl began to lose her hold on life. Kristi was hospitalized and chemotherapy begun. But unlike the first six months of chemo, which she tolerated well, this time it knocked her down hard. By the fifth and last day she couldn't even hold her head up. And her recovery was much slower and more complicated. Two days out of the hospital Carrie was reading to Kristi about Dorcas and how she had been resurrected. Suddenly Kristi became restless, then delirious, and within minutes had stopped breathing. The end came so quickly. But as we've looked back, we marvel at God's timing. Kristi's last thoughts were of the miracle of being raised from the dead.

Living through Kristi's illness, we learned so much that we'd like to share with others who have a seriously ill child. First, take one day at a time. Share your burdens and needs with close friends who can support you. Consciously create memories you can treasure later. Enjoy what you still have. Don't let anticipated loss spoil your fun now. If the disease is terminal, plan ahead, so when the end comes and you're grieving, you aren't burdened with decision-making. And trust in God.

Even through sickness, pain, and death, God is in control.
Are you willing to make Him the Lord of your life and trust
Him with your most valuable possessions—
the members of your family?

PUT MERCY BEFORE JUDGMENT

Kay Kuzma

Speak and act as those who are going to be judged by the law that gives freedom, because judgment without mercy will be shown to anyone who has not been merciful. Mercy triumphs over judgment! James 2:12, 13, NIV.

Addictions of any kind can disrupt the family and destroy relationships, but one of the toughest to deal with is the sexual addiction of a spouse. Don's story was one of innocently picking up a pornographic magazine, followed by adult movies, sexual fantasies, and finally adultery. Then overcome with guilt, he repented, confessed to his wife, and was willing to do whatever was necessary for recovery.

What would you do if you were his wife?

Here's what Sherry says: "I was able to see that Don's sin was not really against me, but against God. I recalled that David in the Bible acknowledged that his sins of murder were not really so much against people as against God [Ps. 51:4]. Once I realized that, the Lord was able to speak to me from Ephesians 4:32: 'Be gentle with one another, sensitive. Forgive one another as quickly and thoroughly as God in Christ forgave you' [Message].

"I knew that Scripture did not require me to remain in my marriage. Therefore, if I stayed with Don, it was because I wanted to, not because anything compelled me to. If I remained with him, I could pursue a high standard—the law of love.

"The thing that hurt me the most was the pain of the broken trust of a Christian marriage. It led me to become insecure, defensive, and suspicious.

"But God gently and persistently dealt with *me*. Exposing my own faults and shortcomings, He kept me humble and dependent on Him. Although I felt utterly crushed and broken, He promised that if I would humble myself under His mighty hand, in time He would lift me up.

"The Lord also began to build in me an identity rooted in my relationship with Him, not in any human relationship. That security gave me the strength and patience to wait on God to work in Don's life. Although Don had previously put success and recognition before our marriage and children, when the Lord changed his heart I discovered a vibrant love in him that was beyond price."

When someone hurts you, remember to put mercy before judgment and be kind, tenderhearted, and forgiving.

REST IN
MEANINGFULNESS

September 13
Niels-Erik and
Demetra Andreasen

There remains, then, a Sabbath-rest for the people of God; for anyone who enters God's rest also rests from his own work, just as God did from his. Heb. 4:9, 10, NIV.

Viktor Frankl survived the concentration camps during World War II and wrote a book about it. In it he described our human search for meaning in terms of the hope we have for a better future. Those inmates who survived were not merely the clever ones, nor the more physically healthy ones, but the ones whose life was filled with meaning. But how can one find meaning in the cruel existence of a labor camp? Only by seeking that meaning in those possibilities held by the future—by hoping. This attitude, a type of stubborn, invincible mental health, kept the inmates alive.

Our daily life bears no comparison to that of the inmates in the Nazi camps, but the fact remains that those who successfully live even ordinary lives live in hope.

Sabbath observers have always been aware of this, but not always as fully as they ought. On the Sabbath day we are to look back to remember a week well lived, God's great gift of redemption, and Creation. But the Sabbath also invites us to look forward, since by definition it always arrives at the end of a working week. Thus on a cold Monday morning in the office we can look forward to Sabbath. After a hard day's work, on Tuesday evening we know that Sabbath is coming. By Wednesday we are rather tired, but fortunately the Sabbath is nearer. As Thursday comes around, we are already preparing for Sabbath. And when Friday arrives, Sabbath is knocking on our door. We open that door simply by stopping our work, and there Sabbath is in our midst. So simple, so profound. Work is finished, tiredness is forgotten, new vistas open to our mind, heart, and body.

Almost no amount of work pressure and stress can overcome the person who finds meaning in life. That meaning comes from hope of better times when work will be complete, stress will subside, and tense relationships will be rebuilt. The Sabbath holds out hope for such meaning in life each week, until it has so changed us that we become people of hope all life long.

Are you a person of hope? What can you do on Sabbath to bring more meaning to your life and strengthen your hope?

Trust in the Lord and do good; dwell in the land and enjoy safe pasture. Delight yourself in the Lord and he will give you the desires of your heart. Ps. 37:3, 4, NIV.

Retirement. As we traveled from Washington, D.C., to Nashville, Tennessee, I frequently said it loudly: "We are going home." After all those years of travel, preaching, and administration, we wondered what lay ahead. We had visions of rose beds, tomato vines, house beautiful, and vacations dancing in our heads.

Dot and I arrived at our new home on Wednesday, August 14, 1991. Days of excitement followed: boxes to unpack, flowers to plant, people to see, and even a visit to the physician for my annual physical checkup. The doctor found no problems—in fact, he was surprised that I was so healthy.

"Keep this up and you'll reach 120," he smiled.

Would anyone be surprised at the doctor's report? After all, I exercised daily, watched my diet, and lived a positive lifestyle. I was always happy. At the General Conference I was heavily involved in a fitness program. In fact, I was known as "Mr. Healthy."

But a big surprise was in store for us. Exactly six weeks later I was recovering from quadruple bypass surgery on my heart. Shock. Impossible. Heredity compounded by stress, the doctor told us.

Recovery was hard for me, partially because I was afraid and partially because I couldn't believe this was happening to me. During those long hours I quoted God's promises. My favorite was Psalm 37.

Little did I know that this was to be the first of five surgeries that would come within two and a half years, including prostate cancer and a gangrenous gallbladder.

Yes, at times I rebelled, but never did my faith fail me. I always knew God loved me and suffered with me.

Today I'm involved in speaking appointments, active in our local church, exercising, and yes, tending the roses. I have greater respect for the laws of health and encourage others to follow them. I sincerely receive each day as a precious gift from God in which I am to bless others as I glorify my Saviour.

Going home has a deeper, richer meaning to me now. And "Straight Ahead" is still my motto and theme.

"Think of Christ. Look to Him in faith, believing His promises. Keep your mind trustful. He will be your stay. Lean on Him, depend on Him. . . . Put your trust in One whose arm will never fail you. . . . But looking to Jesus you will find encouragement" (Selected Messages, book 2, p. 265).

OPENING THE FLOODGATES OF HEAVEN

> Bring the whole tithe into the storehouse. . . . Test me, . . . and see if I will not throw open the floodgates of heaven and pour out so much blessing that you will not have room enough for it. Mal. 3:10, NIV.

God has laid Himself on the line to bless abundantly His children who are faithful first in giving the 10 percent of profits that already belong to Him, and second in giving generous offerings to His cause from the remaining 90 percent.

Instead of putting their trust in God, however, most people choose to put their trust in their mortgage holder, the bank or savings and loan, Visa, MasterCard, and Discover.

Every year tax information researchers total the itemized deductions on Internal Revenue Service data from tax returns. The amounts people reported in itemized deductions during a recent year were very revealing. On average deductions based on adjusted gross income, taxpayers claimed four times more in mortgage or home equity interest paid than they did in charitable gifts! That means for every dollar placed in an offering plate, the average citizen paid out $4 in interest.

The amount people give is also revealing. Those earning $30,000 a year gave approximately 4 percent to charity. In other words, less than half a tithe—less than half of what already belongs to God. Do they think their friendly loan company will open generously the windows of heaven for borrowers, as God has promised to do?

The temptation to plunge into debt is greater today than ever. The result is a shaky pyramid of debt driven by discontentment with one's current income. And little if anything available for God.

Debt seldom brings a sense of well-being. Instead, it's associated with stress-related illnesses, such as ulcers, high blood pressure, and depression.

The solution to the stress problem is to trust in the Lord rather than money. "Do not worry about your life, what you will eat or drink; or about your body, what you will wear. Is not life more important than food, and the body more important than clothes? Look at the birds of the air; they do not sow or reap or store away in barns, and yet your heavenly Father feeds them. Are you not much more valuable than they? . . . But seek first his kingdom and his righteousness, and all these things will be given to you as well" (Matt. 6:25-33, NIV).

Are you giving an honest tithe and generous offerings? If so, pray that God will make it clear to you that His floodgates of blessing are open for you.

ARE YOU LIVING DRUG-FREE?

Aileen Ludington

If the Son sets you free, you will be free indeed. John 8:36, NIV.

Do you boast that you're drug-free? Careful! Nine out of 10 North Americans take a mind-altering drug daily. And you may be one of them.

The culprit? Everyday, ordinary, over-the-counter caffeine. It's found in coffee, tea, chocolate, sodas, and extra-strength pain relievers, just to name a few of the common things we enjoy.

But caffeine isn't addictive, is it? Look in your dictionary, and you'll find that an addictive substance is one that produces measurable physical and mental effects when withdrawn. In this sense, even small doses of caffeine taken regularly produce some degree of addiction.

Check this out for yourself by dropping all caffeine intake for a few days. The most common withdrawal symptom is headache. Fatigue, poor appetite, nausea, and vomiting sometimes occur. And symptoms may last up to five days.

Psychological withdrawal may be even harder. People become accustomed to reaching for their pick-me-up. The urge can be compared to the desire for a cigarette, and it may be just as difficult to resist. Too many people head to the refrigerator for a soda spiked with caffeine.

What's wrong with caffeine? It produces temporary increases in energy by stimulating the nervous system and raising blood sugar. While this extra energy seems desirable, it is eventually followed by a drop in energy, signaling the need for another dose of caffeine. Are you sure you want to be drawn into this endless energy yo-yo?

Continued caffeine use may produce nervousness, tremors, anxiety, and sleep disturbances. In time such symptoms can lead to chronic fatigue and persistent insomnia. Caffeine also aggravates ulcers and other stomach problems.

Sin is something like caffeine. It often looks so harmless—and tastes so good! And immediately after indulging you feel a high—the pleasurable sense of immediate gratification—before the low when the guilt sets in. Because sin seldom destroys its victim immediately, people get sucked in, and it can easily become a habit. But the good news is that Jesus can free us from sin, just as He can give us the willpower to say no to caffeine. And "if the Son sets you free, you will be free indeed."

With the Lord's help, throw out the caffeine and join the truly unhooked generation!

OPERATION
PLANET
EARTH

All this is from God, who reconciled us to himself through Christ and gave us the ministry of reconciliation: that God was reconciling the world to himself in Christ, not counting men's sins against them. And he has committed to us the message of reconciliation. 2 Cor. 5:18, 19, NIV.

I had boarded a ship as a deck passenger leaving Palau, bound for Guam. On our second day out we encountered waters stirred up by a passing typhoon. Perhaps I was too naive to be scared, as hour after nauseating hour I rode the bow of the ship up and down through the crests and troughs of the high seas. One day word leaked out that we had lost radio contact with land. We were lost at sea!

More recently I was asked to see an AIDS patient to insert a central line for intravenous access. He had destroyed every detectable vein by shooting drugs. As I reviewed the man's history, I felt moved to ask him why he used substances that he knew were so devastating. His reply: "I like them."

Two stories. Two examples of people "lost at sea." One not knowing the serious state of affairs at hand. The other knowing it but expressing no desire for rescue.

Lost at sea seems to describe our society today. Many fail to realize that they can have a better way of life, a way offered by a God who created them in love and in love emptied heaven of its most precious possession for their rescue.

I see Jesus, commander in chief of the armies of heaven, sitting at the right hand of God on the throne in Command Central, directing human affairs through this terrible time of judgment. As the world reaps the harvest of its planting, as its armies complete their work of destroying the earth under the command of Satan, every resource at heaven's command concentrates on rescuing the faithful. Every angel, every agent and power of heaven, awaits assignment from Jesus to deliver us.

But that's not all. God has extended to us the high honor of joining the powers of heaven, of serving as instruments in God's hand in reaching out to save our fellow human beings. What a privilege! None of us need be lost at sea in any way.

What part are you playing in helping to rescue those
"lost at sea" on Planet Earth?

TEMPERING
YOUR TEMPER

September 18

Cliff and Freddie Harris

[Love] is not rude, it is not self-seeking, it is not easily angered, it keeps no record of wrongs. 1 Cor. 13:5, NIV.

Although the conclusion that love "is not easily angered" is the heart of the apostle Paul's analysis of love, we tend to look upon bad temper as a harmless weakness. We speak of it as a mere infirmity of nature, a family failing, or merely a matter of temperament, not something to take into serious account in estimating a person's character. Explosions of anger are common, but does its common nature make it acceptable?

No! The Bible condemns bad temper as one of the most destructive elements in human nature. Just look at Proverbs 27:4: "Wrath is cruel, and anger is outrageous."

We've seen the destructive effects of anger in the lives of those who come to our live-in drug alternative program. For example, Joe spent three months with us trying to keep clean, but in the end it was not the drugs that killed him—it was his anger. If he didn't get his way, or if something didn't please him, look out! One day he left our program in a huff, caught a bus to Arizona, and had a confrontation with a man in a bar, and the man stabbed him. He bled to death before help could arrive.

No form of vice, worldliness, greed, or drunkenness does more to degrade society than an evil temper. It embitters life, shatters communities, destroys the most sacred relationships, devastates homes, withers men and women, and takes the bloom off childhood.

But it is not enough to deal with just the temper itself. We must go to the source and change the inmost nature, and the angry symptoms will simply die away. Souls are made sweet not by taking the acid out but by putting something in—a great love, a new spirit, the spirit of Christ. The Holy Spirit penetrating our nature will sweeten and purify us. Only He can eradicate what is wrong by renovating, regenerating, and rehabilitating the inner person.

Willpower does not change a person. Nor does time. Only Christ does! "Let this mind be in you, which was also in Christ Jesus" (Phil. 2:5).

A good temper will improve your health and make you a better witness for Jesus. Won't you invite Christ into your heart today to heal your temper?

293

HOW TO AVOID BRAINRUPTCY

Thou wilt keep him in perfect peace, whose mind is stayed on thee. Isa. 26:3.

Half the people who live to be 85 years of age have some loss of brain function that results in the confusion and memory loss we often call senility, or the mental illness we label dementia.

But it's not because they use up the brain. According to psychologist Elden Chalmers, we are born with 100 billion brain cells, and it's virtually impossible to use them all up in a lifetime. The problem results from either neglect (not using the brain enough) or abuse (not eating the right food).

Paul Giem, of Loma Linda University School of Medicine, analyzed data from the Adventist Health Study that has tracked the diets and diseases of 34,000 Seventh-day Adventists since 1976. He also compared 136 Seventh-day Adventist vegetarians with the same number of meat eaters matched by age and sex. Vegetarians had more than three times less dementia. Plus, none of the vegetarians suffered from stroke-related dementia, whereas five of the meat eaters did. Giem's conclusion? "If you stopped eating meat today, in 10 years you would have half the risk [of dementia] of a heavy meat eater."

Why does Giem believe this? He says the closest diseases to dementia, pathologically speaking, are all transmissible by eating infected meat!

Although eating meat may be linked to brain disfunction, hundreds of other things can effect your brain's health as well. But when I read about Paul Giem's study it reminded me again of the warning Ellen White gave almost 100 years ago: "Again and again I have been shown that God is bringing His people back to His original design, that is, not to subsist upon the flesh of dead animals" *(Counsels on Diet and Foods,* p. 82). "Among those who are waiting for the coming of the Lord, meat eating will eventually be done away; flesh will cease to form a part of their diet" *(ibid.,* pp. 380, 381).

Is now the time?

Lord, You know the way I should go. May Your Holy Spirit convict me to do what is best for my body and brain. Amen.

GOD'S ORANGE JUICE AND BREAD

September 20

Caris H. Lauda

Man shall not live by bread alone, but by every word that
proceedeth out of the mouth of God. Matt. 4:4.

As I began this new day I first thought of a familiar phrase from a
hymn: "Be like Jesus, this my song, in the home and in the throng; be
like Jesus all day long! I would be like Jesus."

And then do you know what? A text from God's Word clearly came to
me. Psalm 3:5: "I laid me down and slept; I awakened; for the Lord sustained
me." And then I read the words of Jesus recorded in John 10:10: "I am come
that they might have life, and that they might have it more abundantly."

Talk about "morning manna"! I am still full of that delightful food. If
you want to get the most out of your day, you've got to start with the best
possible spiritual nutrients.

A hymn is a great way to begin, but that's only like a glass of orange
juice. To really give you a good start, you need the bread of life too. That's
why I advocate that you develop the habit of reading what God says before
you read what human beings say. The more you read it, the more the Bible
will become a part of you.

Here are some statements about the importance of the Bible:

• "The Word of God is the most perfect educational book in our
world" (Review and Herald, Feb. 25, 1896).

• "The whole Bible is a revelation of the glory of God in Christ.
Received, believed, obeyed, it is the great instrumentality in the transformation of character" (The Ministry of Healing, p. 458).

• "The Bible is a field where are concealed heavenly treasures, and
they will remain hidden until, by diligent mining, they are discovered and
brought to light. The Bible is a casket containing jewels of inestimable
value, which should be so presented as to be seen in their intrinsic luster"
(Counsels to Parents and Teachers, p. 421).

I hope you'll find the Bible to be all these things in your life as you start
your day with a song and God's Word.

Have you had God's "orange juice" and "bread" yet today?
If not, sing a hymn of praise and read God's Word.
It's the healthy way to start your day!

295

IS IT TIME FOR NEW SHOES?

September 21

Kay Kuzma

For in his own eyes he flatters himself too much to detect or hate his sin. Ps. 36:2, NIV.

Cleaning out my closet, I found a pair of high heels I hadn't worn in 30 years. Groaning as I remembered how my feet used to hurt after wearing those three-inch spikes with pointed toes, I shook my head. How could I have been so vain to wear them just because someone, somewhere, decided that it was fashionable?

I gave up spikes when the children came along, but I still wore heels.

Then came the accident that severely dislocated my foot, and I had to spend a number of years in shoes with good support. Why had it taken me so long to discover the comfort of a good-fitting flat-soled shoe?

Orthopedists and podiatrists say that in flat-heeled shoes 50 percent of your weight falls on your heel. In high heels only 10 percent does, which means that 90 percent falls on your toes. Is it any wonder women so often find themselves plagued with corns and calluses, flat arches, bunions, and ingrown toenails?

Fashion has a price. And the higher the heel, the more problems. When you stand, the foot is at right angles to the length of the leg, the long axis of the body. Such posture keeps the Achilles tendon in a stretched mode— as it should be. But high heels extend the foot so the Achilles tendon becomes shortened. The ankle is now unable to flex with each step, and in trying to compensate, the arch sags. The result? Fallen arches, flat feet, and more discomfort.

But that's not all. High heels force you to arch backward to maintain balance, or you would tend to pitch forward. The bending calls for an increase in the concave curve of the lower portion of the back, the lumbar spine. Your muscles then have to support this unnatural spinal curvature. An aching back often results.

Sin is something like this. If it's fashionable—and we're vain—we'll do it, even though we know it's not good for us! The root problem, then, isn't really the "shoes," is it? It's vanity!

*Think about it—are there any unhealthful practices or sins
that because of your vanity you are unwilling to give up?*

ALCOHOL
DULLS
THE MIND

Do not conform any longer to the pattern of this world, but be transformed by the renewing of your mind. Then you will be able to test and approve what God's will is— his good, pleasing and perfect will. Rom. 12:2, NIV.

Alcohol causes emotional grief, is devoid of nutritive substances, and leads to early deaths. It stands for everything the devil is. Should we wonder, then, that Satan works hard to tempt us with this substance?

By all definitions alcohol is a drug. Its absorption and distribution in the body follows the same pattern as most other drugs and medications. A dose-response relationship exists between the amount of alcohol consumed and the resulting anxiety and loss of inhibitions. These effects quickly progress to an inability to walk a straight line, impaired reaction time, poor judgment, further lack of coordination, and uninhibited behavior. The overall effect of alcohol is that of a depressant, not a stimulant. In addition to the ethanol content, other substances called congeners found in some alcoholic drinks cause an even worse hangover.

Are there any health benefits to consuming alcohol? To date, no clinical trials using humans have proved that alcohol consumption at any level is beneficial. Any evidence that it raises HDL (good) cholesterol involves the grape used as a basis for wine, not the alcohol itself. The fact is, alcohol destroys life and health.

Alcohol consumption is impossible to control. Some may start with alcohol at meals to create a certain ambience. Soon they need it between meals to handle the rough spots in their lives, depending on it to achieve a certain state of mental numbness. It is this condition that Satan hopes to achieve in our fallen race, because it is during this state of mind that he undermines our Christ-centered resolutions.

Take the challenge and determine to not let anything interfere with the "renewing of your mind" through Christ Jesus.

THE FACTS ABOUT PHYTOCHEMICALS

September 23

Mark and Virginia Messina

These all look to you to give them their food at the proper time. When you give it to them, they gather it up; when you open your hand, they are satisfied with good things. Ps. 104:27, 28, NIV.

During the past several decades the relationship between food and disease has become clearer than ever as scientists have studied the impact of dietary habits on the risk for cancer, heart disease, and other life-threatening conditions.

The knowledge that diet is a powerful way to affect health has spawned an endless array of books and programs that promise "new" secrets to achieving its optimum. Some approaches are expensive; some are not factual; many are confusing. Perhaps most important, though, is that nearly all are superfluous. When all is said and done and all of the data have been analyzed, the truth about how to eat for good health is—not surprisingly—identical to the message that God handed down to His people through the ages in the most authoritative textbook for living—the Holy Bible.

One of the most interesting examples of God's great wisdom appears in relation to some exciting findings of the past two decades. Scientists are discovering a whole bevy of powerful compounds in foods called *phytochemicals*. They have dramatic effects on a host of diseases. Some are powerful inhibitors of cancer and can actually stop cancer cells from growing. Others protect arteries from plaque buildup, and still others prevent bones from breaking down and weakening. Of great importance is the finding that phytochemicals occur only in plant foods. Meat, fish, poultry, milk, and eggs never contain them.

The discovery of phytochemicals has given rise to the concept of designer foods. They are manufactured foods that science has fortified with phytochemicals isolated from other foods. While these foods may provide health benefits, they tend to be overprocessed, overpackaged, and overpriced. They also may contain only a fraction of the existing phytochemicals, since it is likely that science has yet to discover many of these compounds.

But while scientists and food manufacturers struggle to provide us with health-promoting designer foods, we need only to look to nature to see that these foods have always existed. God gave us the only designer foods we need when He created grains, vegetables, fruits, beans, nuts, and seeds (Gen. 1:29, 30; 3:18).

*Lord, help me to remember that Your knowledge and
Your guidance in all things are perfect and complete.*

THE SOLUTION
TO THE
SIN PROBLEM

Elmar P. Sakala

If you live according to the sinful nature, you will die; but if by the Spirit you put to death the misdeeds of the body, you will live, because those who are led by the Spirit of God are sons of God. Rom 8:13, 14, NIV.

S in has a way of bumping us around and squeezing the life out of us. But Jesus has a solution for everything. Just as He solved the problem of how the developing baby could be free to grow within the uterus of a mother, He has a way of dealing with the sin problem.

But first, take a look at how God protects the developing fetus. Since the walls of the uterus stretch only in response to the growing baby, one would think the baby would always be squeezed so tightly it would be unable to move at all. As you might expect, the all-knowing Creator anticipated this problem and prepared a perfect solution—a solution called amniotic fluid (that's not just a pun!).

This water bath, warmed to body temperature by the mother's body, continuously surrounds the baby. The fluid itself is enclosed within a special lined sac called the amniotic sac. The watery space inside the amniotic sac allows the baby room to exercise its arms and legs. The fluid acts as a shock absorber to protect the developing person from being bumped or injured.

The fluid keeps the baby's skin soft and moist throughout the months of life inside its mother's body. Too little or too much amniotic fluid could lead to significant problems for the little swimmer. God has carefully designed that the amount of amniotic fluid will always carefully stay in balance. It is continuously being removed as the baby swallows it, and continuously being replaced in just the right amount as the fetal kidneys produce new fluid.

Our Creator did not leave anything to chance when it came to our requirements as a developing baby. Nor did He leave anything to chance when it came to our needs as a developing Christian. He knew we would need to be cushioned from the onslaught of sin, so His solution was the Holy Spirit. Being bathed in the Holy Spirit, we can be protected from error, cushioned from overwhelming temptation, comforted when discouraged, and led to the truth in Jesus. What an amazing solution to the sin problem!

Each morning ask the Holy Spirit to lead you, and you can be born again each day as a son or daughter of God.

299

A LITTLE
LAUGHTER

Caroline Watkins

---

*Be happy, young man, while you are young, and let your heart
give you joy in the days of your youth. Eccl. 11:9, NIV.*

Bill and Gloria Gaither have a song that refers to the sound of children
at play. Is there anything more refreshing than the laughter of children
as they play?

It's a shame that so many of us lose this joyous "music" as we grow
older and get bogged down in our stress-filled lives. We long for fun and
fulfillment, for satisfaction in our jobs, and for the positive power of peace.
And we end up with distress instead of delight, crisis instead of calm.

In my search for a stress-free lifestyle, I've followed the example of
King David and tried to slow down and get in touch with God through
prayer and meditation.

As the apostle Paul admonished, I had sought to find peace, joy, and
contentment. But there was still something missing. I discovered the answer
one day when my little nephew, Calvin, began laughing as he played with
a plastic toy. Playfully I said "stop," and he laughed louder. It was contagious, and soon both of us were laughing so hard we couldn't talk.

Later Calvin mumbled under his breath, "I didn't know you could
laugh, Aunt Caroline!"

That hit me! Had my daily life become so completely permeated by the
seriousness of just existing that I had forgotten how to laugh?

Dr. Lee Burke, a specialist in preventative care at Loma Linda
University, says, "I think laughter extends life for months, perhaps years.
Happiness is good medicine." Burke, whose work is reviewed in the
Journal of the National Cancer Institute, mentions a dozen scientific stud-
ies showing the Bible's advice to be accurate: "A merry heart does good,
like medicine" (Prov. 17:22, NKJV). Dr. David Spiegel, of Stanford
University School of Medicine, agrees: "It is very possible that happiness is
a factor in longevity."

When we make a conscientious effort to get in touch with God, think
positive thoughts, and to be genuinely happy, eventually these traits will
become second nature to us. I'm thankful for what I've learned from David
and Paul, but I'm most thankful to little Calvin for the music of laughter.

*Today, find something to laugh about. Admire the marvelous
things God has created for your enjoyment. Find joy in just being alive.*

ARE YOU DYING OF THIRST?

"I will restore you to health and heal your wounds," declares the Lord. Jer. 30:17, NIV.

When you think of healing, probably the words "medicine," "hospitals," "physical therapy," and "doctor bills" come to mind. But in many cases the cure might be as close as your kitchen faucet—and it's basically free! Yes, I'm talking about water.

In 1905 Ellen White wrote: "In health and in sickness, pure water is one of Heaven's choicest blessings. Its proper use promotes health. It is the beverage which God provided to quench the thirst of animals and man. Drunk freely, it helps to supply the necessities of the system, and assists nature to resist disease" *(Counsels on Diet and Foods, p. 419).*

But the problem is, most of us aren't drinking it, or at least not enough of it. In fact, your body can be chronically dehydrated and yet you don't realize it because you don't feel thirsty.

If you do not drink at least six to eight glasses of water a day, give or take a little depending on your height and weight, you are dehydrated!

Remaining dehydrated for long periods of time introduces many physical ailments that would disappear with an adequate water intake. Your body needs water to prevent your blood from becoming concentrated, which then draws water from the cells around it. When this happens, you feel thirsty, and too many people satisfy this craving by drinking coffee, tea, or soft drinks. *But these do not count as water.* What your body needs is six to eight glasses of *water* per day if its various organs are to work efficiently.

Here's what Michael Peck said about the merits of drinking eight glasses of water a day: "When I first started this program I was overweight, with high blood pressure and suffering from asthma and allergies, which I have had since a small child. Today, I have my weight and blood pressure under control . . . and the program reduced the frequency of asthma and allergy-related problems to the point of practical nonexistence."

God wants to restore our health to us. Drink freely of the "medicine" He has provided, and see if it doesn't make a difference.

*Don't wait to feel thirsty to drink water for your physical health,
and drink God's Word for your spiritual health.*

SABBATH, A MILEPOST IN TIME

Steven L. Haley

My eyes have seen the defeat of my adversaries; my ears have heard the rout of my wicked foes. The righteous will flourish like a palm tree, they will grow like a cedar of Lebanon; planted in the house of the Lord, they will flourish in the courts of our God. Ps. 92:11-13, NIV.

As you stand in the checkout line of a supermarket, they are difficult to avoid. As hard as you try, every now and then you give in and read the tabloid headlines: "Pterodactyls Invade Backyard Barbecue" or "Elvis Alive and Well, Working as a Bellhop in Toledo."

Stop and consider the incredible popularity of the tabloids. Their appeal lies in their claim of knowing the unknowable.

No matter what great leaps we've taken for more than five decades in the fields of science, medicine, and technology, our human craving to know more is never satisfied. We probe the universe and beyond, and admit that there are still things to be learned and discovered on our own planet. Scientists theorize and Hollywood dramatizes the unknown, and while we have come to understand much about the present world, two places in time remain a mystery for many—the place of our beginning and the place of our end. "Prehistoric Lizard to Swallow New York in '97" hardly satisfies our need to know!

King David knew where to look for answers. He found them in the God He worshiped, and in a time and place called Sabbath. To David the momentary prosperity of the wicked meant little before the promised reality that someday the righteous would be rewarded. "My eyes have seen the defeat of my adversaries. . . . The righteous will flourish like a palm tree." David's peaceful, calm assurance came from a knowledge that he was shaped by the hand of the Creator, and his destiny was nothing less than eternal life in a world made new.

Every week, despite our tendency to forget, God reminds us that we are His family. We are part of His plan. From generation to generation a milepost in time called "Sabbath" invites us to put aside our fears. To lay down our temptation to rely upon great minds for answers, and instead to believe that God alone determines our destination.

May this Sabbath bless you with a reality known across the breadth of the cosmos that the past, the present, and most exciting of all, the future belong to Him. And so do *you!*

God of the universe, thank You for the Sabbath to remind me weekly of who I am—a person created in Your image—and where I am going—life eternal. Regardless of tabloid headlines that could trouble my mind, I can rest in this assurance. Amen.

CHRONO-LOGICALLY ADVANTAGED

September 28

Edwin H. Krick

Being wise is better than being strong; yes, knowledge is more important than strength. Prov. 24:5, TEV.

Solomon implies in Proverbs 24:5 that becoming a senior citizen has some advantages; that the wisdom of age is more important than the strength of youth. Elsewhere he bemoans the passing of time: "So remember your Creator while you are still young, before those dismal days and years come when you will say, 'I don't enjoy life'" (Eccl. 12:1, TEV).

Not much has changed in 4,000 years! Many of my older patients see it as did the Solomon of Ecclesiastes 12. "Don't get old, Doc," they would tell me. "It's no fun." I would ask, "When does 'old' begin?"

How long your cells last is determined in part by your genes, but mainly by the choices you make: how you use your mind and treat your body, which in turn will affect your perception of how old you are.

In these days of "politically correct" language, words such as "handicapped" have been replaced by such expressions as "physically disadvantaged." It would seem appropriate to call "senior citizens" "chronologically *advantaged*"! How can you make that a reality?

When I was in medical school my only physical exercise was limited to summer vacations. My lack of fitness painfully became evident after I descended a mountain peak with a limp lasting several days. Finally I realized that it is important to exercise consistently. Gradually, with regular exercise, my knees have improved to where I can climb mountains with no pain whatsoever. My legs are now "younger" than they were 35 years ago!

Likewise, your mind must be used to keep it young. My mother, in her mid-80s, reads three hours or more a day and continues to teach a wonderfully inspirational Sabbath school lesson. She has taught me a profound lesson about brainpower: the most important aspect of being "chronologically advantaged" is the opportunity to delve more deeply into the Bible and its messages for us, and to share those insights with family, friends, and neighbors.

Solomon was right. "Remember your Creator," and the days of your youth may last well into your "chronologically advantaged" years!

What are you doing to grow "better" as you grow older?

THE HEALING POWER OF FORGIVENESS

Forgive us the wrong we have done, as we have forgiven those who have wronged us. Matt. 6:12, NEB.

Sometimes it feels so good to be driving down a long freeway, mind in semineutral, recalling how another person has done us ill. Our mind wanders through scenes in which we publicly humiliate them, proving that they were wrong and we were in the right. As the miles pass we fantasize about friends taking sides with us against the wrongdoer. We might even miss our off-ramp as we finally picture the judgment in heaven confirming our personal verdict!

Our supposed ability to judge correctly the failings of another makes us satisfied with our own sense of justice and right. Too often we need to nurse a grudge, rehearse a wrong, as a way of feeling OK about ourselves. To build up all kinds of bad feelings about another person, to drain off major energy into dark memories, to ration out little tidbits of forgiveness only when we feel avenged—but what a waste!

We miss the point of how useless it is to judge other people. Perhaps that is why it is so hard for us to grasp God's forgiveness. As human beings we have no experiential reference point, no familiar feeling in our own soul, by which we can make sense of a God who forgives. As a result we think that should we forgive someone who has wronged us, it would be as if we were saying that their wrong really didn't matter.

Lewis Smedes, in his book *Forgive and Forget*, suggests that forgiveness is really for us, not for the one who has harmed us. Forgiving cleanses *us* of all the accusations and built-up animosity we have directed at others. These benefits to us help us sense why God is so eager to make His forgiveness known to us. When we let go of our petty grudges and move on to forgiveness, then we understand that God has indeed forgiven us.

Real growing has nothing to do with announcing other people's failures. Rather, it has to do with helping them learn the lessons from their bad choices and then move on. Learn the lesson and move on—that's all. And that's all for you, too.

Are you nursing a grudge? Is there someone you need to forgive?
Perhaps you need to forgive yourself. How can you allow the
lesson to be learned and move on?

HOLY SPIRIT
TRANSMISSIONS

So, as the Holy Spirit says: "Today, if you hear his voice, do not harden your hearts as you did in the rebellion, during the time of testing in the desert." Heb. 3:7, 8, NIV.

God speaks to us through the Holy Spirit, making impressions in our brains. Sometimes it is so direct we seem to "hear" the message. At other times it is through a dream, insights, or something we hear or read.

Since God's primary vehicle for speaking to us is the brain, it is of vital importance to keep the brain as healthy as possible.

Have you ever had a bad telephone connection and had trouble catching the message? Once I received an important call, but poor reception cut out or distorted parts of the words. I was eager to make a good impression and hesitant to ask them to call me back, so I immediately concentrated my full attention on what the person was saying.

Usually when I'm on the phone, my husband can stand beside me, get my attention, and give me a short message, and I have no trouble catching what the caller is saying while at the same time perceiving my husband's need and nodding or motioning a reply. But with such faulty reception I actually closed my eyes and plugged my other ear to keep out all distraction. When Jan came by, I shook my head vigorously to tell him I couldn't listen to him at that moment. Because of the faulty reception, I had to concentrate totally to catch the message.

That's similar to our reception of the Holy Spirit. There's never anything wrong with the transmission—the problem is always at our end in the receptor equipment that God has given us the responsibility to maintain: our brains. The better our equipment is functioning, the easier it will be for God to get His message through, even if we aren't concentrating completely. But if our equipment is functioning at peak capacity as designed, and if we give our entire concentration to the reception, it will lessen the chances of the devil being able to distort God's message.

How do we keep the equipment functioning optimally so no distortion creeps in? Our brains depend on what we eat and do.

How healthy is your brain?

Think about your brain next time you take a bite of something, and ask, "Is this good brain food?" Remember, God designed our brains to operate on His original diet of fruits, vegetables, nuts, and grains. Junk foods clog the system.

GIVE YOUR "MAW" TO JESUS

October 1

Dane J. Griffin

This shall be the priest's due from . . . them that offer a sacrifice, whether it be ox or sheep; and they shall give unto the priest the shoulder, and the two cheeks, and the maw. Deut. 18:3.

God intended that the sanctuary ceremonies should teach us about the plan of salvation. Each ceremony and sacrifice had double significance. Not only was it to be a foreshadowing of Christ's atonement, but it had a personal application of the sacrifice we, God's people, needed to make if we were to be obedient to God.

For example, when a Jew brought an ox or a sheep as an offering, the priest would receive certain parts. If the person bringing the sacrifice withheld any part, his or her sacrifice was not acceptable. Specifically, the priest was to receive "the shoulder, and the two cheeks, and the maw."

What is the "maw"? It is the stomach.

The stomach? Why would God want the priest to get the stomach?

The sacrifice of the animal was symbolic of us sacrificing ourselves to God. Could it be that God specifically mentioned the stomach because it's the part of our body that we find so hard to control?

Think about it. The first temptation on earth involved Eve's stomach—the eating of forbidden fruit. And the first major test in Jesus' ministry concerned His stomach, when Satan challenged Him to turn the stones into bread. Even today most of us struggle more over physical appetite than any other health-related issue.

The lesson is clear. When we give ourselves to the Lord, our High Priest, we must also give Him our stomachs. We must surrender our perverted, worldly appetites. If we do not, our sacrifice is unacceptable.

Paul says in Philippians 3:18, 19: "As I have often told you before and now say again even with tears, many live as enemies of the cross of Christ. Their destiny is destruction, *their god is their stomach*, and their glory is in their shame" (NIV).

"Eating has much to do with religion. The spiritual experience is greatly affected by the way in which the stomach is treated" *(Counsels on Health,* p. 577).

Have you given the High Priest all that He requires? Are you willing to surrender your "maw" to Him?

What does it mean to give your stomach to Jesus? What specifically could you do today to show you have given your stomach to Jesus?

306

THE DREADED WORD: ALZHEIMER'S

October 2

Connie Coble Starkey

Have mercy on me, O God, have mercy on me, for in you my soul takes refuge. I will take refuge in the shadow of your wings until the disaster has passed. Ps. 57:1, NIV.

Alzheimer's—the word filled my mind with dread, fear, anger, and a chilling sense of hopelessness. The doctor was compassionate yet direct, knowing that my family needed to confront the reality as quickly as possible. Dad had given indications that things had changed—getting lost driving to familiar places, neglecting to finish a project, giving a puzzled glance when conversation didn't flow easily—situations that always came effortlessly for him before. The reality was that we were going to lose him, not in an immediate, physical way, but through a slow and sad deterioration of his mind. An odd sense of urgency came over me. I must live every precious moment I could with the man whom I could always find myself in a debate with, and who loved me dearly.

I questioned God's role in this. How did He fit into our inescapable tragedy? Where did miracles tie in with what we were facing? Why Dad? Tough questions to grapple with, and answers did not come—at least, not for a while.

Dad became carefree, happy, and oblivious to the tragedy, while our family began working through the emotions of shock, denial, and grief, then rapidly moved toward a sense of camaraderie and communication. We would have family councils to talk openly about our fears and together discover our talents and abilities to meet those challenges.

Slowly I began to see God's hand in our little world. He didn't cause Alzheimer's, but He did guide us to Emory University, where Mom and Dad were able to be part of a research team/support group. God didn't move mountains to cure the illness or restore Dad's vocabulary, but He did create opportunity for finding creative talents in our family and friends to meet the specific needs.

Where was God and why did it happen? I don't have all the answers, but I am at peace knowing that He gave us strength and comfort through the actions of family, friends, and the medical professionals who loved Dad. And really, it won't be long until Dad and I can debate once again—only this time it will be on things infinitely more fascinating.

Just as the rainbow follows the rain, smiles follow the pain.
If you look for the blessings in the bad things, you'll find them.
Let God be your refuge.

PRAYER MAKES A DIFFERENCE

October 3

Delbert W. Baker

> Confess your sins to each other and pray for each other so that you may be healed. The prayer of a righteous man is powerful and effective. James 5:16, NIV.

Prayer does make a difference. During the past decade increasing research has examined the efficacy of prayer in the healing process. For centuries Christians have attested to the power of prayer in the context of healing. But for the scientific community to become interested in it is indeed amazing.

Larry Dossey, physician and author, in his book *Healing Words*, corroborates the testimony of Christians on the power of prayer in healing. After graduating from medical school with the belief that prayer was little more than superstition, he confesses that "for many years I'd ignored prayer. I considered it an arbitrary, optional frill that simply was not in the same league as drugs and surgery." However, after years of practicing medicine Dossey discovered a single scientific study that strongly supported the power of prayer in getting well. He describes how his "white-coated scientific" worldview became unsettled and he started on 10 years of research examining the relationship of prayer and healing. After extensive research Dossey found that the majority of more than 100 experiments "exhibited the criteria of good science" and showed that prayer brings about significant changes.

What is Dossey's conclusion? "Prayer complements but does not take the place of good medicine." He describes how prayer has great potential in the healing realm and may be compatible with modern physics. Dossey views prayer not as something that needs "selling" but as "a neglected area of medical science."

One may not agree with all of Dossey's views or conclusions. Others may argue that Christians don't need science to back up what they already know. Nevertheless, Dossey's research focuses attention on the reality of healing from a spiritual perspective.

Prayer is a means for us to communicate with the God of the universe, who has made us and sustains us. It is through this means that God invites all of us, His creation, to take advantage of His wonderful and effective power. As the apostle James says: "The prayer of a righteous man is powerful and effective."

Is there someone you know who is hurting or ill and needs healing? Your prayers can make a difference. Why not talk to God about it right now?

"EATING"
THE BREAD
OF LIFE

Kenneth I. Burke

> While they were eating, Jesus took bread, gave thanks and broke it, and gave it to his disciples, saying, "Take and eat; this is my body." Matt. 26:26, NIV.

"YOU ARE WHAT YOU EAT" reads the sign on the health food store near my home. Health enthusiasts, taking that slogan to heart, sometimes devise innovative dietary plans to ensure good health. They advocate an "all-natural diet"; an "organic diet"; a "juice diet." There are many "diets" and many "cures"! But did you know about the highly recommended diet spelled out precisely by Jesus?

"I am the bread of life," the record quotes Jesus as saying. "Your fathers ate the manna in the wilderness, and are dead" (John 6:48, 49, NKJV). As though eager for every hearer to understand His words, Jesus returned to the thought again and again: "This is the bread which comes down from heaven, that one may eat of it and not die. I am the living bread which came down from heaven. If anyone eats of this bread, he will live forever; and the bread that I shall give is My flesh, which I shall give for the life of the world" (verses 50, 51, NKJV).

However carefully I monitor my eating habits (and I do attempt to eat a variety of foods, simply prepared), my spiritual ancestors did better. They ate manna.

And they are all dead.

What's more, while on the diet they often lacked the positive emotions conducive to health.

In contrast, Jesus says that the person who eats His flesh and drinks His blood "lives" in Him and He lives "in them" too.

And there's more. "He who eats this bread," says Jesus, "will live forever" (verse 58, NKJV).

What a diet! It can be my diet if I take His promise personally: "I did not come to call the righteous, but sinners" (Matt. 9:13, NKJV). "Come to Me, all you who . . . are heavy laden" (Matt. 11:28, NKJV). "The one who comes to Me I will by no means cast out" (John 6:37, NKJV).

It's encouraging to reflect that when we "eat the flesh" in this way, the Father looks at us and sees His Son. To Him we are whole. In this sense, and in His eyes, we are what we eat.

*Invite Jesus to live in you today, and experience
renewed energy and efficiency.*

PRECIOUS
IN HIS
SIGHT

October 5

Blondel E. Senior

God saw all that he had made, and it was very good. Gen. 1:31, NIV.

When Nabo came to Advent Home, a residential facility for hurting boys, everyone knew he was different. He spoke in monosyllables and could not carry on a conversation. Having never played before, he was clumsy and uncoordinated on the ball field. His social skills and hygiene were on the level of a 4-year-old, even though he was 16. His peers described him as a gross couch potato.

His story is a sad one of parental neglect. Both parents were on drugs. When he was 4 his mother left, so his father raised him. When his father went to work he threatened Nabo, telling him not to leave the house or else he would be kidnapped, so Nebo lived on the couch and occupied his time with three things: potato chips, soft drinks, and watching TV and videos. He did not go to school, so his reading skills were at the second-grade level and his math even lower. Nabo was not mentally disabled—just socially and emotionally deprived for too many years.

In the group home it was difficult for Nabo to adjust to the food. A healthy diet was boring. Not being able to watch television made him restless. He could not focus on his classwork. Idleness and indulgence were his daily companions. His brain needed to be reoriented to responsible living.

Starved for attention and stimulation, in counseling and group therapy he was like a sponge absorbing everything. Nabo learned fast, even though he had a poor self-image. His academic performance jumped to the eighth-grade level, and his hygiene and social skills improved. In 15 months Nabo grew into a productive and aspiring teenager. Now 18, he will be finishing high school in two years. He has a girlfriend and aims to go on to vocational school.

I've learned that everyone is precious in God's sight. And irrespective of our backgrounds, God's healing power is available to all. If you've been hurt or neglected in your childhood, ask God to heal you and to help you reach your God-given potential.

Heavenly Father, help me to realize that in Your eyes I am precious. Please heal my feelings of inferiority, and help me reach the potential You created within me.

HEALING THE BROKENHEARTED

Blessed are those who mourn, for they shall be comforted. Matt. 5:4, NKJV.

The Spirit of the Lord God is upon Me, . . . He has sent Me to heal the brokenhearted, . . . to comfort all who mourn, . . . to give them beauty for ashes, the oil of joy for mourning, the garment of praise for the spirit of heaviness" (Isa. 61:1-3, NKJV). If we had none other, this one Bible reference would suffice to tell us that we have a loving God who will light our way through the darkest night.

1. *God will give us beauty for ashes,* radiance after the ashes of the volcanic eruptions that overwhelm our lives. It's well known that the land is renewed after fire blackens fields and forests. Beauty indeed appears after the ashes. Crumbling lava and volcanic ash make the most fertile soil. So God grants us enrichment after we are consumed by a fire that we fear will destroy us. "He lifts [us] from the dust—yes, from a pile of ashes" (1 Sam. 2:8, TLB).

2. *God will give us the oil of joy for mourning.* Jesus often went to the Mount of Olives to pray. I've thought about Jesus' agony that night being the oil pressed out, to become our oil of joy. The garden experience that night was horrendous: "Who, in the days of His flesh, when He had offered up prayers and supplications, with vehement cries and tears . . ." (Heb. 5:7, NKJV). We need not be ashamed of our tears—Jesus wept several times.

3. *God will give us the garment of praise for our spirit of heaviness.* We are to wrap ourselves in praise. It is will, not feeling. The feeling comes *after* we have obeyed and praised, in spite of!

Jesus' "garment was seamless, woven in one piece from top to bottom" (John 19:23, NIV). In His time people indicated great sorrow by tearing their clothes, but His particular garb was left whole. Is this our garment of praise, praise that Jesus comforts and saves us? Come, let us wrap Jesus' seamless garment around us!

If you are mourning, Jesus wants to comfort you.
Read again the wonderful promise in Isaiah 61:1-3.
Write it down and memorize it. He will turn your sorrow into joy!

BETTER
THAN
BIRDS

October 7
Walter Thompson

> Look at the birds of the air; they do not sow or reap or store away in barns, and yet your heavenly Father feeds them. Are you not much more valuable than they? Matt. 6:26, NIV.

I have a friend who helps school kids gain the skills they need to live and grow up in our drug-infested society without becoming dependent on drugs. Much of what she does has to do with building the child's feelings of personal value.

The dearth of self-esteem among us is a major contributing factor to destructive lifestyles and inflated medical care costs. In an effort to change the present course of society, a flood of books and theories attempt to promote and develop self-esteem.

Where does one find self-esteem? Sometimes our youth are encouraged to give themselves pep talks, expounding their own worth. At other times students seek it in scholastic achievement. Many schools use sports in their effort to help the kids. Later, self-esteem comes from a "successful" job or career, or is sought in promotions and bonuses. In the home its absence often shows up as jealousy, sensitivity, or controlling and manipulation.

Human self-esteem sounds good. The theory is rational. But such esteem has no lasting value, no real benefit to the achiever. Like the grass of the field, it may flourish for a moment, but in the end it often fades into disappointment and despair.

Jesus' sermon on the mountainside provides the only real source of self-esteem. It covers all of the bases for meeting our deepest heart longings and personal needs. He says to look at the birds. See the flowers. Study God's activity in nature and note His love for you there. Check out His providential guidance in your life. Watch for answered prayers. Love your neighbor as yourself. And store up your treasure in heaven (see Matt. 5-7).

True self-esteem comes from finding your place in the cycle of love that governs all of God's universe. As we receive the benefits of life, gratefully acknowledge their source, and then add our own unique touch and pass them on in service to others, feelings of value will be a natural by-product.

If you'd like to boost your feelings of value, read Matthew 5 through 7, write down at least three suggestions Jesus makes that you can put into practice, and then just do them!

KIDS, COKE, AND CAFFEINE

Dick Duerksen

I have told you these things, so that in me you may have peace. John 16:33, NIV.

I spent nearly five years of my life as principal of a Christian boarding high school. About 260 teenagers studied there, each of them testing the boundaries and pushing the edges as they grew through adolescence.

One of the rules they pushed the hardest was the "Thou shalt not use caffeinated drinks on the buses" rule. The school used buses and vans to take the kids home on vacations and to transport them to the mall, to snow skiing, on band and choir trips, and anywhere else groups of teenagers could devise to go. But "no caffeine on the trips." Since it was one of the rules I inherited from the previous regime, I asked about it in faculty meeting. The response was swift and direct.

"Caffeine turns these kids into little monsters."

"They'll tear the bus apart."

"You'll go crazy if you're the faculty member on the bus."

Never having heard Coke advertise such responses to its cans of soda, I decided to try an experiment. Who's right, the faculty or the kids?

I was using the old Greyhound bus and driving the band to Sheridan, Wyoming. On Friday, with a busful of hyper kids eager to get off campus, I enforced the rule. No caffeinated drinks. They argued, but drank 7-Up and acted like normal teenagers all the way to Sheridan.

Monday, the bus filled with exhausted kids "eager" to get back to school, I offered to bend the rule. The 7-Eleven manager sure sold a lot of Coke that morning. It was a carefully monitored nonscientific study. Their exhaustion turned to energetic hyperactivity, and the kids just about tore the bus apart. I drove onto campus humbled and more willing to trust the judgment of wiser minds.

A little caffeine does a great job of bringing tired teens awake. It also grants them energy beyond what they are able to control while traveling in confined places. Much caffeine has them bouncing off the walls.

I wonder, what does caffeine do to their hearts that makes their bodies go bonkers?

Could I be taking anything into my body or mind that is making my life go bonkers? God, who created us, knows our bodies run best on healthful food—and noncaffeinated beverages.

WALK YOUR WAY TO BETTER HEALTH

Jan W. and Kay Kuzma

October 9

"But I will restore you to health and heal your wounds," declares the Lord. Jer. 30:17, NIV.

Mavis Lindgren, plagued with severe lung ailments since childhood, finally took responsibility for her own health when she was in her early 60s.

While attending a series of lectures by Dr. Charles Thomas at Loma Linda University, she began to walk every day. She prayed as she walked that the exercise program might help her worsening lung ailment, weakened heart, and weakened skeletal muscles. Decades of inactivity had added 20 extra pounds to her five-foot-two frame. Over the months she increased her walking distance. Before long she took up jogging. She lost the extra weight, and her lung ailments disappeared. "I haven't been sick a day since," she often says.

The running increased. Soon she went on the trail six days a week, five miles at a time—and loved it. At age 70 she entered the Sacramento Pepsi 20-Mile Run. She not only finished the 20 miles but also set a record for her age group. Since then she has gone on to finish marathons (26.2 miles) in which she also set records for her age group, only to come back and reset the record on several occasions. But she says of her races that she doesn't compete with others, she races only against herself. She runs for the love of running, not for the sake of a reward.

Mavis eats a high-carbohydrate vegetarian diet and averages 50 miles of running a week. She believes that although the process of aging is inevitable, it is possible to maintain a higher level of fitness throughout the decline by adhering to simple, healthful habits. Also she suggests that in addition to proper nutrition, sufficient rest, and exercise, the fourth component of a balanced lifestyle is gratitude of heart.

The headline on an article on the sports page of the November 9, 1993, *New York Times* read, "Don't Look Back, Father Time, Mavis Lindgren, 86, Is Gaining on You."

God has designed our bodies to have incredible restorative powers if we treat them right. To renew your health, regardless of how old you are, do as Mavis did. Start walking!

Take the walking challenge: walk 300 more steps today
than yesterday. Do this for two weeks, and see the difference
it makes in the way you feel.

KEEP YOUR HEART WITH DILIGENCE

Harvey Heidinger

Above all else, guard your heart, for it is the wellspring of life. Prov. 4:23, NIV.

I 've often asked the "over the hill" generation if they would like to go back and relive their teen years if they had a chance. The resounding majority agree they'd like to be young, but relive those traumatic, life-changing years? "No way!"

I work with adolescents and young adults at the University of California at Riverside as a pediatrician specializing in adolescent health. On weekends I'm involved in planning programs and activities for the young people in our church. So I'm well acquainted with Generation X. If I could tell them one message that could help them live a long, healthy life, it would be this: "Guard your heart, for it is the wellspring of life."

Adolescence is a time of change. You're developing social skills, making lifelong friends—one of which may become your life partner. Separating from your family of origin, you're learning to assume adult roles, making a career choice, and developing an altruistic giving attitude from immature self-centered thinking. And at the same time your physical body is changing.

But the Lord has not left you alone during this stormy time of change. He has provided you with valuable counsel in a book written especially for those who are developing their own value systems: Proverbs. Follow the advice in this book. Choose good friends, for "a good man out of the good treasure of his heart brings forth good things, and an evil man out of the evil treasure brings forth evil things" (Matt. 12:35, NKJV).

Guarding your heart means watching the input from the computer and television screens, from the language and music listened to, and from the associations and friendships made.

Jesus said: "I am come that they might have life, and that they might have it more abundantly" (John 10:10). Service to others flowing from a healthy self-esteem will be an effective prevention of drug use and illicit behavior.

The exuberance of adolescence, followed by an enriched adult life, is a wonderful preparation for the fulfillment of life eternal with Jesus Christ. Don't waste these precious years.

Are you guarding the avenues to your heart and head?
Don't waste the time God has given you on pleasures that lead to a dead end. Choose life!

DO YOU NEED A HEART TRANSPLANT?

Elmar P. Sakala and
Leonard L. Bailey

And I will give you a new heart—I will give you new and right desires—and put a new spirit within you. I will take out your stony hearts of sin and give you new hearts of love. Eze. 36:26, TLB.

Two babies were both destined to die from fatal congenital defects. One was already born; the other was still in his mother's womb.

Baby Gabrielle came into the world with the major part of her brain and skull absent. Even though her heart was healthy and pumping vigorously, no surgery or transplant could ever correct her terrible brain defect. She was about to die.

Baby Paul was diagnosed before birth with an underdevelopment of his left heart. No problems would develop as long as he remained in the uterus. But immediately after his birth he would need both sides of his heart. He too would die without treatment. The best chance for Paul was a heart transplant. His name went on the heart transplant waiting list.

Gabrielle's grief-stricken parents realized their daughter could not be saved. Perhaps her life could have some purpose if another baby, one who might also die, could be saved by receiving her healthy organs. Her parents decided that just as soon as brain death was apparent, they would give the ultimate gift, the gift of life, by offering her healthy heart to a baby who needed one. Death was declared within another day.

Baby Gabrielle's body and unborn Baby Paul, still in his mother's womb, were flown to Loma Linda University Medical Center, where the decision was made for Paul to receive Gabrielle's still-healthy heart. Baby Paul deteriorated so rapidly after birth that without Gabrielle's heart being immediately available he would certainly have died. Paul became the youngest heart transplant recipient ever attempted up to that time, receiving a new heart at the age of 90 minutes! As of this writing Paul is a healthy 8-year-old, his life made possible by Gabrielle's ultimate gift.

We may each be lost, as Baby Paul would have been, unless we receive a new heart—a new spiritual heart. Sin has flawed our hearts, but Christ offers us a new heart to replace our "heart of stone." Unlike Gabrielle, who had only one heart to give, our Saviour has no limit to the number of recipients He can provide for. While Gabrielle's gift will not last forever, the heart that God gives is designed to last throughout eternity.

Have you taken advantage of His transplant offer?

A LITTLE LOUDER, PLEASE

October 12

Henry C. Martin

Listen to my instruction and be wise; do not ignore it. Blessed is the man who listens to me, watching daily at my doors, waiting at my doorway. For whoever finds me finds life and receives favor from the Lord. Prov. 8:33-35, NIV.

"Pardon me." "Would you repeat that, please?" "I don't hear as well as I would like." Such comments now form part of my vocabulary. I never imagined that I would suffer hearing loss. The audiologist suggests that my high-frequency loss means that I will miss up to 30 percent of a conversation. Communication is especially challenging for me when I am trying to understand someone speaking in a public area, such as a crowded church lobby. I find it is easier to hear when I can see their mouth. That means that even mustaches make hearing difficult! Particularly challenging for me are people who speak quickly or those who don't first alert me they are going to speak. Hearing difficulty can even contribute to elevated blood pressure.

Scripture says: "Behold, I make all things new" (Rev. 21:5). To have new ears with perfect hearing is one more reason I am eager for the Lord to return.

Hearing aids have been a blessing. But even with these sophisticated devices it is still difficult to filter out crowd noises or wind from an open window. Being close enough to hear the chirping of birds is a real treat. Understanding whispering is virtually impossible. Others don't realize that their normal conversation actually goes over my head, because I constantly hear a sound like that of whistling teakettles. I really need to concentrate to understand what people are saying.

Effective communication means that the receiver clearly understands the message. Sometimes loved ones think I'm not listening or don't want to hear. If someone dear to you gives you a blank look after you have spoken to them, try to speak more slowly and distinctly next time. This invisible disability will be removed in "the twinkling of an eye" when the Lord returns in glory. In the meantime, get my attention, speak slowly and distinctly, and a little louder—but don't shout.

And when it comes to the Lord, I want perfect spiritual ears to catch every word! So, please, Lord, if I'm not listening, speak a little louder!

Thank You, Lord, for the ability to hear. So many things we take for granted. And may I always listen to Your instruction.

GET RID OF
HEADACHE
PAIN

Betty Pierson and
Kay Kuzma

The righteous cry out, and the Lord hears them; he delivers them from all their troubles. Ps. 34:17, NIV.

More than 45 million Americans have chronic tension headaches, and 16 to 18 million of them suffer migraines, which have an even uglier reputation. Migraines bring severe, usually one-sided throbbing pain, often accompanied by nausea and vomiting and sometimes tremor and dizziness. What can you do to prevent this debilitating pain? Here's what Betty Pierson writes:

"Headaches have plagued me since adolescence, so I was not alarmed when I developed a 'banger' while on vacation. As I flew home, the headache worsened until I was afraid I would die; then I was afraid I wouldn't!

"I often prayed and asked for deliverance from the pain. My family doctor referred me to a neurologist, who injected me with Sumatriptan, which cut the pain in half, but it was still disabling. Other medications were tried. After three weeks with no improvement I was referred to Johns Hopkins. The neurologist there described himself as a preventative medicine doctor. He took me off all medication and asked me for a period of four weeks to follow a migraine-prevention program that eliminated foods with high amounts of tyramine, an amino acid. This included foods containing caffeine (such as chocolate), citrus fruits, processed meats, nuts, peanut butter, milk, yogurt, sour cream, and cheese. I did not believe this program would work, but with God helping me through each day of the next four weeks of pain without medication, I soon felt better. When I again ate some of those foods and my pain returned within five days, I was convinced. I have followed this program for more than a year and have never had another full-blown headache or menstrual headache! The doctor told me that out of 60 women patients, 40 had responded as I did and 20 did about half as well."

Add to Betty's list a few more items that might trigger migraines: monosodium glutamate (MSG) found in many Chinese dishes, salt, meat tenderizers, soy sauce, yeast extracts, and homemade yeast bread.

But for the biggest headache of the world—that of sin—there's only one solution: the cross of Jesus.

Thank You, God, for the natural remedies for pain, and thank You for the Jesus remedy for sin.

I WAS HUNGRY AND THIRSTY

October 14
Therese L. Allen

For I was hungry and you gave me something to eat, I was thirsty and you gave me something to drink, I was a stranger and you invited me in. Matt. 25:35, NIV.

When will this be over? I kept thinking. *What does God want me to learn from this?* Then I remembered Romans 8:28. Christ says *"all* things." He doesn't say how or when, but *all* things work together for good to those who love Him.

I don't remember the year, let alone the month, that all these thoughts kept going through my head. I only know it happened one summer about six years ago. My attendant walked out on me, and I had nobody to help me. I hadn't lived in this part of Los Angeles for very long and didn't know who to call for help. I phoned some local churches, but found no interest. Then I called everyone I knew, but for whatever reason, the answer was always no.

Lying there alone, a quadriplegic, I kept thinking of Matthew 25:35. I was thirsty and hungry and couldn't help myself. Did Jesus really mean that those people who said no to me were also saying no to Him? Quickly I said a prayer asking Christ not to *ever* let me say no to Him or one of His children in any way.

Finally, I called Joan. We'd met six or seven years previously, but didn't know each other well. Besides, she lived about 30 miles away. For 12 nights straight, at 10:30, Joan came to give me food and water. She'd ask how my search was going and apologize for not doing more. But she did *so* much, for she did *all* she could. Joan was a true light for the Lord.

No, I didn't get a lot of food and water, but my needs were met, just as Paul said in Philippians 4:19: "And my God will meet all your needs according to his glorious riches in Christ Jesus" (NIV).

Joan has moved away, and I don't see her much. But when we do talk and I try to express my gratitude, she says it was just "something that needed to be done." But why was she the only one who saw that I was hungry and thirsty?

Is there someone in your family, your neighborhood, or your church who needs help? Remember, whatever you do for others, Christ says you've done for Him.

AVOIDING EXTREMES

Do not be overrighteous, neither be overwise—why destroy yourself? Do not be overwicked, and do not be a fool—why die before your time? It is good to grasp the one and not let go of the other. The man who fears God will avoid all extremes. Eccl. 7:16-18, NIV.

Most of us are not in danger of exercising too much, but it happened to my sister. She caught jogging fever several years ago, and it seemed to take control of her world. She became a long-distance runner, ran the Boston Marathon several times, even ended up on the cover of *Runner's World* magazine.

Her devotion and commitment put me to shame. While I merely ran 15-20 miles a week, she religiously logged 100 miles a week. She was up at 4:00 a.m. every day to get in her 14-mile run before work, and went to bed every night by 8:30.

I told her that I didn't think you needed to run that much to enjoy a healthy life. In fact, I had heard that too much running could even be bad for you. But she wouldn't ease off. She was clearly possessed.

Of course, she was as lean as a whippet, but not only had she shed all excess weight, she began to shed needed calcium as well, making her bones brittle and dangerously fragile. When she mysteriously broke her arm after a minor fall, her doctor convinced her that she had to make a change.

She still runs more than I, and just completed a marathon in San Francisco, but her training regimen is more moderate and her life more balanced.

As with all things, a line separates the disciplined from the fanatical. Solomon even cautioned us against being "overrighteous," for there is danger in all extremes. For example, until Martin Luther fully understood the biblical concept of righteousness by faith, he denied himself food, sleep, and warmth, and studied and prayed himself to exhaustion and dismay. His "overrighteous" zeal nearly destroyed him.

Balance is certainly the law of nature and a requirement for our physical and emotional health. Our joy will come in finding that balance between work and play, exercise and rest, study and diversion, religious zeal and equally desirable qualities of moderation, patience, and tolerance.

What can you do to live a more balanced life?

I will set before my eyes no vile thing. Ps. 101:3, NIV.

The following paraphrase of Psalm 23 made me stop and think. Just how healthy is TV viewing?

The TV is my shepherd,
I shall want more.
It makes me lie down on the sofa.
It leads me away from the faith.
It destroys my soul.
It leads me in the path of sex and violence for the sponsor's sake.
Yea, though I walk in the shadow of Christian responsibilities,
    there will be no interruption, for the TV is with me.
Its cable and remote control, they comfort me.
It prepares a commercial for me in the presence of my worldliness.
It anoints my head with humanism and consumerism, my covet-
    ing runneth over.
Surely, laziness and ignorance shall follow me all the days of my
    life, and I shall dwell in the house watching TV forever.
—*Author Unknown*

Nancy Larric, a college professor and author, after reviewing the research on how television affects people, identified 10 characteristics of children who watch TV.

1. Short attention spans.
2. Thriving on noise, strife, and confusion.
3. Very worldly in their outlook and attitudes.
4. Little respect for adults (TV so often portrays them as lawbreakers, schemers, swindlers, sexual perverts, drug pushers, and low-IQ females).
5. Regarding of school as irrelevant and as punishment.
6. Filled with hostility or fear and are prone to settle things with violence.
7. Not getting enough sleep, and what they do get being of poor quality.
8. Prone to anti-interpersonal relationship values.
9. Unwilling to cooperate with others.
10. Antidemocratic and prejudiced against minorities.

For the sake of your children's health—and yours—don't make the TV your shepherd. Make the Lord your shepherd, and live a healthy lifestyle.

UNMASKING THE DANGERS OF TOBACCO

Lincoln Steed

No servant can serve two masters. Either he will hate the one and love the other, or he will be devoted to the one and despise the other. Luke 16:13, NIV.

The year was 1994. The place—the congressional hall of the United States government. It was high drama. A nation watched with awe as a bespectacled, somewhat bookish young doctor took on the multinational cigarette corporations. David Kessler, Food and Drug Administration commissioner, was angry and wanted all America to hear his charges against tobacco.

"Nicotine delivery systems" was the pointed phrase he used to show that cigarette manufacturers actually manipulated cigarette nicotine content for maximum addictive result.

Committee chair Henry Waxman nodded along in agreement and summoned the chief executives of the major tobacco manufacturers to answer the charge. When they claimed to be innocent of any manipulation, you could almost hear the collective boo from across the nation. David Kessler had the facts, the detailed findings of three surgeons general to add force to his statements.

Ellen G. White took the unmasking of the tobacco trade a giant step further than even Kessler when she wrote: "In fastening upon men the terrible habit of tobacco use, it is Satan's purpose to palsy the brain and confuse the judgment, so that sacred things shall not be discerned. When once an appetite for this narcotic has been formed, it takes firm hold on the mind and the will of man, and he is in bondage under its power. Satan has the control of the will, and eternal realities are eclipsed" (Temperance, p. 60). The amazing thing is that she wrote this in 1893, more than 100 years before Kessler's charge rocked the tobacco industry.

Ultimately the battle against tobacco, as with other addictions and addictive behaviors, comes right down to the struggle between good and evil, allegiance to Satan or allegiance to God. Cigarettes are indeed nicotine delivery systems. And Satan is indeed in the business of the delivery of sin and destruction to all who play with his toys.

How wonderful to know that God's power can protect us from all of the mind-benumbing plots of Satan.

Dear Lord, give me the clarity of perception to see Your ways always in a world offering so many false and ultimately destructive alternatives.

322

THE LAMP OF THE BODY

The eye is the lamp of the body. If your eyes are good, your whole body will be full of light. But if your eyes are bad, your whole body will be full of darkness. Matt. 6:22, 23, NIV.

The eyes reveal the innermost feelings, or emotions: love, joy, and hope, but also anger, grief, and fear. Such emotions release hormones, particularly epinephrine, norepinephrine, and cortisone, from the adrenal glands just above the kidneys. Exposure to cold, hunger, disease-producing organisms, injury, lack of sleep, etc., all produce the same reaction. The experimental animal (or person) adapts by their adrenals enlarging and secreting more hormones. If nothing happens to reduce the stress, the excessive hormones become harmful.

The typical modern lifestyle with its ceaseless striving and self-imposed demands makes chronic anxiety seem healthy. Such "lack of joy" triggers many diseases, such as hypertension, angina, peptic ulcers, irritable bowel, migraines, insomnia, and other stress-related diseases.

Nor is the inside of the eyes immune. Central serous chorioretinopathy (CSC) is one disease strongly linked to the type A personality. These people are highly motivated, impatient, and ambitious. The typical patient is a healthy business executive with very blurred vision. Special tests show a small leak in the back of the eye, with clear fluid collecting like a blister under the retina. CSC is rarely serious, nor does it usually require treatment. Often the change in lifestyle compelled by poor vision allows the leak to seal, and the fluid reabsorbs. Science further proved the link with stress when epinephrine injections produced CSC in experimental animals.

Interestingly, today's text is from the Sermon on the Mount, appearing between "storing treasures in heaven" and "not worrying about food, clothes, or life." The commandment against coveting in reality decrees that we be satisfied. Happiness lies not in getting what you want, but in wanting what you get.

God's instructions do not limit our joy or restrict our freedom, but provide the best guidance to achieving complete contentment. "The precepts of the Lord are right, giving joy to the heart. The commands of the Lord are radiant, giving light to the eyes" (Ps. 19:8, NIV). A large outdoor sign at a local church says it all: "When Have You Last Read Your Owner's Manual?"

Even the inside of the eyes will show it.

If someone checked your physical or spiritual health by looking into your eyes today, what might the "lamps of your body" reveal?

A GIFT FROM THE HEART

Each man should give what he has decided in his heart to give, not reluctantly or under compulsion, for God loves a cheerful giver. 2 Cor. 9:7, NIV.

Ashley was just 3 years old, and it had been a very difficult few weeks for her. The diagnosis of an extremely rare condition and the need for immediate surgery were tough to handle.

Her surgery went according to plan, but fear and uncertainty filled the days following it. The painful treatments were difficult to understand, and her budding faith in God suffered some painful setbacks.

Two days after surgery Ashley got a new hospital roommate. Hillary was 8 years old and wore a worn-out baseball cap to hide her bald head. She was in the hospital for her chemotherapy treatment for bone cancer. Her mother was not able to stay with her, because she had five other small children to take care of. During the night Hillary received her dose of chemotherapy, and by morning she was feeling very ill. Ashley noticed the change in Hillary's condition and was concerned about her new friend.

Sometime during the next morning Ashley received a large bouquet of mylar balloons with a card saying "Get Well Soon." She had never seen so many large and shiny balloons together before. "Are these for me?" she asked tentatively.

"Why, of course!" I answered. "Your friends are thinking about you and wanting to cheer you up while you are in the hospital."

A short time later Ashley requested some help to get out of bed. She asked if she could share her balloons with Hillary, because the other girl was sicker. It took quite an effort to help the frail little girl down from her bed and get her tubes and IVs arranged. Tears rose in my eyes as I watched my child make that walk to the next bed. She was in pain but was able to muster the strength to visit with her new friend and present her with a selection of balloons from her bouquet. I will never forget the joy Hillary expressed as she realized that the balloons were for her.

The incident reminded me of the beauty of unselfishness. "Freely you have received, freely give" (Matt. 10:8, NIV).

What gift have you received that would bring cheer to someone else if you were to pass it on?

WHAT'S THE SCOOP ON SALT?

You are the salt of the earth. But if the salt loses its saltiness, how can it be made salty again? It is no longer good for anything, except to be thrown out and trampled by men. Matt. 5:13, NIV.

What's the scoop on salt? First of all, Americans eat 20 times more than they need.

Second, medical science blames salt for high blood pressure, heart failure, and other problems related to fluid retention.

And third, not everyone is salt-sensitive. That's right, some people can eat all the salt they want without ill effects. The problem is that we have no satisfactory test for identifying which half of the population is salt-sensitive and which is not. That's why it's a good idea to be on the safe side and control your salt intake.

If you don't think you can live without salt, remember, you weren't born relishing its taste. Saltiness is something you've learned, and eating salty food fuels the craving. (Have you ever eaten one potato chip?) Plus, salt masks natural flavors that you could be enjoying if you'd leave off the salt.

Why not live on the safe side, lowering your salt intake and your chance of heart disease? Give yourself three weeks on a lower-salt diet. You can retrain your taste buds.

Just as too much salt in our bodies creates problems, so in the spiritual sense does salt that has "lost its saltiness."

God's people "must receive the saving salt, the righteousness of our Saviour. Then they become 'the salt of the earth,' restraining evil among men, as salt preserves from corruption (Matt. 5:13). But if the salt has lost its savor; if there is only a profession of godliness, without the love of Christ, there is no power for good. The life can exert no saving influence upon the world" *(The Desire of Ages,* p. 439).

Our effectiveness of witnessing to our family and loved ones depends on our receiving His Spirit. "If you are salt, saving properties are in you, and the virtue of your character will have a saving influence" *(Testimonies,* vol. 6, p. 259).

What can you do to lower your salt intake?
What can you do to be "the salt of the earth"?

MIDGES
AND
CAMELS

> Alas for you, lawyers and Pharisees, hypocrites! . . . Blind guides! You strain
> off a midge, yet gulp down a camel! Matt. 23:23, 24, NEB.

'm going to be healthy if it kills me!" Sound ludicrous? Not to the person who has made a healthy lifestyle into a substitute god. We call that addiction. Even good things can become a trap if they separate us from our sources of spiritual strength.

According to Jesus, the two greatest commandments were first to love God above all else, and second to love your neighbor as you love yourself. When persons have strong, committed relationships to God (vertical) and to close friends and family (horizontal), they are rich in spirituality. But when something—even religious behavior—becomes the centerpiece of their lives, spirituality vanishes. Gradually such people lose the ability to think and act according to their conscience and values. We observe that they have become addicted to an activity or object and have lost control of their lives.

The danger is that we may become addicted even to good and positive things. Following a prudent diet or getting proper exercise has many benefits. But when one becomes obsessive-compulsive about such practices, then the addiction can be very destructive. To make things worse, addicts rely on denial and create self-delusions in order to protect their addictions. The Pharisees were religious addicts. Christ described the results of their obsession with the letter of the law, and called them hypocrites and blind guides.

I once heard a zealot say, "I'm going to be healthy if it kills me!" He was arguing with a nutritionist concerned by his pallor and emaciated frame—evidences of the deficiencies of his extremely narrow dietary regimen. He had become so rigidly compulsive about avoiding minor dietary indiscretions that he ignored matters of greater importance. In the process he was alienating his children and other family members and creating disunity in his church by demanding a fat-free vegan potluck line to accommodate his dietary "standards." In addition, he discouraged new members by preaching his dietary doctrine. While endeavoring to "strain off" the midges of dietary imperfection, he was gulping down camels wholesale! The man had become a religious addict—in this case addicted to dietary behaviors.

Lord, please stay in the center of my life today, and save me
from any danger of swallowing camels!

BLOOD
OF THE
OVERCOMER

Tim Crosby

And so Jesus also suffered outside the city gate to make the people holy through his own blood. Heb. 13:12, NIV.

John Hendee, in his book *Ambassadors for Christ*, tells the story of Dr. Felix Ruh, a Jewish physician in Paris, whose granddaughter died of diphtheria. Vowing that he would find out what killed his granddaughter, Dr. Ruh locked himself in his laboratory for days. He emerged with a fierce determination to prove, with his colleague Louis Pasteur, that the "germ theory" was more than a theory. The French medical association had disapproved of Pasteur and had succeeded in getting him exiled, but he did not go far from Paris. He erected a laboratory hidden in the forest in which to continue his forbidden research.

As scientists, doctors, and nurses watched, Ruh opened a steel vault and took out a large pail filled with black diphtheria germs, which he had cultured carefully for months. The pail contained enough germs to kill everybody in France. The scientist went to each of 20 beautiful horses and swabbed their nostrils, tongue, throat, and eyes with those deadly germs. The scientists waited several days to see the outcome. Every horse developed a terrific fever, and all but one soon died. Most of the doctors and scientists wearied of the experiment and did not remain for what they thought would be the death of the last horse. For several more days the final horse lingered, lying pathetically on the ground. One morning, though, the horse's temperature began to drop, and by night the fever was gone entirely. Soon the animal was able to stand, eat, and drink.

Then Dr. Ruh took a sledgehammer and struck that beautiful horse a death blow between the eyes. The scientists drew all the blood from the veins of the animal that had developed the disease but had overcome it. After driving rapidly to the municipal hospital in Paris, they forced their way past the superintendent and guards and into a ward where 300 babies had been segregated to die from diphtheria. With the blood of the horse they forcibly inoculated every one of the babies. All but three recovered completely.

They, like us, were saved by the blood of the overcomer. Unlike those infants, no one forces the choice upon us. Accepting the blood of Jesus is a choice we must freely make today.

Have you let the Holy Spirit fill your life with
the blood of the Overcomer?

327

A DIFFERENT
PERSPECTIVE

But whatever was to my profit I now consider loss for the sake of Christ. What is more, I consider everything a loss compared to the surpassing greatness of knowing Christ Jesus my Lord, for whose sake I have lost all things. I consider them rubbish, that I may gain Christ. Phil. 3:7, 8, NIV.

On April 14, 1994, Elaine wrote her last entry in her diary:
"Lord, You may grant to heal me,
    or in the grave have me lay.
But I press this one petition,
    to be faithful every day."

Three months later Elaine, only 42 years of age, died. For 10 long years she had suffered with cancer. The nearness of death had constantly overshadowed her life.

Why do the faithful young have to suffer and die? Could it be that God has a work to accomplish that otherwise would never have been done? Could it be that the Christian who manifests patience and cheerfulness under bereavement, suffering, and even death accomplishes for the gospel more than he or she could have effected by a long life of faithful labor?

The following words made me see death from a different perspective: "Patience as well as courage has its victories. By meekness under trial, no less than by boldness in enterprise, souls may be won to Christ. The Christian who manifests patience and cheerfulness under bereavement and suffering, who meets even death itself with the peace and calmness of an unwavering faith, may accomplish for the gospel more than he could have effected by a long life of faithful labor. . . .

"Let not the follower of Christ think, when he is no longer able to labor openly and actively for God and His truth, that he has no service to render, no reward to secure. Christ's true witnesses are never laid aside. In health and sickness, in life and death, God uses them still. When through Satan's malice the servants of Christ have been persecuted, their active labors hindered, when they have been cast into prison, or dragged to the scaffold or to the stake, it was that truth might gain a greater triumph" *(The Acts of the Apostles, p. 465).*

So whether sick or well, a Godlike patient, cheerful attitude is the key to life. Therefore, be of good cheer—God has overcome the world (see John 16:33).

God, in times of crisis and pain, may I hold on to the fact that You have overcome the troublemaker of this earth, and with Your power, may I be able to maintain a patient, cheerful attitude. Amen.

YOU'RE NOT A GRAZING MACHINE

I praise you because I am fearfully and wonderfully made; your works are wonderful, I know that full well. Ps. 139:14, NIV.

Not even the most sophisticated electronic computer can come close to matching the "machine" God made when He created human beings. But we've pretty well disregarded His instruction manual about how to maintain optimal performance. Instead we put into our bodies whatever tastes good, whenever we feel like it. And we've turned ourselves into grazing machines. Like cows, we munch a little here and a little there. In fact, studies estimate that most people get approximately 30 percent of their food each day through snacking.

What's wrong with snacking? Dr. John A. Scharffenberg, health consultant to the General Conference of Seventh-day Adventists, gives five reasons not to snack:

First, demineralization of the teeth occurs for two hours after eating, then remineralization takes place. So continual eating increases the risk of tooth decay.

Second, blood triglycerides (fats) go up when we eat. The blood fats increase the stickiness of the platelets and red blood cells, increasing the risk of a clot being formed that could result in a heart attack.

Third, blood sugar rises as we eat, which stimulates a need for insulin. Continual stimulation causes hyperinsulinemia, and this increases the risk of heart attack.

Fourth, when we eat two or three large meals, we burn about 40 calories more per day than the same amount of food eaten in six to eight smaller meals, which has implications for weight management.

And finally, we face an increased risk of developing ulcers, since grazing generates more frequent gastric juice production.

Maybe it's time to go back to the instruction manual. Here's what God inspired Ellen White to say about snacking. "Regularity in eating is very important for health of body and serenity of mind. Never should a morsel of food pass the lips between meals" *(Counsels on Health,* p. 118).

That's pretty strong, isn't it? I don't know about you, but it makes me feel a little guilty about the way I've treated God's marvelous machine. I think it's time to quit acting like a cow. Quit grazing, and start following God's instruction manual.

What changes should I make to more closely follow God's instruction manual for my body?

HIS EYE
IS ON
THE SPARROW

Elmar P. Sakala

> Are not five sparrows sold for two pennies? Yet not one of them is forgotten by God. Indeed, the very hairs of your head are all numbered. Don't be afraid; you are worth more than many sparrows. Luke 12:6-8, NIV.

With a heavy heart I entered the cesarean birthing suite to deliver Cindy's tiny baby almost four months prematurely. After trying to conceive for many years without success, she saw her pregnancy as truly an answer to prayer. How could Cindy and Greg consent to this delivery, a virtual death sentence for Tara Jo, the baby they had anticipated for years?

For weeks Cindy's blood pressure had been gradually creeping upward to now-hazardous levels. Her kidneys showed profound injury from the worsening pre-eclampsia. Her severely swollen body showed the effect of gaining 30 pounds in 30 days. And now the dreaded headaches indicated changes to her brain's circulation that threatened her very life. Yet not only was Cindy's life in the balances, but so was Tara Jo's. Cindy's high blood pressure had so diminished the flow of vital nutrients to her uterus that Tara Jo had stopped growing in the womb. Both mom and babe would die! The delivery must take place.

Tara Jo weighed only 1 pound 1 ounce at birth. I had never seen any baby survive who was so tiny and so immature. The air sacs in her lungs had barely started to form. Her intestinal tract would not be ready for oral feedings for many months. The fragile blood vessels in her brain could so easily bleed, resulting in blindness, deafness, and cerebral palsy. Germs could easily overwhelm her immature immune system, resulting in a fatal infection. "Lord," I prayed, "You worked a miracle in her conception. Don't let Tara Jo die!"

After 100 days of intensive special nursery care and multitudes of intensive prayers on her behalf, Tara Jo left Loma Linda University Medical Center needing only low-flow oxygen.

Today, as I held Tara Jo in my arms at her dedication service, my mind went back to that agonizing night nine months ago. With eyes alert, hearing intact, and developmental landmarks on course, Tara Jo is a living testimony to the partnership of dedicated, highly trained health-care professionals working together with an infinitely loving Creator, who takes note of even the littlest sparrows that fall.

Praise You, Lord, for miracles great and small.

WHEN
MARRIAGE
GETS ROCKY

I, the Lord, have called you in righteousness; I will take hold of your hand. I will keep you and will make you to be a covenant for the people and a light for the Gentiles, to open eyes that are blind, to free captives from prison and to release from the dungeon those who sit in darkness. Isa. 42:6, 7, NIV.

Most thought our marriage was doomed from the start. We were too different. Ron's childhood had led him to crime and prison. Mine was filled with love, overprotection, control, and isolation from worldly influence.

Our introduction, in a courtroom on the day Ron was released from prison, was no coincidence. Our instant attraction was more like a psychological sense of destiny than mere chemistry.

Looking back now, after 30 years of marriage, we can see God's leading in every circumstance, even though marriage was "hell on earth" for 10 years! While our love was strong, our pain was deep. Previous wounds blinded us to the tools we needed for healing.

At one time, desperately hurting, both of us considered suicide. We feared God had rejected us. I was lying awake, crying out to God, angry and needing resolution. Looking for His answer, I fearfully opened the Bible and determined that I'd believe whatever verse my thumb landed on. That text, Isaiah 42:6, 7, has now become the covenant and commission of our Life Skills ministry to help others who are hurting.

First, God declares that He is creator of the universe—He is in charge and can do *anything!* Then the passage speaks of the covenant He wants to have with us to save others. I latched on to this as God's commission for our lives. I agreed to cancel my planned suicide and begged God to act quickly. He did! Our healing came as we submitted ourselves to Him and began to help others.

While I don't recommend arbitrarily picking Bible passages as a way of problem solving, God knew that in my desperation I needed an answer and chose to reward my feeble faith. When I think about how God gave direction to our lives, I realize we don't have to fear the future if we just remember how God has previously led us.

Now we thank Him for the pain of the past. We've learned that God sometimes allows us to come to the brink of destruction so that we can become submissive and teachable. Our joy is full each time we are able, through God's power, to release others from the chains of their past.

Challenge: do whatever it takes to become teachable
and submissive to God's will.

GOD IS
A FRIEND
OF DREAMERS

Robert Kuczek

And I—in righteousness I will see your face; when I awake, I will be satisfied with seeing your likeness. Ps. 17:15, NIV.

The blue-gray water, the sunset gleaming on the waves—it was a picturesque background for my dreaming along Lake Wigry's shore in northeastern Poland. In sleep during the period of rapid eye movement (REM) baffling nerve impulses shoot up the cerebral cortex from the lower brain. Some studies suggest that dreams result from the brain's effort to organize the impulses into tangible images. But I was awake, and it was an array of real ideas in kaleidoscope-like patterns that bewildered me. I needed a wedge to break through the impenetrable walls of prejudice surrounding the hearts of the people I had come to witness to. My thoughts raced as I kept asking myself, "How can I share Jesus?"

A sick feeling stirred my stomach as I pictured the vivid faces of my uncles suffering with cancer. Later, their deaths intensified my dream and my sorrow. Could anything have prevented their deaths?

A young woman who attended one of my health seminars did not protest when I offered more than health principles when I offered her Jesus. Joy filled her, and she gave her heart to Jesus. Health work, I realized, was that needed wedge.

Seven years have passed since that evening on Lake Wigry's shore. As from a dream, I awake to see what God has created from nothing. A series of miracles led us to a farm from which we could launch a health program in Poland, a country where tobacco, alcohol, and ignorance of nutritional facts rob millions of their health and their dreams.

Now three health food stores, a small publishing house and press, and plans for a school testify to God's willingness to transform dreams into reality. At least 1,000 people have attended our various health seminars, and we have sold more than 150,000 copies of recipe books. Many have found Christ and been baptized.

Just as our early church leaders discovered, I also have found that God is the friend of dreamers. "He is well pleased when they [His people] make the very highest demands upon Him. . . . They may expect large things if they have faith in His promises" *(The Desire of Ages, p. 668)*.

My dream keeps demanding, "How can I share Jesus?"

What large things are you expecting from God? Remember, He is the friend of dreamers.

LEPROSY
OF THE
CHARACTER

David Grellmann

He poured water into a basin and began to wash his disciples' feet, drying them with the towel that was wrapped around him. John 13:5, NIV.

I recall one particular Communion service at Masanga Leprosy Hospital. When it was time for the foot-washing service, I selected a leprosy patient who was part of the Masanga Town community. In times past he had been a thorn in the flesh for the hospital administration by organizing opposition to certain hospital plans.

I washed his feet first. He wore custom-shaped sandals, because his entire forefeet, including toes, had disintegrated because of his leprosy. When I knelt to wash his feet, he informed me I could wash only the left foot, because he had an ulcer on the right foot. The experience was sobering.

Leprosy is an interesting disease. For some reason the body's immune system turns a blind eye to one single germ—*Mycobacterium leprae*. It is unlike AIDS, which destroys the body's ability to fight any germ or tumor. The leprosy bacteria prefer cooler areas of the body, i.e., skin, mucous membranes of the eyes and nose, and superficial nerves throughout the body. Because of incomplete or no response from the immune system, the bacteria multiply unhindered.

Fingers and toes don't simply fall off, but they lose the ability to feel because of nerve damage. Without sensation there is no pain, and without pain there is no alarm to the brain that a thorn has penetrated the foot or that the hand is holding a pot so hot that it burns the flesh. These injuries and the subsequent infections don't hurt, so they tend to be neglected, resulting in further damage that eventually leads to gangrene and loss of toes, fingers, and more.

The spiritual lessons are many. It is not just total yielding to sin (broad immune system defeat, as in AIDS) that damages our characters. A single vice or pet sin (single bacterium immune deficiency, as in leprosy) can be equally devastating. With Holy Spirit insight we can perceive sin and get rid of it before it destroys us. But when our conscience is dulled and we experience no immediate consequence or pain, we're often not aware of the tragic results of our sinful ways until it's too late.

Lord, give me Holy Spirit insight to discern the little temptations that Satan wants to use to destroy my chance for living a more vibrant life.

NATURAL PAIN REDUCTION

October 29

Vivian Raitz

I am the Lord, the God of all mankind. Is anything too hard for Me? Jer. 32:27, NIV.

I can't thank you enough. I'll never stop singing the praises of this class!"

Phyllis, age 77, had been plagued by painful arthritis in her hands, knees, and back for years, and it was getting progressively worse. Then she attended a series of health classes featuring a total vegetarian diet and other natural remedies.

"This food tastes like the abomination of desolation!" she exclaimed. But Phyllis was ready for some drastic changes if it would reduce her pain. So she jumped in with both feet, cleaned out her kitchen cupboards, and no longer frequented the supermarket meat counters or ice-cream parlors.

"I have so much more energy," she told me, "and my arthritis is much better. My children even tell me I sound more lively on the phone."

"That's wonderful, Phyllis, but you must start walking. You don't get enough exercise."

"Vivian, I can't do that. My knees aren't *that* much better."

A few weeks later Phyllis informed me that she had gradually started walking and could now go up to a mile without difficulty.

However, Phyllis had forgotten to monitor her blood pressure. Because it had been so high she was on potent blood pressure medication, and she had continued taking it even though she had changed her lifestyle. She fainted on a visit with her son in the Northeast and was taken to the emergency room, where expensive tests were run on her. The diagnosis? Her blood pressure was too low! The program had been successful, all right. The physician took her off all blood pressure medication.

Now Phyllis is hopping around like a young woman and wouldn't go back to the old lifestyle for anything. "And," she said, "the food even tastes delicious!" She's now tasting the true flavors of the food without salt and grease masking them.

During the years Phyllis was living with pain, the promise "Fear thou not; for I am with thee" (Isa. 41:10) kept coming to mind. Since she started living a healthy lifestyle, she feels she's a living testimony to the truth of Jeremiah 32:27, that there is nothing too hard for the Lord.

Nothing is too hard for the Lord if we will cooperate with Him, and treat our bodies according to the instruction He has given.

BATTLING
BUSYNESS

Remember the Sabbath day by keeping it holy. Ex. 20:8, NIV.

Do you sometimes feel you're losing the battle with busyness? Take advantage of God's winning weapon: the Sabbath.

The fourth commandment says: "Six days you shall labor and do all your work, but the seventh day is a Sabbath to the Lord your God. On it you shall not do any work" (Ex. 20:9, 10, NIV).

During the six days of labor each week you may feel you're coming apart at the seams. But one day each week you receive permission—yes, are commanded—to come apart in a different way.

• Come apart from the noise of alarm clocks, machinery, traffic, telephones.

• Come apart from the information-bearers: newspaper, radio, TV, fax machines, and computers.

• Come apart from the rush: schedules, Day-Timers, freeways, airports, taxis, watches.

• Come apart from the clamoring for decisions: those endless committee meetings and conference calls.

• Come apart from the busyness of life—and rest in the assurance of God's love, His salvation, and the value that He places on *you*—not on what you do.

The Sabbath commandment is more for us today than for any people in human history. Of the Sabbath, Abraham Joshua Heschel writes: "There is a realm of time where the goal is not to have but to be, not to own but to give, not to control but to share, not to subdue but to be in accord. Life goes wrong when the control of space, the acquisition of things of space, becomes our sole concern."

During the week our very self-image becomes embroiled in our busyness. The Sabbath, however, rests on a revolutionary concept: we have value beyond what we produce. God values us just for being us, for being His children. That's what the Sabbath is all about.

As Tilden Edwards notes: "Stopping work tests our trust: will the world and I fall apart if I stop making things happen for a while?"

The busyness of modern life cripples our stamina, wounds our self-image, shatters our joy. But the Sabbath celebrates the wonder of being totally alive.

Lord, thank You for the Sabbath. How wonderful it is that You have created that day for us so we can rest from the busyness of life.

335

THE ILLUSION OF "WHOLISTIC" HEALTH

Ever since God created the world his everlasting power and deity—however invisible—have been . . . there for the mind to see in the things he has made. That is why such people are without excuse: they made nonsense out of logic and their empty minds were darkened. Rom. 1:20, 21, Jerusalem.

L iving in a New Age community, I felt compelled to find out about my neighbors' philosophies. A college class on wholistic health seemed a way to find out, so I signed up.

Each session followed the same format: a philosophical talk about human connections with universal energy (often demeaning Christianity), a mind-altering activity, then personal testimony as to how each person felt as a result of the activity.

I would listen to the instructions, observe or leave during the activity, then listen to the evaluations.

During one session the instructor asked the students to lie on the floor and hyperventilate for 90 minutes. A yoga expert, with her phenomenal breath control, was among the first to have a reaction—a grand mal seizure. Later she said it was the highest high she had ever had. One third of the class had "out of body" experiences, half were "visited by their personal spirit guides." All felt enlightened by their "spiritual" experiences. The rest of us were Christians and hadn't participated.

This "rebirthing" activity, as well as meditation, visualization, and many other mind-altering activities, is touted as a way of "getting in touch with the god within," a seeking for universal "wisdom." In reality, all they were doing were activities that would affect the brain's wave patterns and chemical balance that almost certainly induce hallucinations and self-hypnosis.

We think of this as a modern phenomena, but in 1890 Ellen White warned: "Satan tempts men to disobedience by leading them to believe they are entering a wonderful field of knowledge. But this is all a deception. Elated with their ideas of progression, they are, by trampling on God's requirements, setting their feet in the path that leads to degradation and death" *(Patriarchs and Prophets, p. 55).*

I came away from this experience grateful for a God who is my personal Saviour, a God whom I can trust to speak to me words of truth through His Holy Spirit. It's frightening what Satan can put in our minds when we lose control by doing unhealthful things that affect our brain's wave patterns and chemical balance.

Our personal Saviour and Creator promises that our meditation on Him is mind-renewing and strengthening.

REACH OUT AND
TOUCH SOMEONE
THROUGH PRAYER

November 1

Dianne Affolter

Be joyful in hope, patient in affliction, faithful in prayer. Share with God's people who are in need. Rom. 12:12, 13, NIV.

One evening in November 1992 a stranger on the phone notified me of an accident. My sister Kay and my mother had been hit head-on by someone driving in the wrong lane. Kay had an almost-severed foot, and my mom had multiple injuries. The prognosis didn't look good.

An hour later I ran into the emergency room to find it full of strangers praying for my mom and sister. Kay was already in surgery, and Mom was ready to be wheeled into the operating room.

At midnight Kay was back in her room, awake from the anesthetic, groggy, but coherent. A few seconds later the telephone rang, and to my astonishment, someone from a prayer circle in California was calling to give us encouragement and comfort. I was amazed.

July 1993 our plane landed in Atlanta, ending a wonderful vacation. As we arrived a message told us that our 16-year-old son, Brett, was in the coronary intensive-care unit at Emory Hospital. We were shocked to learn that when Brett was waterskiing he had experienced severe chest pains. Fearing a torn aorta, they had flown him to Emory for surgery.

Brett's story is full of amazing, unusual, and scary facts. But while we were staying in hotels and at the hospital, people called us from all around the world to tell us they were remembering him in prayer. How the word got out to such places as Canada, Singapore, and England I'll never understand, except to know that there is a special bond between Christians all over the world. A warm, comforting feeling comes from knowing that people are lifting you and your problems to the Lord through prayer.

Recently I learned about 10-year-old Nicky, from Canada, who had fallen from a horse. She was in a coma. As I started a prayer circle for her in Georgia, I was reminded how wonderful prayer is. And there's no long-distance rate. We can reach out and touch someone instantly with prayer, whether they're next door or across the ocean.

Do you know someone who needs healing, comfort, or strength?
Prayer is the answer, and it's even cheaper than that highly touted
10-cents-a-minute rate you see advertised on television!

PAIN—FRIEND OR FOE?

Wounds from a friend can be trusted, but an enemy multiplies kisses. Prov. 27:6, NIV.

Profoundly, without a sound, pain speaks. Its message requires immediate action and seeks to preserve and protect more than to offend, yet we seldom willfully invite its presence into our lives. Pain comes to us because God created us to think and to feel.

The nervous system, like an intricate telecommunication system, relays messages about the environment around us and inside us. Though unwelcome, pain is one of its necessary signals. Pain tells us if a pot is too hot to touch so that we will remove our hand at once. It lets us know if something is wrong and gives us good reason to find out what that something is. If we eliminate the cause, the pain leaves—its benevolent purpose accomplished.

If nothing else, pain at least lets us know we are alive. Whether it be fleeting or lasting, physical or emotional, pain has a purpose. Its wounds are faithful—it is a friend and not a foe.

Herod, tetrarch of Galilee, was unaware of his life-threatening problem until the message of John the Baptist arrested his attention. John rebuked Herod's sins, especially that of taking Herodias, his brother's wife, for his own (Luke 3:19). The Baptist's reprimand was a signal, like pain, demanding change. But instead of choosing life, Herod silenced the messenger and forfeited the blessings of obeying God's Word.

From the foundation of the world pain has asserted itself. Tears first rolled from the all-seeing eyes of God. His heart first throbbed and ached over pitiful, vulnerable, disloyal humanity, and His pain demanded immediate action—the life of the only-begotten Son of God. The Scriptures say: "Although he was a son, he learned obedience from what he suffered" (Heb. 5:8, NIV).

Pain teaches us, and as we experience it today, it will remind us that Christ understands exactly what we are feeling. "And with the stripes that wounded Him we are healed and made whole" (Isa. 53:5, Amplified).

Lord, when I hurt, let me not limit Your purpose, but allow
You to strengthen my faith and give me the fullness of Your joy.

" 'If you can'?" said Jesus. "Everything is possible for him who believes." Mark 9:23, NIV.

Leslie Lemke has the ability to reproduce on the piano anything he hears. But the incredible thing is that not only is Leslie blind, but he's also crippled with cerebral palsy and severely disabled mentally! Here's his story:

Leslie was born prematurely and abandoned as hopelessly disabled. He had already lost his sight when May Lemke, a 52-year-old nurse, decided to quit her job to raise the pathetic 6-month-old child everyone thought was hopeless. Everyone, that is, except May. As the days of her patient, loving care stretched into years, she saw few signs of improvement.

But May didn't give up. She knew God had given Leslie a gift, and she prayed she would have the wisdom to help him find it.

May carried him everywhere until he was too heavy to lift. Then she stood him beside the backyard fence, hoping he would hang on and stand by himself, but he just crumpled into a heap. Eventually he did stand, and then walked. But he still didn't talk.

The boy did one thing, however, that seemed out of the ordinary. Whenever he touched a piece of taut string or wire, he would pick at it with his fingers. The day May found him strumming rhythmically on the bedsprings she suspected Leslie might be musical. So she and her husband bought a used piano and put it in Leslie's bedroom.

Then came the task of teaching him to play. She had him listen to classical music by the hour. Then she placed his fingers on the keys and explained the sounds he heard. And finally, after years of "practice," he began picking out simple tunes.

Early one morning, when Leslie was 16, May woke up to a flawless performance of Tchaikovsky's Piano Concerto No. 1. She rushed into Leslie's room and found him sitting at his piano reproducing perfectly the music he had grown to love. Three years later he said his first word.

It's an incredible story, isn't it? But every person has God-given possibilities, if we will just look for them in ourselves and in others!

Dear Lord, help me to see possibilities in myself and others. Amen.

FLOGGING A TIRED HORSE

> Unless the Lord builds the house, its builders will have toiled in vain. . . . In vain you rise up early and go late to rest, toiling for the bread you eat; He supplies the need of those He loves. Ps. 127:1, 2, NEB.

The cart horse had toiled in the midsummer heat from early morning. It had had no rest from pulling the heavy loads. As its walk slowed from fatigue and thirst, the driver became impatient. The more haulage accomplished, the more money to be made. So he began to apply the whip. At first the lash seemed to create a burst of energy—the pain-induced adrenaline gave the horse renewed strength. But as the whip descended more and more frequently, the horse responded less, then began to stumble and waver. Finally the animal collapsed—no longer able now to feel the lash at all.

We may condemn with horror such brutality to a dumb beast. But might we also sometimes use similar behavior? Are we sensitive to our body's need for rest? Or do we "flog" our tired nervous system with chemical stimulants in order to "keep going" just a little longer, get a little more work done by staying up later—all in the name of accomplishing some goal that seems more important than balancing work with rest?

Caffeine is the most popular whip that people use on themselves. Some people become tolerant of its stimulation and believe it has no effect on them. Stimulated by the chemical, we cannot even sense our fatigue burden, and as a result our abnormal body function now feels normal.

I have a friend who consumed large quantities of caffeinated sodas each day to enable him to work harder and longer. When he realized the effects of overworking on his life, and caffeine's role, he endured the drug withdrawal in order to break free. Later he admitted that after a few days with no energy, he began to notice more his need for rest. And as he responded to the body's normal signals for rest, he began to get back in balance and break the overworking habit he had created through the caffeine whip.

God does not expect us to overwork to please Him. He made us with certain laws of physiology. When we cooperate with our Maker, He will bless the house we are building of our life.

Are you building your house on a healthy foundation, or on the sand of drugs and artificial stimulants?

PREPARE
TO MEET
THY GOD

Show me, O Lord, my life's end and the number of my days; let me know how fleeting is my life. Ps. 39:4, NIV.

Robert Spangler, longtime director of the General Conference Ministerial Association, tells of a time he faced his life's end.

"Not many sunsets ago my devoted wife, Marie, and I were walking the halls of our Washington Adventist Hospital, where I was unexpectedly admitted as a heart patient. An angiogram had revealed severe blockages in four leading heart arteries, a condition requiring bypass surgery. The next day, scheduled as I was for surgery, Marie cautiously questioned me about any fears I might have over facing such a crisis. . . .

"In that connection, let me just note here that I was fully aware that my heart would be purposely stopped, while its functions would be taken over by a blood-pumping machine. I was also aware that there was no guarantee that I would not join the society of the dead in a few hours, as happened to my roommate a few days later.

"With these and other thoughts chasing each other through my mind, I finally answered in a way that may seem presumptuous: 'No, Marie, I have no fears.' For in that moment I knew that defective and limited as it sometimes is, my belief in Jesus' love for me and my love for Him would sustain me in this crisis, regardless of the outcome."

The genius of Adventism is in the reality of the future. Eternity with our Saviour in heaven and in the New Earth is real and tangible. Eternity is as touchable as the scars Thomas saw and felt in the hands and side of Jesus!

It's a real wake-up call to realize that eternity can be only a moment away. It can be measured in the hesitant beat of the heart, the sickening crash of steel and glass on the highway, or the slow breathing of the terminally ill. But could eternity be closer to all of us than we might imagine? The end of this world—the fulfillment of Bible prophecy is imminent.

Do you have any fears about facing the future crisis? What will sustain you? What could you do today to prepare to meet your God?

A LESSON
IN HOPE
AND HEALING

Linda Willman Johnson

May the God of hope fill you with all joy and peace as you trust in him, so that you may overflow with hope by the power of the Holy Spirit. Rom. 15:13, NIV.

Children with cancer certainly have much to feel discouraged and hopeless about. Daily they suffer many painful experiences, and the side effects of chemotherapy and other treatments affect their body image and self-esteem. Yet most children and adolescents with cancer face their situations with a positive outlook and cheerfulness that amazes those who work with them. I believe the key is their faith and hope in the future.

Ann is an example of this. She was diagnosed with sarcoma at the age of 13, then treated with radical surgery, radiation, and two years of chemotherapy. With no relapses for more than 10 years, she is now classified as a long-term survivor.

Rather than blaming God for her illness, Ann saw Him as the source of her strength. Her faith in God grew stronger through her therapy. As a result of her experiences undergoing treatment for cancer, she made a decision to dedicate her life to helping others. She is now enrolled in graduate study in medical ethics and plans to become a hospital chaplain.

Ann acutely believes her experience as a cancer patient was the most positive experience of her life. She is convinced her faith and hope enabled her to become a survivor. As she expressed it: "I believe the experience fundamentally changed who I am. I value life more. I take joy in the little things, like the smell of a flower or the color of a sunset. I think a lot of people make their own lives difficult. Each of us needs to enjoy each day God gives us."

Whenever I feel overwhelmed or discouraged by the stresses and problems of my life, I think of Ann. I am simply unable to feel sorry for myself when I reflect on her courage. Her life is a powerful lesson in hope and healing.

With God's help, we, like Ann, can learn to view all of life's experiences as positive. If we let Him, God can turn the bad things that happen to us into positive things that strengthen our faith, deepen our trust in Him, and fill us with joy and hope.

Make Romans 15:13 your personal prayer: "May the God of hope
fill me, [your name], with all joy and peace as I trust in Him,
so that I may overflow with hope by the power of the Holy Spirit."

THE INCREDIBLE
POWER
OF MUSIC

Because you are my help, I sing in the shadow of your wings. Ps. 63:7, NIV.

Music was my salvation. Going through a difficult time with my parents and experiencing a lot of stress, I had feelings that I didn't feel free to express. Although I always liked music, it hadn't played an important part in my childhood. Then when I was 12 I went to a concert and heard a violin solo. It was a magical moment! From that time on I had a passion to play, although I didn't have a chance to do so until more than a year later, when the violinist who had made that magical moment happen for me became my teacher. She inspired me. And the violin gave me a purpose in life I didn't have before.

I found that through music I could now express feelings deep inside me that I couldn't bring out before. At the same time that I expressed those feelings, I felt a healing come over me, and I became happy—for the first time in my life! But not only was I happy, I was making others happy through my playing. My joy doubled! It was the beginning of my lifelong journey with my violin.

Music has an incredible emotional power. My husband, who is a pianist, and I were asked to play for the funeral of a friend's husband. The couple had been married many years, and the widow was deeply grieving. After the funeral she said to me, "I was dreading this funeral so much and didn't see how I was going to make it through the ordeal. But you played such beautiful and hopeful music that I was transported away from the circumstances to a better place."

Music has the power to express every human emotion. David played and sang all types of mood music and found healing in them. God even instructed the Israelites to go into battle with trumpeters and singing. And every time they did, they won!

Every day we face a battle with our emotions. Allow the power of music to soothe, energize, uplift, and inspire you, as it does for me.

Researchers have found that children who listen to Mozart get better grades. Why don't you play a little Mozart on your stereo or CD player, and see what it might do for you?

A DAY IN GOD'S DWELLING PLACE

November 8

Niels-Erik and
Demetra Andreasen

Better is one day in your courts than a thousand elsewhere; I would rather be a doorkeeper in the house of my God than dwell in the tents of the wicked. Ps. 84:10, NIV.

A few weeks ago at dinner we discussed a request for prayer an employee had made of us. A similar request came a week later. We prayed, not knowing the precise nature of the problem. Was it something at work? at home? a concern for children or spouse? Before long the mystery was solved. Two more Christian marriages went on the rocks, leaving spouses in despair, children lost, careers ruined, financial hardships, and doubts about God and His calling to Christian service.

It would be foolhardy to explain precisely what went wrong, but the reasons offered sounded like a familiar litany. Missing attentions, children growing up, the pressures of finances, careers, advanced study, house and home, and church and community. Trying to have it all and to do it all became too overwhelming, until what was once a healthy family became a sick one.

What is the remedy for such illness? May we suggest a serious consideration of Psalm 84:3, 4: "Even the sparrow has found a home, and the swallow a nest for herself, where she may have her young—a place near your altar, O Lord Almighty, my King and my God. Blessed are those who dwell in your house" (NIV). Here the psalmist portrays God's house, which means His presence, as a lovely place. Sparrow and swallow find safety near God's altar so they can build nests and raise their young.What a picture of family health! Mother and father building a home and feeding the young in God's presence. Every living person longs for such fulfillment, and sings in heart and body for joy once it comes.

Remarkably, this remedy is available to all who linger in God's presence long enough to watch the birds fly back and forth building nests and feeding their young. How much lingering does it take? Just one day in God's courts is better than a thousand elsewhere. Have you ever wondered what that day is? God's day of rest is the remedy for family illness. It comes once each week and is ours if we simply stop the thousand other things we have been doing and enter His dwelling place.

Think about your family and how you spend your time. Are you dwelling in the tents of the wicked, or are you a doorkeeper in the house of your God?

344

AVOIDING THE YO-YO EFFECT OF DIET

November 9

Jan W. and Kay Kuzma

Why spend money on what is not bread, and your labor on what does not satisfy? Listen, listen to me, and eat what is good, and your soul will delight in the richest of fare. Isa. 55:2, NIV.

I've lost hundreds of pounds and I'm still fat," the frustrated dieter exclaimed. The problem was that she lost four or five pounds at a time, then regained it, only to have to lose it again. We call this the yo-yo effect. And it's the reason diets don't work.

It's not hard to lose a few pounds during the first couple weeks of a diet. You watch your calories and eat significantly less. But your body doesn't know you are trying to lose weight and it thinks you're starving, so it kicks into "starvation mode." Your metabolism slows so you use less energy, which means you burn fewer calories. Once your metabolism slows, it's difficult to lose any more weight. The bad news is that your metabolism can stay depressed for a couple months after you return to normal eating. That's why after you diet, it's very easy to gain weight again.

Researchers have demonstrated the yo-yo effect in animals. They fatten them, and then place them on a restricted-calorie diet. The animals lose weight, but their bodies become more efficient at storing fat, so after they resume the original high-fat diet, they regain their lost weight easily. The second time the researchers restrict their diet, it takes them substantially longer to lose weight. And when the animals start to regain weight the second time, they do it much faster and end up gaining more.

The answer to your weight problem is not to starve yourself. Instead, get on a good lifestyle program. The combination of fewer fat calories and more exercise will keep your metabolism up, and the pounds will drop off and stay off.

Think about it in still another way: if the yo-yo effect has such a negative influence on your body, what kind of an effect will a yo-yo spiritual life have on your soul? Wouldn't a steady diet of God's Word be better than dieting one day and trying to make it up the next?

*Lord, grant me the self-discipline to maintain a
healthy lifestyle, physically and spiritually.*

THE ROYAL
WATER CURE

November 10
Raymond and
Dorothy Moore

> Jesus answered, "Everyone who drinks this water will be thirsty again, but whoever drinks the water I give him will never thirst. Indeed, the water I give him will become in him a spring of water welling up to eternal life." John 4:13, 14, NIV.

A few years ago in Africa a tribal king became seriously constipated. He vainly explored the world for relief. Medical authorities prescribed a variety of cures, but his digestive tract had become so fragile nothing worked. A Christian servant suggested he visit an Adventist clinic, famous for its treatment of the country's poor. The king's desperation for relief finally overcame his pride, and he rolled up to the mission in his Rolls-Royce with his secretary and stacks of medical records.

The clinic staff knew of the monarch's unfriendliness to Christian missions. The physician nevertheless greeted him. As the doctor looked over his records, the king sighed and said he came as a last desperate resort.

"How much water do you drink?" the physician asked.

The king looked at him with furrowed brow, "What is this you ask?"

The king's secretary explained that "the king has other things to drink." The physician knew this all too well. Many African royalty drank blood.

"In the morning," continued the physician without hesitation, "please drink two to four glasses of lukewarm water at least a half hour before breakfast. Drink a half hour before meals or at least an hour after meals so as not to dilute your digestive juices. Boil your water thoroughly to be sure it is pure."

The monarch had expected an exotic cure. His mouth dropped. "Only water? Is that all?"

"One more thing—for the next several weeks eat only fresh fruit, whole grains, and vegetables moderately cooked with little or no oil. My wife will help your cook, if that's necessary."

The doctor walked His Majesty to his limousine, adding, "Please let me know how you feel."

Six weeks later the king again rolled up to the clinic, bounced out of his Rolls-Royce, and his servants followed, loaded with gifts.

"So simple! So wonderful!" he exclaimed. "I am cured."

Like the simplicity of the water cure for constipation, so is the Jesus cure for sin. Just let Jesus flood your system—getting as much of Him as possible before breakfast, and you'll be amazed at what this simple remedy can do for your life.

Have you had enough water—and Jesus—today to keep physically and spiritually healthy?

WILLING
YOURSELF
TO LIVE

November 11
George Kuzma

[At the Pool of Bethesda] . . . One who was there had been an invalid for thirty-eight years. When Jesus saw him lying there . . . he asked him, "Do you want to get well?" . . . Then Jesus said to him, "Get up! Pick up your mat and walk." At once the man was cured; he picked up his mat and walked. John 5:3-9, NIV.

I once had a fiercely independent patient who had been ill for many years with adult onset diabetes and heart disease. She finally ended up in the hospital, where it became apparent that the only way to save her life was to amputate her infected leg.

I presented her with the options. The first was that she could go on the way she was and end up living in a nursing home, where someone could take care of the progressive gangrene that would eventually take her life.

The second choice was to amputate her leg before it got to that point, which would mean that she could live a satisfactory life.

Her response was an emphatic, "No. I will not have it amputated, and I won't live in a nursing home!"

I tried to reason with her, but she just turned away. Reluctantly, I left. Later I was shocked to learn that a few hours afterward she died. There was no acute reason for her immediate demise. She was in poor health, yes, but I had expected her to live from six weeks to two years longer.

I'm convinced she willed herself to die. A person's thoughts can be incredibly powerful!

And then I discovered something Ellen White wrote on the power of the will. "By the exercise of the willpower in placing themselves in right relation to life, patients can do much to cooperate with the physician's efforts for their recovery. There are thousands who can recover health if they will. The Lord does not want them to be sick. He desires them to be well and happy, and they should make up their minds to be well" *(The Ministry of Healing,* p. 246).

If only she had used her willpower to live, and had exercised and eaten a healthy diet so she could have avoided obesity and its consequent health problems. Nothing forced her to adopt the unhealthy lifestyle of her parents, but she did. And in the end, instead of willing herself to live, as did the paralytic who picked up his mat and walked, she willed herself to die!

How can you use the power of your will to live a more vibrant life?

MAKE A COVENANT WITH YOUR EYES

Izak Wessels

I made a covenant with my eyes not to look lustfully at a girl. For what is man's lot from God above, his heritage from the Almighty on high? Is it not ruin for the wicked, disaster for those who do wrong? Does he not see my ways and count my every step? Job 31:1-4, NIV.

More than 60 percent of the cranial nerves, which enter and leave the brain directly, have to do with the eyes. Visual input exceeds all the other senses combined, explaining the eyes' profound influence. Even the amount of light seen has a powerful effect on the body. Poultry farmers use fluorescent lights at night to fool a chicken's hormones, through its eyes, into thinking that it is still summer and to continue producing eggs. The chicken simply cannot help it. Humans seem to respond more to a lack of light. The short days and gloom of winter in northern countries make many people depressed and even suicidal, a condition known as "Seasonal Affective Disorder." They simply cannot help it.

The content of what we see is even more influential. Our age is spectacularly visual, assaulting our eyes and therefore the mind with almost overwhelming propaganda. Large-screen cable TV, computerized video games with virtual reality headsets, 3-D IMAX movie theaters with screens 10 stories high, glossy full-color magazines, and books with more illustrations than print all continue the barrage. Permitting the eyes to dwell on what is wrong or evil will overcome any restraints. Only after Eve looked again, and saw that the fruit was "pleasing to the eye," did she sin (Gen. 3:6).

As a visual reminder of guarding their eyes, God instructed the Jews to sew blue tassels to the corners of their garments. "You will have these tassels to look at and so you will remember all the commandments of the Lord, that you may obey them and not prostitute yourselves by going after the lusts of your own hearts and eyes" (Num. 15:39, NIV). It was the lingering glance back to the condemned cities that cost Lot's wife her life.

The revealing fashions so provocatively flaunted by many women are powerful visual stimuli. These, and magazines or videos with suggestive material, make men respond with their hormones, just like a chicken under light. They simply cannot help it.

If only the chicken realized it did not have to look at the light, but could close its eyes.

Are you sometimes like the chicken? Lord, give me the willpower to shut my eyes to the temptations of the world.

FOR WHAT DO YOU STRIVE?

I will not leave you as orphans; I will come to you. Before long, the world will not see me anymore, but you will see me. Because I live, you also will live. On that day you will realize that I am in my Father, and you are in me, and I am in you. John 14:18-20, NIV.

It made no sense. He'd spent four years diligently turning himself from an overweight, heavy-smoking, hypertensive borderline alcoholic into an almost physically fit individual. He scheduled himself and his wife for comprehensive physical evaluations from which he received an excellent report. Physically he was in the best shape he'd been in for years. Eight weeks later, under the pressure of financial reverses, he thrust a knife into his chest and died.

Here was a man who'd worked so hard to please *somebody*—maybe a parent, maybe himself, maybe a God he didn't understand. I had the task of preparing records for the insurance adjusters that required me to review each entry in his chart over the past 10 years. That, with a small degree of personal knowledge of him, created a haunting picture in my mind of a terribly lonely person. He must have had some unattainable image of what he must be, what he must do, and what he must obtain and maintain in life in order to be acceptable.

Most of us have experienced loneliness and the desire for acceptance. For some it's a transient thing brought on by circumstances like moving or the loss of a loved one. For others it's a gnawing need that eats at the very core of their existence. It seems that nothing can satisfy until they meet the demands of that emotional core.

God has an answer to meet even this. Do you long for a father's love? Read Jeremiah 31:3, NIV: "I have loved you with an everlasting love; I have drawn you with loving-kindness." Do you miss a mother's love? Read Isaiah 49:15, NIV: "Can a mother forget the baby at her breast and have no compassion on the child she has borne?" Claim this love as your own—for it truly is.

Then examine your life. Is what you are doing an effort to gain acceptance? Or is it because you are God's and you are accepted and loved, and you are availing yourself of privileged opportunities?

Are you aggressive and fearless on the outside, but hurting and empty inside? Open that pain to Jesus. He waits for you with love.

KEEPING YOUR MOUTH SHUT

If anyone considers himself religious and yet does not keep a tight rein on his tongue, he deceives himself and his religion is worthless. James 1:26, NIV.

The task of putting together a devotional book in three months, from the contacting of various individuals with a story or an inspirational message to the final editing, has meant that I have thought of little else. Every time I see a friend, I ask if they have a story that would help people live a more vibrant life. And so a few weeks ago, when I ran into Harry, I said, "I need a health devotional from you." He looked bewildered. "Tell me how you keep healthy," I continued.

Harry laughed, and with a twinkle in his eye replied, "I've learned that the best things I can do for my health are to keep my wife happy and my mouth shut!"

We both laughed at that. But there is truth to what Harry said. If you want to have a healthy relationship that brings personal satisfaction and happiness, you can't hurt others by spouting off everything that pops into your mind. Happiness comes as a by-product of making others happy, not by looking out after number one. Each of us, in our own relationships—whether it be with our spouse, our parents, our children, our roommate, or our friends—needs to figure out what we could do to contribute to another's happiness, and then do it. And sometimes this means we're going to have to change.

As I was waiting at the checkout counter one day, my eyes caught the headlines of a tabloid: "Hubby glues gabby wife's mouth shut!" I smiled. But I wonder how many husbands or wives read that headline and thought, *I wish I could do that!* I sometimes wonder if King Solomon felt that way when he said, "Better to live in a desert than with a quarrelsome and ill-tempered wife" (Prov. 21:19, NIV).

If you have trouble taming your tongue, if you find yourself having said things that you wish you hadn't, if your words sometimes hurt the one you love, let me suggest you do what Harry does: count to 50 before speaking. You might just find that taming your tongue is good for your health!

What is it that you could do to make others happy?

UNCLOGGING
THE BRAIN

> But Daniel resolved not to defile himself with the royal food and wine, and he asked the chief official for permission not to defile himself this way. . . . "Please test your servants for ten days: Give us nothing but vegetables to eat and water to drink." Dan. 1:8-12, NIV.

A number of years ago my mom gave me a tape by Dr. Elden Chalmers about how to make better grades. One of the things he mentioned was not to eat any sweets for five to 10 days prior to exams. But I never tried it.

Then when I was a physical therapy student studying for my written comprehensive exams, I was really scared. I had so much material to cover, so much I had to learn. Plus I've always had a tough time expressing myself on exams. So I asked myself, "What could make a big difference as I study and complete these exams?"

Then I came across the story of Daniel resolving not to eat the rich food served at the king's table, and I challenged myself not to eat sweets and desserts until I had written the exams. What made things really tough was that it was during the time we celebrated Thanksgiving, Christmas, and New Year's, with all the traditional rich holiday foods and sweet desserts!

I prayed for God's strength, because I really love good-tasting food. My husband encouraged me and never once tried to entice me to sample what I had chosen to not eat. Just sticking to my resolve was an incredible miracle, since we received invitations to many special occasions serving scrumptious homemade cookies, candy, cakes, and pies.

But the biggest difference I felt was that my mind was clearer and I was able to concentrate on my studies for longer periods of time. How I wish I had taken Elden Chalmers' advice before!

You're probably wondering if it made a difference in my exam scores. I'm sure it did. I went into the exams with a confidence I had never possessed before, and passed them all.

Ellen White said: "The free use of sugar in any form tends to clog the system" (*Counsels on Health,* p. 154) and "A great amount of milk and sugar . . . clog the system, irritate the digestive organs, and affect the brain" (*Testimonies,* vol. 2, p. 370).

Now I'm a believer!

Do you have a sweet tooth? What could you do without today to have a clearer mind for the Holy Spirit to impress?

THE LIGHT
OF THE
WORLD

Walter Thompson

You are the light of the world. A city on a hill cannot be hidden. Matt. 5:14, NIV.

A lone man walked down the streets of the old city of Gdansk, Poland, where he had come to do business. As he finished his business and prepared to return to his home, he noted a meeting going on inside the building he happened to be passing. Curious, he stepped in and sat down. What he heard captured his heart at once.

For the next two weeks he returned night after night to listen and learn as the gospel worked its subtle changes in his heart. When at last the meetings ended he returned to his home, not now to pursue his business, but with a burning desire to share the beautiful things that he had seen and heard about this God who he discovered was out to rescue the world from sin. Nothing was more important now than to open the door of his soul temple and invite the Spirit of his God to come to dwell within.

When he arrived at his home village and began to share the glories of the gospel with his neighbors, it dawned upon him, *Wouldn't it be nice if this temple, this body of mine, were more effectively suited to be a lighthouse to the world? Wouldn't it be nice if the lights inside were bright, and the windows huge with beautiful pictures in colored glass portraying the saving truths for the whole world to see?*

And then it was that he realized the value of the simple laws of health that God has so graciously given to His people and the reason for them. By the grace of God he would make something of his body that would witness to the world.

Soon a whole company of family and neighbors worshipped together each Sabbath day. And as the light of the love of Jesus radiated out from these believers into their community by word and deed, many "miracles" of health and healing accompanied them. The light shining from one ignited another and another, and grew brighter and brighter and lighted the whole community and beyond.

Take Jesus' challenge: "Let your light so shine before men, that
they may see your good works, and glorify your
Father which is in heaven" (Matt. 5:16).

Above all else, guard your heart, for it is the wellspring of life. Prov. 4:23, NIV.

After King David committed adultery with Bathsheba, he begged for God's mercy and pleaded, "Create in me a pure heart, O God, and renew a steadfast spirit within me" (Ps. 51:10, NIV). Although we understand that David wasn't requesting a literal pure heart, in modern terms he was asking God for a pure mind. As we read about the heart in the Bible, we find that typically the writers are referring to our thoughts and attitudes—our minds.

Neuropsychologists studying the mind and the brain have begun to understand that every action and thought we have exists only in the neurons and neurochemicals of our brains. Thoughts transfer through neurons and across synapses, forming pathways and networks intimately involved in everything we do, from recognizing a word or a sound to recalling what it means, where we have seen or heard it before, and how we might respond to it. Our brains store our memories and experiences, what we have learned, and what we have done. New neuronal connections and pathways that at first sent only rivulets of electrochemical signals can potentially become well-used rivers sending torrents of information.

What this meant for King David is still true for us today. Every act or thought, anything that we perceive, makes changes in the structure of our brains, however small, and over time those things we become most familiar with create stronger connections and well-traveled pathways in our brains. Knowing this, it is understandable that being "heart smart" involves careful consideration of the kinds of patterns we establish in our lives, as well as the experiences we involve ourselves and others in. As the old familiar words prompt us: "Finally, brothers, whatever is true, whatever is noble, whatever is right, whatever is pure, whatever is lovely, whatever is admirable—if anything is excellent or praiseworthy—think about such things" (Phil. 4:8, NIV).

Lord, my prayer is that I will be "heart smart," and that
You will create in me a pure mind. Amen.

INTOLERANCE

November 18

David J. DeRose

> Why do you spend money for what is not bread, and your wages
> of what does not satisfy? Isa. 55:2, NKJV.

June came into my office complaining of serious abdominal difficulties. After taking a careful history and performing her exam, I told her that she might have a lactase enzyme deficiency. Her stomach did not properly digest dairy products, causing bloating, cramps, gas, or watery diarrhea. Consequently, I recommended that she avoid all dairy products for the next three weeks.

June was skeptical. However, a short time later she was back in the office convinced that we indeed had identified the problem. A dairy-free diet had caused her symptoms to vanish.

The irony of June's story is that she no doubt had many good reasons for using dairy products. Perhaps she felt it was a good source of calcium or protein. Or perhaps she just simply liked the taste. Nonetheless, no matter how good they seemed, they were causing her untold misery.

Although there are growing concerns about the health effects of dairy products, my focus is not to condemn, but to recognize that it is a food group that commonly causes acute problems often not recognized by the people afflicted.

This provides us with an illustration. Even though we've grown up with something—for example, dairy products—it doesn't mean that it's necessarily good for us. In some cases it can even undermine our health.

In contrast, another "dairy product," "the pure milk of the word" (1 Peter 2:2, NKJV), can be digested by all who are willing to receive the Spirit's illumination. In the physical realm a food may cause problems for some individuals even if the majority classify it as not all that bad or even good or excellent. So in the spiritual realm, the Spirit through the Word may convict you to cut certain things out of your life. These things may not be bad in themselves—they may be all right or even desirable for others to do. However, because of your nature and tendencies, the only route to your total health—spiritually or physically—involves leaving that practice out of your life.

*Are you willing to ask God to search your lifestyle to see if you
need to set aside some things that may be OK or even good for others?*

HEALTH IS
WHOLENESS

> Do you not know that your body is a temple of the Holy Spirit, who is in you, whom you have received from God? You are not your own; you were bought at a price. Therefore honor God with your body. 1 Cor. 6:19, 20, NIV.

One of the major myths in modern society is the passion for fitness as an end in itself. I have a friend who is totally caught up in the fitness craze, working out at a fitness palace virtually every night. Vitamins and supplements that promise to give her greater energy and help her eliminate deposits of fat (of which a casual look would suggest she has few) clutter her desk. She subscribes to body-building magazines that display sculptured bodies that seem almost inhuman in the extremes of muscle definition. She even had dreams of competing in such contests herself.

On the surface it would seem that she has a passion for health. Surely, trying to look good and feel good are positive things. But health is more than muscle definition. And fitness is more than the relationship between weight and body fat.

In her pursuit of the perfect body, my friend has chosen to exclude from her life many other elements that contribute to overall wholeness. Her marriages have ended painfully, and the relationship she's in now is quite unconventional. She has selected for her preferred social setting the bars and clubs that cater to the mindless, pleasure-seeking crowd, most of which is a generation younger than she is. She no longer attends church or finds anything appealing in the spiritual dimension of life.

The real problem with what she is doing, however, isn't so much the elements she's brought into her life (though others might choose differently), but the elements she's excluded. A life in balance is one that places the physical aspect in proper perspective with the others, including the social, the intellectual, and the spiritual. Health is wholeness, a life in which all the parts work together in a symmetry that exceeds just that of a sculpted body. And in so doing, we honor God with our bodies, not self.

I know "man does not live on bread alone" (Matt. 4:4, NIV) but it must also be said that we should not live by exercise alone, either!

Remember that "holiness is wholeness for God; it is the entire surrender of heart and life to the indwelling of the principles of heaven" (The Desire of Ages, p. 556).

TOO LITTLE, TOO MUCH

November 20
Patricia K. Johnston

> Behold, this was the guilt of your sister Sodom: she and her daughters had pride, surfeit of food, and prosperous ease, but did not aid the poor and needy. Eze. 16:49, RSV.

We use the term *malnutrition* most often to describe circumstances in which there is too little food or nutrients to supply the body's requirements. We are all acquainted with emaciated faces peering out at us from the TV screen, asking for help. The malnutrition of too little.

On the other hand, we also find the malnutrition of too much, most often called overnutrition. The percentage of the U.S. population classified as overweight or obese is growing. Many have too much food, but not all.

The world's food distribution is not equitable. Several visits to Haiti served to underscore in my mind what happens in too many places. The shelves of stores where the simple people shop are empty, or what little food is there is priced beyond their meager funds, but the storehouses of the wealthy are full.

I cannot forget the man standing just outside the circle of mothers and children waiting to receive a small package of dried milk. Obviously he didn't qualify for the food, so he just stood and watched others receive theirs. His tattered shorts were the remnants of once-longer pants. His T-shirt had more holes than cloth. He carried a broken machete, a few sticks to start a fire, and one breadfruit.

I couldn't help thinking of the statement: "If men today were simple in their habits, living in harmony with nature's laws, as did Adam and Eve in the beginning, there would be an abundant supply for the needs of the human family. But selfishness and the indulgence of appetite have brought sin and misery, from excess on the one hand, from want on the other" *(The Ministry of Healing*, p. 47).

Too little and too much. It's not a new problem. The question is What can you do about it? Which side will you be on when "the King will say to those on his right, 'Come, you who are blessed by my Father; take your inheritance, the kingdom prepared for you since the creation of the world. For I was hungry and you gave me something to eat" (Matt. 25:34, 35, NIV)?

Think of someone in your town, neighborhood, or church who is struggling financially and may benefit from something healthful to eat. What can you do to meet that person's need?

356

CLOSE THE DOOR, BUT NOT SO HARD

All this is for your benefit, so that the grace that is reaching more and more people may cause thanksgiving to overflow to the glory of God. 2 Cor. 4:15, NIV.

When I was a little girl and my mother wanted to teach me not to slam the door, she would often make me open and close the door and say out loud, "I will not slam the door closed."

This memory for some reason came to mind when I hung up the phone after being told I had a breast lump that would need immediate surgery. I asked God why He was slamming the door on a new job and move I was about to take.

I was absorbed with my private memory for only a few minutes when I heard a page for another outside call. It was the adoption agency with a boy, and my husband and I had been matched with him. I had three days to decide and commit to taking him or turn down the opportunity.

That afternoon I talked a long time with my husband. As we spoke to the social worker and held the child's picture, we knew we wanted him. But what if God wanted to slam another door?

The surgeon was most reassuring and positive. "I'm sure everything will turn out fine, so don't put your life on hold just because of this. If you want to adopt, then do it, but it probably would not be a good idea to move and take a new job in the middle of an unknown health crisis." I knew what he was saying was true!

I had the surgery, and we adopted Christopher. As I was leaving the surgeon's office on my return postop visit, I overheard him telling another patient not to worry. "I am sure everything will turn out fine."

I thought to myself that maybe this woman would be as blessed as I have been and discover that just because one door slams doesn't mean the hand of God won't open another.

None of us likes to have doors slam on what we want to do. But I've learned God holds our lives—and the doors of this world—in His hands. And He never shuts one door without opening another. Why then should we worry?

Thank You, God, for knowing which doors in my life should be closed, and for opening the ones that You know are best for me.

He went away again the second time, and prayed, saying, O my Father, if this cup may not pass away from me, except I drink it, thy will be done. Matt. 26:42.

I've relived the accident hundreds of times—cresting the hill, the terror of seeing the van in my lane, the immediate impact, my exposed leg bone protruding through my sock as my foot dangled to the side, and no sound from the passenger seat. "Mom, talk to me," I cried. Silence. I hopped around the car to get to my mother. Mom, doubled over and squashed between the seat and dash, was now groaning in pain, "I can't breathe." I had to straighten her or she would suffocate. Pulling her out of the car, I placed her on a pillow on the pavement, fell down beside her, cuddled her in my arms, willed her to breathe, and prayed for help.

The following days were a blur. The miracle was that the surgeons could reattach my foot and I would walk again. But within a week my mom's chances of surviving narrowed to 10 percent, then 5 percent as infection set in and her kidneys and liver began to fail.

I called the pastor to have Mom anointed. "You know, Kay," he said, "an anointing is as much for the family to say 'Thy will be done,' as it is for your mom's healing."

I hung up, sobbing bitter tears. "No," I screamed. "Mom has to live." I couldn't say the words "Thy will be done." Mom couldn't die like this— an innocent victim of a senseless accident in which I had been the driver. I wept. For two hours I pleaded with the Lord for her life. Then, emotionally spent, I gave up my fight and between sobs of resignation finally uttered, "Thy will be done." At last peace came.

Later as I told the pastor about my struggle, he said, "Do you think it was easy for Jesus to say "Thy will be done" in the Garden of Gethsemane when He knew in a few short hours He was facing his own painful death?"

Suddenly I realized that through this experience I had been to Gethsemane with Jesus and found God there, and now with peace in my heart I could say "Thy will be done."

Twenty-two days after the accident Mom died.

What is your prayer? Can you say "Thy will be done,"
or are you still saying "My will be done"?

A SOUND
MIND

November 23

Pat B. Mutch

God hath not given us the spirit of fear; but of power, and of love, and of a sound mind. 2 Tim. 1:7.

Fear is a normal human emotion. We can't control it or avoid it. It just happens—especially when we are uncertain about the future. But fear was not in God's plan, and He does not leave us helpless as we face it.

The stifling heat and humidity of a tropical night did not help in my battle with mindless panic. For two weeks a physician from the division office had escorted me around the Philippines. I had felt secure. Now his schedule compelled him to return to Singapore, leaving me to complete my first overseas itinerary alone. My last destination was a small town in the politically tense island of Mindanao. But in spite of our many efforts, we had been unable to discover if a seminar was actually planned. The local conference office had no phone or telex, the union health/temperance secretary was away, and no one else knew.

My thoughts whirled in circles. What would I do if no one met me? I had been warned that as a white woman traveling alone I should not go outside an airport terminal unless I recognized someone as being there to meet me. Was I being foolhardy to take the risk? What was the Lord's will?

"What shall I do, Lord?" I asked. "I'm so afraid." Then softly came His first gift—a sound mind to reason through the situation. I realized that if no one did meet me, I could always buy a return ticket back to Manila! Then came love—a guiding motivational force keeping me aligned with God's will. I began to want to go on the trip. And finally there was power—the strength to make the decision. I would go. My anxiety had vanished. God's power would uphold and protect me. With those gifts to help me, I fell asleep.

The next morning as I deplaned to view two smiling faces holding a huge banner proclaiming "Welcome to Mindanao, Dr. Mutch," I knew that God had indeed given me His gifts to conquer fear: the spirit of power, of love, and of a sound mind.

When you're frightened, hold on to the promise that God will give you a sound mind, love, and power.

359

TRAITS OF A STRONG, HEALTHY FAMILY

Unless the Lord builds the house, its builders labor in vain. Ps. 127:1, NIV.

Researchers have found that the majority of strong, healthy families have the following traits in common:

1. **Commitment:** Put God and your family first, and commit to helping each other become everything God designed you to be.

2. **Appreciation and affirmation:** Give positive attention and affirm each other, letting each family member know they're special. Strong families focus on the strengths of each other, not the faults.

3. **Time together:** Healthy families enjoy being together. Work together, play together, and enjoy leisure times together. Family members may be busy, but they don't let jobs, school, or personal hobbies steal family time.

4. **Communication:** To understand each other a family has to be willing to invest the time necessary to share their feelings and opinions. Each day you are a new person. Without sharing those experiences with each other, family members can soon become strangers.

5. **Religion:** Sharing a religious faith and having similar religious values and standards is extremely important. Worshipping together is a bonding experience. But most important is a commitment to God, the foundation of the family.

6. **Play and a sense of humor:** Happy families have fun together; they play together; they laugh together. Having a sense of humor during troublesome moments is like pouring oil on restless water. It defuses the tension and has an immediate calming effect.

7. **Sharing responsibilities and roles:** If family members will do whatever is necessary to meet each other's needs, even if the task doesn't happen to be on their priority list, everyone is happier. Be flexible and responsible.

8. **Common interests and goals:** The more a family has in common, the more its members tend to do together. Having similar interests and getting behind common goals gives the family something to look forward to, to plan, and to experience together.

9. **Service to others:** Just as a pond grows stagnant if it has no outlet, so does a family. Reaching out and helping others bonds families together.

10. **Admitting to and seeking help with problems:** Healthy families aren't problem-free; they just admit to problems and get the help they need to solve them!

How does your family measure up? For a little bit of heaven on earth, make God the foundation of your family and add these 10 essential traits.

PRAYER'S POWER OVER ADDICTION

He will respond to the prayer of the destitute; he will not despise their plea. Ps. 102:17, NIV.

ears spilled from 15-year-old Vicca's soft brown eyes. Her story was all too familiar to me as a health evangelist in Russia. Luda, Vlad, and Tamara had the same story. Their parents were alcoholics, a common problem among those with no hope.

Vicca was afraid. Her father was leaving to work in Germany, and she felt she would never see him again because of his heavy drinking and poor physical condition. "What can I do?" she wondered.

I also wondered what I could do! I had little firsthand knowledge of alcoholism. Despite the many hours of seminars, college classes, and visiting Alcoholics Anonymous meetings, I was still unsure how to handle such a situation. With no local support groups to help, I had only one answer. If Vicca's father would come to our evangelistic meetings, I could pray with him.

To Vicca's surprise, he came. Every night for four weeks he sat front row, center. Together Vicca, our translator, and I prayed with him after three of the meetings. He was appreciative, but that was all I knew.

One of the great disadvantages of such meetings is the loss of contact with those who attend. However, I was fortunate enough to have a visit with Vicca two years later. She is a baptized believer and active as a church member. Her father has not joined her, but since the third time we prayed, by the power of God, he hasn't had a drink of alcohol. She considers it a miracle, and so do I.

I'm reminded of this story every time I read Psalm 107:17-21: "Others, the fools, were ill because of their sinful ways. Their appetites were gone and death was near. Then they cried to the Lord in their troubles, and he helped them and delivered them. He spoke, and they were healed—snatched from the door of death. Oh, that these men would praise the Lord for his lovingkindness and for all his wonderful deeds!" (TLB).

When you are tempted and tried, hold on to this picture that Ellen White paints in The Desire of Ages: *"God is bending from His throne [on high] to hear the cry of the oppressed. To every sincere prayer He answers, 'Here am I'" (p. 356).*

THE GIFT
AND THE
GIVER

Jesus said: "Were not all ten cleansed? The other nine, where are they?" Luke 17:17, NEB.

I magine that as you get up every morning and look into the mirror, you see yourself covered with blotchy, decaying skin and deformed tissue. In Jesus' time thousands of people had this experience—leprosy—and they knew it to be an isolating, painful, and ultimately fatal illness.

Even worse, people told them that the disease was far more than a physical problem—it was a religious problem, a public sign of God's judgment and disapproval. It was a disease that, in the view of the religious authorities of the day, enabled the rest of society to see one suffering under punishment from God for some major sin. And because one languished with leprosy in a steady, downhill slide into death, it was clear to them that God's condemnation and punishment were both permanent and fatal.

No wonder, then, that Jesus never encountered a leper without healing him or her. For not only was Jesus moved by their physical suffering; He also protested against the twisted and tragic view of His Father the disease was thought to represent.

On one occasion He even healed 10 lepers at the same time. Then the story takes an interesting turn. Nine of them were so taken with their fresh skin that they rushed down the road to embrace their friends and forgot all about the One who made them well. Only one former leper recognized that the power of the moment was not in his clean skin, but in the One who made it whole. And he returned and bowed at the feet of Jesus.

Our old instincts would likely have approved should God have allowed the leprosy to return to those nine ungrateful wretches as they scampered down the road so self-absorbed in their gift that they forgot the Giver. But that would have missed Jesus' larger point. Though forgiveness is offered to all, only those who *love* the Forgiver have entered into life.

Have you entered into life?

GIVING
GLORY
TO GOD

> Then I saw another angel flying in midair, . . . He said in a loud voice, "Fear God and give him glory, because the hour of his judgment has come. Worship him who made the heavens, the earth, the sea and the springs of water." Rev. 14:6, 7, NIV.

Discussing the meaning of the verse "Whether therefore ye eat, or drink, or whatsoever ye do, do all to the glory of God" (1 Cor. 10:31), my public health professor startled me with his words. "Health is part of the three angels' messages," he said.

Now, wait a minute, I thought, *how could that possibly be?*

He continued, "In Revelation 14:7 the third angel says, 'Fear God, and give glory to Him.' How do you give glory to God? Well, 1 Corinthians 10:31 says we do that by what we eat and drink and anything else we do."

Well, I thought, *that's a real revelation from Revelation! The health message is a part of the three angels' messages!*

We can give glory to God by what we eat and drink. Take Daniel and his companions, for example. After 10 days on a vegetarian diet everyone could see how God had blessed (Dan. 1).

The Lord is also glorified if an expectant mother follows the simple rules of health. Judges 13:4 says an angel told Samson's mother not to drink wine or strong drink, or eat any unclean thing. An angel notified Zacharias, John the Baptist's father, that his son was never to drink alcoholic beverages (Luke 1:15). John followed a simple diet and gave "glory to God" in a spectacular way. His clear brain, through the Holy Spirit's insight, was able to recognize the Messiah and announce, "Look, the Lamb of God, who takes away the sin of the world!" (John 1:29, NIV).

The number of years we live and our quality of life can also glorify God. "The silver-haired head is a crown of glory, if it is found in the way of righteousness" (Prov. 16:31, NKJV).

I'm way past 70 and actively traveling, giving Bible studies, coordinating retreats, and involved in the lives of my children and grandchildren. Every time the retired church workers obituary list is published, I'm amazed at the number of those who have lived far beyond three score and 10! To God be the glory!

> *Do people notice what you eat or don't eat? Do they notice what you drink or don't drink? Does that embarrass you, or do you seize the opportunity to glorify God?*

GIVING UP
THE BULGE

Raymond O. West

Come to me, all you who are weary and burdened, and I will give you rest. Take my yoke upon you and learn from me, for I am gentle and humble in heart, and you will find rest for your souls. For my yoke is easy and my burden is light. Matt. 11:28-30, NIV.

Six of us had entered the deep Virginia cave a few hours before on the dangling end of a stout rope. We had ambled, crawled, and crouched our way through tunnels and crawlways from caverns to vast stalactite-strewn rooms. Then we had eaten lunch by the shore of a tiny lake. Yes, it had been a spelunker's day of delights. Somewhere up there on the surface the winter afternoon had waned and it was past time to exit.

Now again, with the aid of our trusty rope, four of our group were already on top. Bob, my stocky spelunker friend, crouched with me on a narrow shelf of solid rock, with 80 feet of dark vertical passageway below and a shaft of wintry light slanting down from above.

Unfortunately, we had a problem—we were stuck just below a narrow confinement. As Bob had clawed his way upward, I had pushed from below. But he was simply too stocky and the defile too narrow. On the way down Bob had been assisted by gravity, but going up, it was like a cork stuck in the neck of a bottle. Several times we had heaved and shoved. Now, breathless and fatigued, we considered our options: a pound of butter for grease? a jackhammer? even a minor earthquake?

In frustration Bob exploded, "You'll just have to leave me here."

With just the breath of a prayer we rallied our strength for a final try. As Bob heaved on the rope, I shoved from below. Nothing! Then, curiously, I noted for the first time a bulge in Bob's back pocket. "Bob," I exulted, "slide back down here and take out your wallet!"

That was it. In our anxiety we'd missed the cause of the jam-up. Bob's wallet had been the plug. With another hefty shove we were soon on top and headed for home.

Concerned over health-related burdens? Why not decide today to give them over to Jesus? Hand Him your anxieties and stress. Trust Him with your empty calories and adipose pounds—and all the rest.

He has promised to make our burdens easy and light.

What is the bulge in your life that is keeping you from reaching your desired goals? Give it to Jesus and expect a miracle!

THE GIFT OF A DISABILITY

Kay Kuzma

> But he said to me, "My grace is sufficient for you, for my power is made perfect in weakness." 2 Cor. 12:9, NIV.

The apostle Paul was a choleric, type A committed doer. He met every assignment with great enthusiasm, total conviction, and utter determination. Paul was an influential teacher, dynamic evangelist, and dedicated missionary. But he had a disability. Some feel that he never fully recovered from the blindness that struck him on the way to Damascus. Others think that maybe he suffered from malaria. Here's what Paul says:

"I will say this: because these experiences I had were so tremendous, God was afraid I might be puffed up by them; so I was given a physical condition which has been a thorn in my flesh, a messenger from Satan to hurt and bother me, and prick my pride. Three different times I begged God to make me well again. Each time he said, 'No, But I am with you; that is all you need. My power shows up best in weak people.' Now I am glad to boast about how weak I am; I am glad to be a living demonstration of Christ's power, instead of showing off my own power and abilities. Since I know it is all for Christ's good, I am quite happy about 'the thorn,' and about insults and hardships, persecutions and difficulties; for when I am weak, then I am strong—the less I have, the more I depend on him" (2 Cor. 12:7-10, TLB).

None of us would choose to have the gift of a disability. But many have no choice. For example, consider Mike Boyd, who fell when his scaffolding collapsed and is now a quadriplegic. Yet his testimony remains strong. "If I can be a better witness for God from my wheelchair, then I would not want anything else."

As long as we live in this world of sin, we are targets for accidents, chronic pain, and debilitating disease. Hopefully, we can learn to say as Paul did: "I have learned the secret of being content in any and every situation. . . . I can do everything through him who gives me strength" (Phil. 4:12, 13, NIV).

In what way are you "disabled"? How are you allowing God to use your "disability"?

365

A REMEDY
FOR GUILT

November 30

Lois (Rittenhouse) Pecce

> All that the Father gives Me shall come to Me; and the one who comes
> to Me I will certainly not cast out. John 6:37, NASB.

The headline virtually screamed the word "GUILTY." The photo beneath it could break a heart. It showed a mother and father bidding farewell to their beloved 18-year-old daughter before guards led her away to serve the next 10 years or more in prison for the alleged murder of her newly born infant.

The love and pain mingled in their faces strikes to the heart of anyone who has loved a child—to the heart of anyone who has loved anyone. What true parents have not dreamed dreams and hoped hopes for their children? What parents have not labored and sacrificed to help these hopes come true? College . . . music lessons . . . ball games . . .

Such a scene reminds one that for all of us, when called to stand before God, the righteous Judge, and answer for our lives, the verdict will be guilty! The Bible tells us that "*all* have sinned" (Rom. 3:23).

But in our hurting love for a straying or troubled child another picture comes to mind—a picture of God, our Father, who emptied all heaven on our behalf and spent His most cherished possession to redeem us. God did something for us that the young girl's parents were unable to do for her. Isaiah 53:5-9 tells how He took our punishment! "But he was pierced for our transgressions, he was crushed for our iniquities. . . . We all, like sheep, have gone astray, each of us has turned to his own way; and the Lord has laid on him the iniquity of us all" (NIV).

Our way of dealing with another's guilt (or supposed guilt) is to throw stones and to separate the troubled person from the very sources and community that might render aid. Someone has referred to it as "shooting our wounded."

The Lord does not let the guilty go free, but He does offer a solution— a solution that, were it practiced among us as family, friends, community, and church, would restore many a troubled, hurting soul. With heart and arms wide open, He pleads, "Come unto me" (Matt. 11:28). His promise is that He will not cast out any who do so (see John 6:37).

*Is there someone who needs your example
of God's love and acceptance?*

THE HEALTH BENEFITS OF GENEROSITY

Command them to do good, to be rich in good deeds, and to be generous and willing to share. In this way they will lay up treasure for themselves as a firm foundation for the coming age, so that they may take hold of the life that is truly life. 1 Tim. 6:18, 19, NIV.

When John D. Rockefeller was in his 50s he was broken in health and ready to die as the richest man in the United States. It was said that the veins in his arms were as hard as lead pipes. He was a driven man—driven to satisfy his lust for material wealth—and had used every possible means available to him to make money and destroy his competitors.

As Rockefeller faced death he began to see himself for the greedy fool he really was, and to fear his encounter with God. Maybe if he used his money to meet the needs of others, he thought, God would forgive him for the way he had acquired his wealth.

He resolved to become kind and benevolent, and began giving away millions. Instead of dying, he steadily improved in health. He was also far happier in his money-giving days than he had been in his money-making days. When he died at the ripe old age of 97, it was said that the veins in his arms were as soft as a baby's.

Long before Rockefeller, the Bible illustrated the health principle of generosity with the story of two rich farmers.

The farmer in Luke 12:16-21 had a problem. His harvest was so bountiful his barns weren't large enough to store it. In a purely selfish but very logical decision, the man ordered larger grain elevators built, and then stretched out in his recliner and gloated over how lavishly he had provided for himself for years to come so he could take it easy, eat, drink, and be merry. Jesus called him a fool, because that night the man died and someone else inherited his wealth.

The second was Boaz. In contrast, Boaz allowed the poor to glean in his fields. He was particularly generous with a foreign-born widow, Ruth, and later married her. Because of his generosity he became the great-grandfather of King David and a forerunner of the Saviour Himself (Ruth 2-4).

When you're tempted to accumulate things for yourself, remember the scriptural health principle: "It is more blessed to give than to receive" (Acts 20:35).

What more could you do to practice the health principle of generosity?

CLEANING UP MY KITCHEN

There is a way that seems right to a man, but in the end it leads to death. Prov. 14:12, NIV.

It all started when I began skimping on my sleep, eating on the run, and pushing myself to renovate a halfway house for prisoners. Lack of funding forced me into full-time fund raising and full-time construction. After six months of abusing my body, moving became painful. I couldn't get out of the car without Al's help. I kept thinking, *All I need is a good night's rest, and I'll bounce back.* But I didn't. Instead, I began taking Advil to kill the pain.

While at a board meeting at Weimar Institute, Dr. Vernon Foster noticed me trying to get up out of the chair and asked, "What's wrong?" After a quick exam, he said, "You'll have to see a doctor and have tests, Jane, but it looks like polymyalgia rheumatica."

I went back home, found a specialist, and started drug therapy. But month after month I got no better. When the dosage was increased and another drug given to prevent hemorrhaging, I became convicted that this was not the way to go, so I called Dr. Foster. He agreed, and instead of prescribing drugs, he asked me to walk three miles a day for five days a week, drink more than 2 quarts of water daily, sleep eight hours a night, rest with my eyes closed one hour in the middle of the day, and eat no dairy products or refined fats or sugars.

Do you know what that does to the "good old Adventist diet"? It gets you back to nature. Almost everything you buy has animal products or hydrogenated fat or sugar in it. I put a 30-gallon trash container in the middle of my kitchen and filled it with what I cleaned out my refrigerator and cupboards.

Within 10 days I felt better. In 30 days the change was significant. By the end of 90 days I could hardly remember I had been sick. Now I can tell within an hour if I eat things that aren't good for me.

I'm convinced that there is a way that may seem right to us, but in the end is pain, sickness, disability, and eventually death.

Just to know and not to do is not good enough, either in the area of our physical health, or in our spiritual lives. "Lord, help me to walk the walk, and not just talk the talk."

> But a Samaritan, as he traveled, came where the man was; and when he saw him, he took pity on him. He went to him and bandaged his wounds, pouring on oil and wine. Then he put the man on his own donkey, took him to an inn and took care of him. Luke 10:33, 34, NIV.

Dale Shields fell into a deep depression after having seven bypass operations. He thought he had nothing to live for and abandoned all hope in himself and in life. Then one day as he was fishing at a wharf in Florida, he saw a pelican trapped and dying in the rocks. He rescued the pelican, took it home, and cared for it until it was well again. Since then Dale Shields has dedicated his life to the rescue of thousands of birds wounded by helicopter rotors or fishing nets and lines. They call him "the pelican man."

The amazing fact is that in aiding others, he helped himself and discovered the "double healing effect." In saving helpless birds, he ended up saving himself. He found a reason to live. "Those birds need me," he says. "Someone has to help a bird in need."

If only more people would discover the double healing effect and reach out to others instead of focusing on themselves and their miserable condition. Abraham Lincoln expressed it well when he said that by relieving the pain of another, one relieves their own.

Dr. Karl Menninger, the famous psychiatrist, once gave a lecture on mental health and was answering questions from the audience.

"What would you advise a person to do," asked one man, "if that person felt a nervous breakdown coming on?"

Most people expected him to reply, "Consult a psychiatrist." To their astonishment, he said, "Lock up your house, go across the railway tracks, find someone in need, and do something to help that person."

I like the thought that Ellen G. White expresses: "Doing good is a work that benefits both giver and receiver. If you forget self in your interest for others, you gain a victory over your infirmities. The satisfaction you will realize in doing good will aid you greatly in the recovery of the healthy tone of the imagination. The pleasure of doing good animates the mind and vibrates through the whole body" *(Testimonies,* vol. 2, p. 534).

I challenge you to begin serving others and experience for yourself the double healing effect!

Lord, give me the good Samaritan's heart to serve others unselfishly.

TEACH THEM TO LOVE MY SABBATH

"I said, 'You are my servant'; I have chosen you and have not rejected you. So do not fear, for I am with you; do not be dismayed, for I am your God. I will strengthen you and help you; I will uphold you with my righteous right hand." Isa. 41:9, 10, NIV.

Several years ago depression overcame me. In addition, I am in constant, excruciating pain from a herniated disk, vertebral spondylosis, and bone spurs. I became convinced I was too crippled, too ugly, too fat for anyone ever to care about and began to believe I couldn't do anyone any good. I was ready to give up. What was the point of going on? But God had put two wonderful nephews in my life—Joel and Chad. I thought if I could make a difference in their lives and their friends' lives, then maybe there would be a reason to go on. So I prayed, "Lord, what can I do for You and them?"

God responded with "Teach them to love My Sabbath." But I had no idea what to do. So God provided me with two wonderful books: *From Dilemma to Delight*, by Gerita Garver Liebelt, and *A Love Song for the Sabbath*, by Richard Davidson. Here I found a wealth of ideas. I decided to plan a typical Jewish Shabbat celebration and welcome the Sabbath with these young people.

God helped me gather Bible texts that took symbols of salvation in the Old Testament and linked them to their fulfillment in Christ. The service is simple, but full of meaning. Everyone participates.

Early in the service the "father" or person in charge places his hands upon the head of every child and pronounces blessings. It is a very solemn and moving experience. During dinner we give our testimonies, and end with a call for rededication to God.

Friday evenings have become the most special time in the week for us. The young people show up early to help prepare the meal and set the table with our best china, silver, and crystal to welcome the King of the universe. They stay late into the evening talking about their spiritual concerns and blessings.

I am living proof that a person can "come again from the land of the enemy" (Jer. 31:16). Now I have a reason to live: to help every young person I meet to love the Sabbath and the Lord of the Sabbath.

Why not invite the Lord of the universe to dinner next Friday evening and celebrate Shabbat with Him!

ARISE
AND EAT

Betty M. Hoehn

And as [Elijah] lay and slept under a juniper tree, behold, then an angel touched him, and said unto him, Arise and eat. 1 Kings 19:5.

It had been a long, trying, and tiring day. Elijah had had little or no time to eat, and certainly no time to rest. He had to keep a vigilant eye on the priests of Baal.

More than 12 barrels of water had been hauled up that mountain, probably from the sea below. Following the dramatic display of fireworks from God, Elijah had given the order to execute justice, killing all the priests of Baal. It was a physically and emotionally draining time.

Elijah prayed intensely seven times for rain, and when it finally came, he ran ahead of King Ahab's chariot for about 25 miles through a torrential downpour to the gates of Jezreel.

He was totally exhausted, physically and emotionally spent, when a messenger notified Elijah that he was on Jezebel's hit list.

Immediately he and his servant fled down the 95-mile stretch to Beersheba, and then another 20-some miles out into the desert. Ancient Palestine had no Taco Bells or Subways. Just a juniper tree. There Elijah collapsed, asked God to let him die, and slept.

Then an angel touched him. The being offered no scathing rebuke, no "Where was your faith?" criticism, no "Don't you think if God could protect you from all the priests of Baal, He could shield you from Jezebel?"

No, the Bible record simply states that the angel provided him with fresh bread and a jug of water and said, "Arise and eat."

Elijah ate. He drank. He slept.

Then enters the angel again and says, "Arise and eat; because the journey is too great for thee" (1 Kings 19:7). God knew it was going to be a 40-day-and-night journey of about 200 miles to Mount Horeb, the next rest area.

God knows we can't deal with spiritual conflicts until we get our physical bodies back in balance.

How is it with you today? Have you been overstressed, overworked, overburdened? Rest, then "arise and eat" the food and drink of angels.

Thank You, God, for meeting all my needs: for rest, for food,
and for drink. And Lord, help me to remember,
when I'm stressed out, that You don't require me
to go on until my life is back in balance. Amen.

"WHAT ARE YOU DOING HERE?"

So he got up and ate and drank. Strengthened by that food, he traveled forty days and forty nights until he reached Horeb, the mountain of God. There he went into a cave and spent the night. And the word of the Lord came to him: "What are you doing here, Elijah?" 1 Kings 19:8, 9, NIV.

Elijah was in the depths of depression. He saw himself a target for execution because he had defended God before the whole rebellious nation. The prophet considered himself the only one left on earth loyal to God. It didn't look like there was much use for him to continue his witnessing.

The Lord told him to stand in His presence, then offered a demonstration of power. A mighty wind hurled rocks and shattered the mountains. But God was not in it.

A mighty earthquake heaved the ground beneath his feet. But God was not the earthquake.

Then came the fires. But God was not there.

Finally a quiet, tender voice. That was God!

"What are you doing here, Elijah? You are important to Me. I have some vital work for you to do. First, I want you to anoint Hazael to be king over Syria. Second, anoint Jehu to be king over Israel. Third, anoint Elisha to be a prophet after you. And, by the way, Elijah, 7,000 have not bowed the knee to Baal. Come, let us be going."

God did not chide Elijah, just used some dramatic events to change the focus of Elijah's attention.

No harsh words—just affirmation. "You are still My prophet. Go, return to do the work of a prophet, Elijah."

Elijah must have taken a deep breath, squared his shoulders, and walked back toward Damascus. He had seen scarier things than an angry Jezebel, but God had preserved him again.

Let us remember, as we work for Him, that we too are not alone. He will be guiding us by the still, small voice of His Holy Spirit.

We do not need to fear furious Jezebels. And somewhere out there 7,000-plus loyal members also work along with us for God.

And if we get discouraged and think our efforts are ineffective, and run away to hide, be sure God will ask, "What are you doing here?"

Think about your circumstances, where you are at this time. If God asked you "What are you doing here?" what would you answer?

BOUNDARIES

Paul and Carol Cannon

There was strife between the herdsmen of Abram's cattle and the herdsmen of Lot's cattle. . . . Then Abram said to Lot, "Let there be no strife between you and me, and between your herdsmen and my herdsmen; . . . Is not the whole land before you? Separate yourself from me." Gen. 13:7-9, RSV.

The Bible offers many examples of healthy boundary-setting, of setting limits beyond which we can refuse to permit ourselves to be pushed against our wills. For example, Jesus set boundaries, even with his own parents (Luke 2:49). When His mother attempted to dominate and control Him, He told her not to tell Him what to do (John 2:4). As Peter tried to manage Jesus' behavior, Jesus replied, "Get away from me, Satan! You are an obstacle in my way" (Matt. 16:23, TEV). Yet many Christians feel guilty if they define a psychological boundary, or defend themselves when they feel they are taken advantage of or hurt.

What is a boundary? It is the means by which we protect ourselves from others who would hurt or control us in some way, yet without offending others. It is a barrier beyond which we will not go, and behind which we will not allow others to come.

Our boundaries define who we are and what is important to us. In order to let others know how we want to be treated, we have to be willing to tell the truth and set limits. Trying to relate to a person whose boundaries are blurry is like trying to play volleyball on an unmarked court. You can't tell when the ball is out of bounds. Lack of boundaries causes all kinds of personal conflicts.

In the interest of better relationships and greater intimacy we need to learn how to set boundaries.

Boundaries keep bad, negative, undesirable stuff out and hold good, positive, helpful stuff in. The bark on a tree protects it from disease (bad stuff). The peel on an orange keeps the juice in (good stuff). Our immune system works similarly. It is the physiological barrier that protects us from illness.

In most cases sickness indicates that our immune system has broken down. When our boundaries aren't working—boom. We get sick! Likewise, when our personal relationships become messed up, it indicates that our social and emotional boundary system needs attention. We must learn to set boundaries as Abram and Lot did in order to maintain healthy relationships.

Dear Lord, help me to learn to speak up when I feel someone is trying to control me, and on the flip side, Lord, help me to be careful not to control others with my anger, jealousy, moodiness, or fear.

THE FOUNTAIN OF YOUTH

December 8
Edwin H. Krick

> Who satisfies your desires with good things so that your youth
> is renewed like the eagle's. Ps. 103:5, NIV.

For hundreds of years humanity has dreamed of finding a "fountain of youth" whose healing waters would make the old young, cure disease, and prolong life. I'd like to propose that we have found the elusive fountain of youth but haven't realized it. One important secret to longevity lies in protecting and maintaining a healthy immune system.

We have more control over it than medical science previously realized. The Creator has built into the body tremendous capacity for maintaining and restoring health. Therefore, good habits maintained and bad habits discarded may help us discover the legendary fountain of youth.

You should know that during the next 24 hours you will probably get cancer! The wildly growing cells we know as cancer develop frequently in the body, perhaps even several times a day. A healthy immune system detects and eliminates the cancer cells before we have a chance to know they're present.

Other areas of disease in which the immune system plays a role include infections, certain types of autoimmune diseases including arthritis and lupus, and the major killers: heart attack and stroke.

The good news is that you can *choose* to have a healthy immune system. Exercise regularly (a minimum of 20 minutes every other day), eat a balanced diet (avoid the high fat and protein of animal products), get seven to nine hours of sleep a night, and be optimistic and laugh a lot. And *avoid* the damaging effects on the immune system of obesity, alcohol, tobacco, marijuana, and other "street drugs," as well as unbridled stress and negative emotions.

Solomon may not have been an immunologist, but his statement in Proverbs 17:22—"A merry heart doeth good like a medicine: but a broken spirit drieth the bones"—shows great insight into the immune system, a major portion of which originates in the bone marrow. Science confirms that a merry heart does good, probably better than a medicine, while a broken spirit damages the bone marrow (immune system).

If you make healthy choices daily, avoid harmful substances, and keep a song in your heart, you may have taken a big step toward discovering your own fountain of youth.

Dear Creator, thank you for my immune system. May I determine to make healthy choices to keep it strong and vigilant. Amen.

ON WINGS
OF PRAISE

> For the Lord takes delight in his people; he crowns the humble with salvation.
> Let the saints rejoice in this honor and sing for joy on their beds. Ps. 149:4, 5, NIV.

I was just recovering from having partially ruptured a lower disk in my spine. I had spent three weeks in bed trying to allow it to heal with gentle, conservative treatment.

My husband, Dan, had purchased a motor home so that I could lie down as we traveled about 2,000 miles to our next evangelistic assignment. I was just rejoicing that I was doing so well when we stopped at an RV park to take a shower. The hot water in the shower suddenly turned ice cold, causing the muscles in my back to go into painful spasms. Muffling a cry of pain, I feared the disk had slipped out again.

We spent the night in a motel, thinking a hot tub bath might give me some relief—but it was in vain! I was alone now, lying in pain on the couch in our motor home, anxious and depressed, when our teammate John gave me some much-needed advice. "Don't let your physical condition get you down," he said.

His quiet admonition aroused me, and I lifted my thoughts to God. "Father, I really am getting more and more depressed. Please lift me up on wings of praise and fill my heart and mind with joyful songs and promises from Your Word, for when the Holy Spirit has control, there is peace and joy."

I began singing songs of praise and happiness in my mind, and as I sang, Jesus removed the depression. The spasms lessened! Now I really praised Him! "O thank You, Lord, that the disk is not out, and that it's just muscle spasms!" The more I praised Him, the better I felt.

It reminded me of the admonition: "Let the saints . . . sing for joy on their beds." When do you go to bed? It's when you're tired, sick, or depressed. You go to bed when you least feel like singing. But on beds of pain, whether spiritual, mental, or physical, is also the very time you most need to sing and ask God to lift you up on wings of praise.

What better time than now to sing a praise song to the Lord?
"Rejoice in the Lord always, and again I say rejoice."

THE ENVIRONMENT AND HEALTH

Max Torkelsen

The nations were angry; and your wrath has come. The time has come
. . . for destroying those who destroy the earth. Rev. 11:18, NIV.

Consider these facts:
- In 1960 the average U.S. citizen produced three pounds of trash per day; today five pounds per person per day go into the trash.
- Ten thousand people die each year from pesticide poisoning, and another 40,000 fall ill. The rapidly increasing use of such chemicals throughout the world threatens water quality and poses risks of increased cancer and birth defects.
- Each year human beings clear an area of tropical forest the size of Scotland; the soil then erodes, the climate begins changing, and the forest's replenishing resources have vanished.
- Scientists estimate that as many as one million species of plant and animal life will have become extinct from the human destruction of forests and ecosystems by the end of the twentieth century.

The beginning of Hosea 4 describes the Lord's "controversy with the inhabitants of the land" (verse 1). He says that they lack kindness and faithfulness, replacing it with lying, stealing, cheating, adultery, and murder. And what is the result? "The land mourns, and all who live in it waste away" (verse 3, NIV) and the beasts, birds, and even fish disappear.

The Bible clearly laments the deterioration of the environment. When you contrast it with the wondrous pictures of creation's intended harmony and wholeness given in Scripture, you realize that environmental ruin is an offense against God.

At Creation God gave humanity "dominion" over all the earth (Gen. 1:26-28). However, the biblical term *dominion* does not mean arrogant domination. The biblical concept of dominion is connected to two other key ideas—covenant and stewardship. The Bible expresses not only God's covenant with humanity, but also His covenant with all of nature (see Gen. 9:13-15). Dominion implies the responsibility to serve nature in what is essentially a stewardship relationship. God calls upon the Christian to exhibit dominion over nature without being destructive.

Unfortunately, God's command to "subdue" the earth (Gen. 1:28) has served as a sweeping rationalization for mindless exploitation of natural resources. Christians, of all people, should not be the destroyers. We should treat nature with an overwhelming respect.

*What can I do to help preserve the national resources that
God created for our use and management?*

AVOID
HALT

Pat B. Mutch

> Be most careful then how you conduct yourselves: like sensible men,
> not like simpletons. Eph. 5:15, NEB.

Through the writings of Paul we find woven the thread of self-control as a Christian virtue. He writes: "This is the will of God, that you should be holy: . . . each one of you must learn to gain mastery over his body, to hallow and honour it" (1 Thess. 4:3, 4, NEB). The implication is that we must respect the Creation laws. The context is often one of avoiding lust—that is, craving for illicit pleasure.

Recovering alcoholics and addicts have much wisdom to share about such physical battles. An alcoholic may be "dry," that is, not drinking, but still have strong cravings to "feel good" by drinking. Only through surrender to God's power can the alcoholic learn true sobriety and obtain victory. But God's power isn't like a magic wand that instantly solves any problem—living in connection with God involves making wise choices every day.

Some of these choices have to do with respecting the powerful influence of those places and people that can lure a person back into drinking. It means staying away from such places and people. The 12 steps of recovery offer practical guidelines for building spiritual strength. Other choices involve participation in a fellowship of recovering people, such as Alcoholics Anonymous (AA), which offers encouragement and spiritual strength for working through these steps. AA teaches a helpful motto—"Avoid HALT"—that has merit for any person seeking to live a positive Christian life.

"Avoid HALT" stands for "avoid becoming hungry, angry, lonely, or tired (HALT)." Irregular or skipped meals result in low blood sugar levels, often leading to irritability and emotional imbalance. Anger is a normal human emotion, but nursing it and rehearsing our reasons to be angry lead to depression and often actions we regret. Isolation from other human beings, whatever the reason, weakens us socially and spiritually. God made us to be interdependent with others (Gen. 2:18). When we become overly tired, short of sleep or rest, it impairs our ability to think clearly. Our emotions become less stable.

"Avoid HALT" offers a practical self-monitoring tool for life balance because it honors the laws of the body.

How would you rate yourself on avoiding HALT
(being hungry, angry, lonely, or tired)?

OUT OF THE ASHES OF MY LIFE

J. Rita Vital

To appoint unto them that mourn in Zion, to give unto them beauty for ashes, the oil of joy for mourning, the garment of praise for the spirit of heaviness; that they might be called trees of righteousness, the planting of the Lord, that he might be glorified. Isa. 61:3.

How many times had I been the one listening to the heartbreak of a wife going through a divorce she never dreamed would happen? Now it had happened to me! The shock and disbelief left me numb. My mind reeled as I tried to sort out this cataclysmic emotional trauma from the already heavy pressures of wife, mother, daughter, worker, and church and community volunteer. Dad was ailing and nearing death. Mother was trying to be courageous after a recent leg amputation. Both needed loving support and care. I felt as David did when he mournfully sang, "Faint and badly crushed I groan aloud in anguish of heart" (Ps. 38:8, REB).

Broken under the weight of it all, I staggered outdoors into the mild August evening air. There I found myself in the midst of my vegetable garden, furiously weeding the bean patch. Each clump of weeds felt like an enemy evicted. As I stepped back to view the weeded row with a sense of satisfaction and relief, a sudden pleasing aroma surrounded me. Wondering about its source, I glanced downward. In disbelief I realized I had trampled on my basil plants!

Standing motionless as the quiet fragrance enveloped me, I was impressed that it took "crushing" and "brokenness" to produce the sudden fragrance that had proved such a blessed experience.

Yes, Christ's body was broken for *me* and sin crushed Him, bringing forth the fragrant gift of salvation for *me!* With a deeply thankful heart I prayerfully walked from the garden, nurtured by the object lesson that God could take my "crushed" and "broken" life and make me a fragrance for Him.

After my divorce, while my friends were retiring from work, I found myself enrolled in graduate school, prayerfully pursuing a master's degree in public health. During this same time a prayer band was praying for someone to start a van ministry in Boston. A week after my graduation the Boston Van Ministry was born out of the ashes of my life, perfumed with crushed basil!

When you feel broken and crushed, remember that God has promised beauty for ashes!

WHO TAUGHT ME TO FEAR?

> In love there can be no fear, but fear is driven out by perfect love: because to fear is to expect punishment, and anyone who is afraid is still imperfect in love. 1 John 4:18, Jerusalem.

Perhaps millions of people have bowed down on their knees in sincere prayer to the God of the universe . . . but for a terribly wrong reason. Fearful at having discovered flaws and stupid choices in their lives, they have a deep inner dread that a powerful and righteous God is going to do to them what they deserve. That He is going to punish them, inflicting some kind of pain on them to show His extreme displeasure. And they fear Him.

Fear—that anxious dread of pain to come—makes people pay attention. It starts their adrenaline flowing, and they begin to negotiate with God. Maybe they can give larger offerings or serve on a church committee. Perhaps if they pray longer, with a tighter feeling in their throat and more sweat on their palms, they can appease God's anger. Or maybe they can throw some good deeds onto the other side of the scale and make up for the bad deeds.

In fact, the fear of God's punishment produces so many "good" behaviors that it lets us overlook how unhealthy fear really is. To begin with, fear is a physical destroyer, pumping stomach-eating acids and inducing nerve-wrenching anxiety. Fearful people live tense, risk-averse lives, flying at very low altitudes and missing the greater adventures of being alive.

What is more, fear is the poorest form of motivation for doing good things. It keeps us from seeing that right choices carry their own rewards. Fearful people become victims of whoever makes the loudest threats of pain. And fear blinds us to the presence of genuine unconditional love. We can't get close to people we fear. When we fear failure, rejection, or loss, we end up missing some of life's greatest joys and adventures.

Most tragically, fear of God is a primitive, immature, wholly unnecessary, and soul-destroying response to Him. He is our teacher, not our slave driver. God unfolds reasons across our understanding rather than cracking whips across our backs. Truly knowing Him—knowing His love—drives out all fear.

How do you see God? As someone to fear? a judge? a shepherd?
If you were to paint a picture of God, what would you depict?

WAS I GOING TO DIE?

December 14
Jill Kennedy

Peace I leave with you; my peace I give you. I do not give to you as the world gives. Do not let your hearts be troubled and do not be afraid. John 14:27, NIV.

was scared. Was I going to die? Would my boys be motherless? And would my husband love me less if I had to have a mastectomy?

I had just received news of a mass in my left breast. It was our twenty-first wedding anniversary. A hushed reserve hung over us as we ate our special dinner together, and later, as we sat in our hotel room, we talked about what the future might hold.

By Friday, without our anniversary celebration to think about, the depressing "what if" feelings crept in. I prayed constantly, and forced myself to sing and be happy. But the next day in church, thoughts of possible death and despair overwhelmed me, and I broke down. The statistics kept ringing in my ears. After lung cancer, breast cancer is the leading cancer killer of U.S. women.

On Sunday we both went to see the surgeon, and we were encouraged. He felt that it was possibly a fibrocystic nodule. Saying that he wanted to see me in two months, he put me on a strict diet and increased exercise. According to research findings, an extra 15 pounds increases the risk of breast cancer by 37 percent, and with an extra 20 pounds the risk rises to 52 percent. That means that a 10-pound difference may be significant when it comes to lowering your cancer risk. And according to Dr. Noreen Azid, of the Lee Moffit Cancer Center in Tampa, Florida, of all the decades of life you should lose that extra weight, it's the third one.

The weeks passed, and I had lost 12 pounds. Allan went with me to see the doctor. Following an ultrasound and mammogram, the doctor reported: "There is no mass." After comparing the reports and seeing the mammogram, we sighed in relief and sent a prayer heavenward in thanksgiving.

From that experience we learned how precious is our health, and how its threatened loss can suddenly and markedly rearrange our priorities. Continually I resolve to appreciate each day the Lord gives and to be glad and rejoice in it.

What should you do today, in case there is no tomorrow?

IN MY MOST EMBARRASSING MOMENTS

But he said to me, "My grace is sufficient for you, for my power is made perfect in weakness." 2 Cor. 12:9, NIV.

Father, today I tried to take out my patient's teeth to wash, only to discover that they weren't dentures. One of my confused patients thought his water pitcher was a urinal, and I ordered two meal trays for the same patient and both were the wrong diet.

That's not all.

I embarrassed myself by asking my patient's wife if she was his daughter. The student nurse asked me a simple question, and I didn't know the answer.

Days like this make me feel inadequate. Help me, Father, not to be critical of myself.

Remind me that Your followers of old had days like this too. Peter failed at walking on water and Jonah jumped into the belly of a whale.

Their "bad" days passed. Mine will too.

Do your prayers sometimes sound like mine? Do you sometimes have days when nothing seems to go right? You get up early and have a neat devotional time with the Lord, get dressed in your new outfit, and head off to work, thinking the day will be great, only to end up getting a traffic ticket on the street all your colleagues take coming to work. Or at the end of the day find the sales tag still on the jacket you've been wearing!

I'm convinced that sometimes I'm more the bull in a china closet trying to get through the day than a neurosurgeon cauterizing tiny blood vessels in the brain. My blundering ways cause more embarrassment than I care to endure.

That's why I need that devotional time with the Lord. God can't keep me from making a fool of myself, but He can remind me each morning that even though He lives in a high and holy place and will never make a mistake, He lives with those who do—"with him who is contrite and lowly in spirit, *to revive the spirit of the lowly and to revive the heart of the contrite*" (Isa. 57:15, NIV).

Many days I am contrite—broken, crushed—and need a heart revived by God.

Thank You, Father, for Your daily reminder that You will never laugh at my mistakes, but will proudly stand by my side in my most embarrassing moments.

WHAT'S YOUR SACRIFICE?

Dane J. Griffin

> Does the Lord delight in burnt offerings and sacrifices as much as in obeying the voice of the Lord? To obey is better than sacrifice, and to heed is better than the fat of rams. For rebellion is like the sin of divination, and arrogance like the evil of idolatry. 1 Sam. 15:22, 23, NIV.

People are willing to give up anything to get their health back." Dr. Bruce Hyde looked me squarely in the eyes, then leaned back in his chair. "They'll give up their car, boat, plane, vacation, house—*any-thing!*" The young physician shook his head and sighed. "Anything except the very cause—their poor lifestyle habits."

Can what we eat or don't eat, can what we do or don't do, make a difference between health and sickness? Listen to the words of a few "experts":

"A healthy diet could dramatically reduce your chances of getting cancer of the colon, prostate, and breast."—Dr. Sushma Palmer, Georgetown University.

"The dietary factors responsible for cancer are principally fat and meat intake."—Dr. Gio B. Gori, National Cancer Institute.

"We can say with almost total certainty that the diet we eat is leading to heart disease."—Dr. Scott Grundy, University of Texas.

"Diet change . . . , not drugs, should be the first treatment for people with high cholesterol."—Dr. Dean Ornish, University of California, San Francisco.

"Many of the people I see in my office probably wouldn't be needing my help if they had learned the principles of low-fat living at an early age."—Dr. Steven Van Camp, Alvarado Hospital Medical Center, San Diego, California.

God's people face a serious question today: Will we continue to be governed by appetite, refusing to obey either God or science, or will we submit to God's counsel? What will we sacrifice as we obey God's health principles?

The choice is clear. According to what Samuel said to Saul in 1 Samuel 15:22, to rebel against God on any point is like divination or witchcraft, and to stubbornly refuse to change is like worshiping idols.

"If [those who have had insight on diet and dress] blunt their consciences to avoid the cross which they will have to take up to be in harmony with natural law, they will, in order to shun reproach, violate the Ten Commandments" *(Testimonies,* vol. 3, p. 51).

If you refuse to obey, you may be sacrificing more than you think!

*Lord, help me to sacrifice the unhealthy food that I love so
I can have good health to serve You better.*

WALKING AND "TOGETHERING"

Dick Duerksen

Blessed are all who fear the Lord, who walk in his ways. Ps. 128:1, NIV.

Getting out of bed is the hardest thing I do. When I'm horizontal, warm and comfortable between the sheets, I'm about as peaceful as a guy can get. Then Brenda stands beside the bed and asks the daily question, "Are you going to go for a walk with me?"

The correct answer is "Yes, I'll bounce right up and be with you." Instead my lips give her an inarticulate grunt that promises action, while my body still clings to the bedspread. Then, since I have promised to get up today, I pour my eager body onto the floor, where Drinian's doggy kisses remind me of the value of standing on my feet.

Five minutes later I'm in front of the garage doing 50 jumping jacks in an attempt to activate at least a few of my dormant red blood cells. Brenda joins me, and "the walk" begins. Our track leads through the neighborhood, down a couple hills, back up past the Wilsons, down the Cresses' long cul-de-sac, past two lovely flower gardens, around the corner, and back up Tuckahoe Lane. The whole trip takes about 30 minutes and covers most of two miles. I know we should probably take an hour and dash lightly across many miles of God's earth. But this is working wonderfully for us right now.

While on the trail we walk quickly and talk softly. We remember good times from yesterday, review the day's calendar, and wonder together about the lives of those we love the most. Although the conversation helps us maintain a brisk pace, that's not its greatest benefit. The conversation/walk is our way of breathing a new vitality into our relationship each morning. It is a daily reconnecting and recommitting to God and each other. Yes, there is healing in the walking, but the "togethering" has even greater value.

Getting out of bed is still the hardest thing I do. But the walk that follows has become one of the easiest. And one of the best.

Are you getting the best out of life? What about a little walking and "togethering" with someone you love?

SPIRITUAL GLAUCOMA

Izak Wessels

> Woe to you, blind guides! You say, "If anyone swears by the temple, it means nothing; but if anyone swears by the gold of the temple, he is bound by his oath." You blind fools! Which is greater: the gold, or the temple that makes the gold sacred? Matt. 23:16, 17, NIV.

Glaucoma is a serious eye disease, too often resulting in blindness. It is a slow and insidious atrophy of the optic nerve that follows a too-high pressure inside the eye. A normal pressure keeps the eyeball just firm enough for it to function. Loss of the delicate balance between secretion of the aqueous fluid and its absorption results in increased pressure that damages the nerve connecting the eye to the brain. This causes loss of the peripheral vision so important for not bumping into things. However, a small central spot (like looking down a tube) remains up to the end. Only after severe and irreversible damage has occurred does the victim begin to notice a problem.

More than half of the 2 to 3 million Americans over 40 with glaucoma have no idea that they are slowly going blind. Unfortunately, it has no cure. Regular daily use of special eye drops with surgery, if necessary, can prevent further damage. Because timely diagnosis and therapy is critical, one should have regular eye exams. Individuals especially at risk include those who have a close relative with glaucoma, have used cortisone for a long time, have had previous surgery or injuries to the eye, or have diabetes or nearsightedness.

The Pharisees and Laodiceans both seemed to have spiritual glaucoma. An arrogant, too-high self-opinion slowly but irreversibly damages the connection between the soul and heaven. This results in narrow vision, not seeing the bigger picture, and constant focus and emphasis on insignificant minor issues. Unfortunately, such individuals do not realize their predicament, which can be learned only from regularly consulting the True Physician. Evil relatives or friends, critical cynicism, as well as past hurts make a person more likely to develop this spiritual disease. Fortunately, God has a divine remedy that restores spiritual eyesight, but only if its victims regularly apply it, and if treatment starts before too much damage has occurred.

"But you do not realize that you are wretched, pitiful, poor, blind and naked. I counsel you to buy from me . . . salve to put on your eyes, so you can see" (Rev. 3:17, 18, NIV).

Are you in danger of developing spiritual glaucoma?
What can you do to prevent it?

WHEN NOTHING IS EVERYTHING

David Beardsley

If ye then be not able to do that thing which is least, why take ye thought for the rest? Luke 12:26.

Right from the beginning God gave us a clue as to one of His favorite mediums to create out of—little or nothing. As we read through the Bible it becomes apparent that God is at His best when He is working with nothing. It all started at Creation, when God fashioned the beautiful earth which we enjoy—from nothing.

All through the Bible we find stories illustrating the same principle. When a widow was about to have her boys taken from her because she was not able to pay her bills, Elisha told her to take the only thing she had, a small flask of oil, and with it fill all the containers she and her boys could find. She then sold the oil and paid her creditors.

Sarah bore a son when she was physically unable to have a child, and from that child came descendants numbering as the stars of the sky.

After reducing Gideon's army to little or nothing, God then used it to defeat the Midianites.

With only a little stone David, with no sword or spear or armor, defeated the strongest warrior in Palestine.

God provided food for more than 40 years to the Israelites in the desert, where there was no food. Also, in the desert when there was no water God issued a stream of water from a rock.

When the man had no strength, Jesus told the paralytic to take up his bed and walk. When there was no sight, He enabled the blind to see. When there was no life, He raised Lazarus from the grave. When there was no hope, He gave the thief dying on the cross confidence in a future life. When His disciples had no vision, He gave them a mandate that would send the gospel to the then-known world.

It is when we feel our emptiness that we can be filled. The Bible says it best in John 4:14: "But whosoever drinketh of the water that I shall give him shall never thirst; but the water I shall give him shall be in him a well of water springing up into everlasting life."

Give God your emptiness today, and allow Him to make something beautiful of your life.

SUGAR
IN THE
MORNING . . .

Jan W. Kuzma

Woe to those who call evil good and good evil, who put darkness for light and light for darkness, who put bitter for sweet and sweet for bitter. Isa. 5:20, NIV.

Remember that jingle about sugar in the morning, evening, and suppertime? Well, most of us, including children, take the jingle literally and stuff ourselves with sugar—120 to 150 pounds a year. Of course, we wouldn't think of going to the sugar bowl and eating a spoonful. And most of us have no idea we're even consuming sugar, because it's deceptively hidden away in our favorite foods. Take an apple for example. If you would eat a ripe apple as God intended it to be eaten, it would have natural sugars in it, but no refined sugar, and would contain only about 70 calories. When you concentrate the apple into apple juice, the calories increase to 120. But put that apple into a slice of apple pie, and the number of calories zooms to 350, because that pie is filled with sugar.

Did you know that manufacturers use more than two thirds of refined sugar by adding it to food products? They even put sugar in salt! And every tablespoon of regular catsup contains a teaspoon of refined sugar!

Here are a few of other popular food items laced with sugar: peanut butter, pickles, canned fruits and vegetables, mayonnaise, breads, many juices, soups, cereals, cured meats, hot dogs, lunch meats, salad dressings, spaghetti sauce, crackers, tomato juice, and pasta products.

Most people eat a third of a pound of sugar a day—600 calories of health-destroying sweetness. The results show in epidemic tooth decay, overweight, and diabetes, as well as other diseases that scientists are beginning to link to high sugar consumption.

These facts probably shock you, because you don't see the sugar you're eating. Like Satan, it's deceptive. A typical satanic strategy is to gain control of innocent people by making deadly things look good, taste good, or feel good. Gambling begins with a lottery ticket. Lung cancer starts with a glamorized Virginia Slim or Marlboro. And obesity commences with the hidden sugars in your favorite foods.

Begin reading labels and discover the hidden sugar.
Don't let Satan deceive you.

PREVENTING
DECEPTION

December 21
Fred Hardinge

False Christs and false prophets will rise and show great signs and wonders to deceive, if possible, even the elect. Matt. 24:24, NKJV.

Have you ever wondered how it could be that Satan could deceive "even the elect" before Christ returns?

Today modern scientific research on the brain reveals how this could happen. Dr. Gregory Belenky and his colleagues at Walter Reed Army Institute of Research have demonstrated that fatigue primarily impairs the function of the frontal lobes of the brain. Using advanced test methods, they have demonstrated that even relatively small losses of sleep significantly reduce the amount of blood flow to this crucial area of the brain.

It is in the frontal lobes that we carry out the highest mental processes, such as judgment, reason, initiative, and forethought. Judgment and reason involve discerning, evaluating, and comparing relevant information to make a correct decision. Forethought is the process of making judgments and plans relating to future events, and initiative is the mental power to begin doing necessary tasks. Fatigue dramatically impairs these important processes.

Have you ever been in a situation in which you were trying to take notes but the speaker was going too fast? Even after the speaker repeated it, you still couldn't get it all. A fatigued brain responds in a similar way. As it tries to handle the first information, it can't process what follows afterward, so important information gets lost, and consequently the person makes decisions on partial information, creating mistakes.

Fatigue selectively targets the highest mental functions. Careful thinking and reasoning become impossible. Because our spiritual life is the highest of all mental functions and requires our very best discernment, thought, and reasoning processes, it is extremely important that we not fall into the trap of not getting enough sleep. It doesn't matter how motivated you are, or how good you are at your profession, or even in your walk with God, a tired brain does not function well and cannot make good, clear decisions, and therefore is easily deceived!

Ellen White wrote: "Whatever detracts from physical vigor, weakens mental effort. . . . We cannot maintain consecration to God, and yet injure our health by the willful indulgence of a wrong habit" *(Review and Herald,* June 15, 1886).

Don't let your lifestyle trap you into fatigue. If you do, you will be much more easily tempted and fooled by the devil!

DIAMONDS AT
CHRISTMAS

December 22
Therese L. Allen

*But when you give a banquet, invite the poor, the crippled, the lame,
the blind, and you will be blessed. Luke 14:13, 14, NIV.*

Emotionally the holidays can be either a joyous occasion or a sad,
lonely, and difficult time.

I was looking forward to Christmas Day, because I was going to
be spending it with my "big sis" and her family. Then Darilee called and
said some friends had invited her family to spend the day with them. She
had told them about me, and they had invited me to come along.

I didn't know these people, so I wasn't sure how welcome I'd feel.
Some people aren't comfortable with my wheelchair. Others give me tons
of unwanted sympathy. I just wanted to be with my family so I could be
myself—no airs, no prim and proper behavior, and no dressing up. But
since I didn't want to be alone, I decided I'd go.

Instantly I felt at home. I received no sympathy, and even though there
were a number of steps into their home, no big deal was made about the
need to carry me up and down them.

They had a delicious meal without too many spoons, knives, and forks
to make me feel uncomfortable. And later in the afternoon we all went
down to the beach. Since there were so many stairs, they could have easily
left me home, but they insisted that I was no trouble, and carried me and
my chair right down to the sand.

Sitting on the beach may not be your idea of an ideal white Christmas,
but it was one of the brightest days in my life! The sky was a brilliant blue
and the sun shone on the water, making it sparkle like diamonds from the
windows of Cartier's or Tiffany's, but no window separated me from
God's treasures. I was right there! It was awesome, as if God was smiling
on a beach full of diamonds. The entire day was wonderful—a gift of peace
and tranquillity with people who loved the Lord, a little heaven on earth.

God has His diamonds in this world who open their hearts and homes
to people like me, to bring an extra sparkle to an otherwise lonely life. You
too can be a diamond.

*As you plan for this Christmas, what can you do to bring an extra
sparkle into lives that might otherwise be sad and lonely?*

WHEN WORDS CANNOT EXPRESS IT, MUSIC CAN

Carlos Pardeiro

Where were you when I laid the earth's foundation? . . . On what were its footings set,
or who laid its cornerstone—while the morning stars sang together and
all the angels shouted for joy? Job 38:4-7, NIV.

Music was made to serve a holy purpose, to lift the thoughts to that which is pure, noble, and elevating, and to awaken in the soul gratitude and devotion to God" *(Patriarchs and Prophets*, p. 594).

I've been a musician for more than 30 years, playing classical music, switching to secular, and back to classical, and in my experience the above quote is the best description I've found for the purpose of music.

God in His love and mercy "made" music. It is a part of His creative work, and its purpose is to take us to the highest level of adoration and gratitude to Him. *When words can't express it, music can.* As the holy angels sense God's love, and they cannot restrain their unmeasurable bliss, they strike a higher note and burst into song (see Ellen G. White, in *Review and Herald,* July 15, 1909). No words or physical expression can surpass the sound of music that comes from a grateful, reverent, joyful heart.

In addition to the creation of the world (when the angels sang together), the two events that mark the highest hope of all ages, the birth of Christ as the Messiah and the second coming of Christ, were and will be accompanied by the sound of "pure, noble, and elevating" music (see Luke 2:13, 14 and 1 Thess. 4:16).

You may feel inadequate to sing or play a musical instrument, but you can still express your song to God in your heart. "Singing is as much an act of worship as is prayer" *(Education,* p. 168). The Holy Spirit will translate your song to God into the most magnificent rhapsody of thanksgiving imaginable. Just approach the throne of Jesus with a humble, repentant, and grateful heart, and He will heal and restore your soul, and the angels will sing for joy.

*Sing a chorus or hymn of praise to God right now, and see
if it doesn't make a difference in the way you feel!*

HOMECOMING

December 24

Kay Kuzma

In my Father's house are many rooms; if it were not so, I would have told you. I am going there to prepare a place for you. And if I go and prepare a place for you, I will come back and take you to be with me that you also may be where I am. John 14:2, 3, NIV.

As we crested the hill, I saw hometown lights aglow with the shimmer of softly falling snow. Christmas Eve. To the left was the huge lighted star on the Flatiron. And to the right, lights stretched far beyond the city limits that we had known as children.

Boulder was beautiful. But it was not the glistening lights that held the meaning—it was the love that was waiting for us in that double-wide mobile home where we would find family.

Our other siblings, Dianne and Richard, and their families were going to be with our parents for Christmas, so Joanie, my other sister, and I, who were living in California, decided to surprise everyone and just show up with our families.

At last we pulled up in front of the house. A soft light filtered through the frosted windows. Our parents were home. All nine of us (two sisters, our husbands, and five children) piled out of the van. We pulled our woolen hats down over our faces and turned up our collars so as not to be recognized too quickly, rang the doorbell, and started singing, "Silent night, holy night, all is calm, all is bright . . ."

We finished the verse and started the second, but no one opened the door. We could hear voices inside. "What shall we give the carolers, cookies or money?" At last my mom opened the door with a plate of cookies in her hand. Suddenly she recognized us. "Daddy," she yelled, "the kids are home."

I'll never forget those next few moments. Daddy jumped out of bed, and in his bright-red ski pajamas ran right out on the porch and gave us all bear hugs. What a homecoming!

And we have never been sorry we drove more than 1,000 miles to get home for Christmas. It was the last Christmas Daddy was alive. He died of a heart attack the next Thanksgiving.

Now I'm looking forward to another homecoming, when our family will be reunited in a land even more beautiful than Boulder, Colorado, with its glistening snow on Christmas Eve. I'll be watching for you there.

Family homecomings are marvelous occasions.
Why not start planning for one today?

THE MAGIC MOMENT OF CHRISTMAS

December 25
Kay Kuzma

The time came for the baby to be born, and she gave birth to her firstborn, a son. She wrapped him in cloths and placed him in a manger, because there was no room for them in the inn. Luke 2:6, 7, NIV.

Every woman, as she nears her time, wonders, *How will it be?* Those who have gone before talk about the intensity of pain, the breathing, the pushing, the exhilaration of anticipation, and finally, the birth of the baby itself. Although each birth is special, something about the first especially tugs at the heart and body of each mother.

I remember my first—remember exactly where I was standing, and what I was wearing when I felt that first contraction of my abdominal muscles. Then 18½ hours later, the final push, the cry, and the announcement "It's a girl!" Fulfillment!

But the magic moment was when I held this 7½-pound miracle to my breast and felt the bonding knot the two of us together in a relationship that only a mother can understand.

As I ponder the magic moment of that first Christmas, when the angel announced to the shepherds, "For unto you is born this day . . . a Saviour," and the angel choir sang "Glory to God in the highest," what was that young mother experiencing at that moment when she first held "God in the flesh" to her breast? I wish the scene had been recorded. But God the Father in love allowed this intimate moment to be shielded from public view. There was no doctor, midwife, or attending family, at least that we know of—only Mary and the Baby, and the earthly father God had chosen for His Son.

God loves families. And God has provided a means by which they can become bonded. Touch! Mary through the Baby's touch to her breast. And Joseph? . . .

As her contractions intensified, I see Joseph ready himself for a task women were expected to perform. I visualize him reaching for the head of that Baby as it emerged, and then with the final contraction, his hands become the first to touch the world's Saviour.

Touch is what Christmas is all about. Touch is what Christ did coming to this earth. Touch is why families come together at Christmas. And touch is the magic moment of Christmas.

Thank You, Jesus, for touching me with Your love.
Which person should I touch for You today?

391

Linda Bell

Let them praise the name of the Lord, for he commanded and they were created. Ps. 148:5, NIV.

A professor of theoretical physics at Cambridge University by the name of Stephen Hawking describes himself as "unlucky" for being diagnosed with amyotrophic lateral sclerosis when he was in his late 20s. Now he is confined to a wheelchair, has a permanent tracheostomy, and communicates with the help of a computer-generated voice synthesizer. He is dependent on others for all the activities of daily living.

But he says he feels fortunate that his chosen field is not one requiring physical abilities. He has been blessed with a mind that roams the universe, testing the limits of time and space. People frequently discuss his theories in context with other great minds such as Galileo, Newton, and Einstein. He continues to lecture in the university setting and has written books about his theories.

I am a healthy adult with full physical capabilities who has freely chosen to be a couch potato on a routine basis with only occasional forays into "weekend warrior" types of activities (hiking, swimming, or whirling through the shopping malls). At times when I am angry about my minor physical limitations I resent others who remind me that regular exercise improves health and longevity.

I am far more likely to exercise my verbal capabilities than my physical ones, many times to my detriment. My mind usually centers on my own small universe and rarely wanders beyond my own egocentric space. Nor have my thought processes generated any theories of time or space. No one could make any comparisons between me and the great ones in my chosen field.

To the casual observer, Stephen Hawking would appear to be disabled. However, he has found ways to use the abilities he was given rather than focus on what he cannot do. Those of us who can roam freely on our own, care for ourselves and others, and have a reasonable expectation of privacy, tend to disable ourselves by our attitudes and behaviors.

We all have disabilities. The secret is to turn our disabilities into capabilities, and focus on what we can do rather than on what we can't.

Father, thank You for creating me as I am. Help me to focus on what I can do, rather than what I can't, and to turn my disabilities into capabilites.

SKATE FOR
THE JOY
OF SKATING

December 27
Kay Kuzma

Let all those rejoice who put their trust in You; let them ever shout for joy, because You defend them; let those also who love Your name be joyful in You. Ps. 5:11, NKJV.

Winter Olympics, 1988. Calgary. The headlines blared: "Going for the Gold: East Germany's Katarina Witt v. Debi Thomas From the United States." Who would win the gold metal in women's figure skating?

The final competition fell on Saturday night. Our family watched TV with breathless silence as Katarina skated a perfect performance. She took no chances, skating only the requirements, no extra spins or jumps, and no mistakes.

Debi was to skate at the end, and since I really wasn't interested in the other skaters, I went to take a shower.

Suddenly I heard the kids scream, "Mom, come quickly. You won't believe this!" Throwing a towel around myself, I raced to the TV and stood there dripping wet as Elizabeth Manley, an "unknown" Canadian, electrified the crowd. The possibility of obtaining the gold medal was out of her hands. Not worried about perfection, she pulled out all the stops and whistles and skated merely for the joy of skating—and for her country. She put her whole heart into the performance of a lifetime. The crowd erupted in spontaneous cheers.

You know the end of the story. The pressure was too much for Debi. She fell twice and finished third, with the silver going to Elizabeth and the gold to Katarina.

We live our lives much like those three skaters. Some are so focused on "going for the gold" that they follow the rules to the letter of the law. Terribly correct, their goal is perfection. And they make most of the people around them miserable—and probably themselves too.

Others find the pressure too much. They stumble, fall, and may even give up their faith.

Then there are those who pull out all the stops of life's possibilities. They realize that on their own they can never do enough to deserve the gold. It's a gift from Jesus. So they skate not for perfection, but for the joy of skating—and for their God.

Which skater are you?

Are you praying for the joy of praying, studying the Bible for the joy of studying, and keeping His commandments for the joy of obedience, or are you so busy being terribly correct that you're in danger of slipping, or of making yourself and others miserable? God wants you to be joyful in Him.

BORN FOR
SUCH A
TIME AS THIS

December 28

Pat Nordman

And who knows but that you have come to royal position for such a time as this? Esther 4:14, NIV.

Our oldest son, Chuck, died during the Christmas holidays. Since he chose of his own free will to die, I decided to share with our four younger sons the verse in Esther 4:14 that has had great meaning to me personally.

A few days after his death I took them back to Chuck's bedroom and asked them to sit with me on his bed. Then, after a silent prayer for wisdom to guide their little hearts, I tried to explain to them about God and His purposes for us. I told them that we are born neither too soon nor too late—that we are born at *this* time because God has purposes for *us* and no one else. We have jobs to do that no one else on earth can do.

I could have chosen hundreds of verses that might have been more relevant. But I still believe, years later, that the Holy Spirit prompted me to share this particular verse at that time: "And who knows but that you have come to royal position for such a time as this?"

Chuck's death, especially the fact that he chose to give up what we think would have been a good life, had a profound impact on my blasé attitude about life, its mysteriousness, its urgency—and its preciousness!

As I tried to explain, suddenly I saw my treasured sons in a new light. I realized that God knows the right time and place for us to be born, and He wants us to make use of our talents and our strength right where we are and at that time. He doesn't want us dreaming of other times and places and what we could have done there. It's senseless, useless, and hopeless, and can drive us to despair.

My other sons have gone on to lead caring and giving lives. They have happy marriages to wonderful women, and now we are grandparents. Life, that dear gift, goes on. How I thank God for our sons and daughters who choose to live and love and use their God-given gifts so others may be blessed!

*Ellen White says: "No one but you yourself can do your work.
If you withhold your light, someone must be left in darkness
through your neglect" (Testimonies, vol. 5, p. 464). What is
the royal work that God needs you to do at this time?*

Sing and make music in your heart to the Lord, always giving thanks to God the Father for everything, in the name of our Lord Jesus Christ. Eph. 5:19, 20, NIV.

Like many women, I grew up believing that if I was a very good girl, followed all the rules, and loved God enough, life would turn out pretty well. What a disappointment, therefore, to wake up one morning in adulthood to discover that the formula had failed. My health had taken a decided dip. I was a walking combination of burnout, disappointment, frustration, and midlife crisis.

In frustration I turned to a more in-depth study of the brain and the immune system. Emerging research provided some practical tools that changed my life. For example, I learned that although we often use the terms *emotions* and *feelings* interchangeably, they are not the same. Emotions arise in the brain's limbic system (pain-pleasure center) and are simply little flags designed to get our attention. Information about the physiological changes these emotions cause in the body travels to the cerebrum (thinking portion of the brain). There we assign weight to these flags, and our interpretations then become our feelings.

Practically, this means that while we may not always have complete control over our initial emotions, within six or seven seconds of becoming aware of our thoughts we can begin to take control of our feelings.

First I learned to identify the entire range of emotions God has placed in the human brain. Next I honed the ability to translate those flags into feelings more accurately. Gradually I gave myself permission to feel all my feelings until eventually I accepted complete responsibility for managing my emotions and feelings.

Often we handle them with faulty screens we have absorbed early in life. I actually did some very helpful family-of-origin work to discover some of the generationally transmitted response patterns that had been operating among the members of my family.

The bottom line? If we want to change the way we feel, we need to change the way we think. It is our choice to maintain a given feeling, to choose a different feeling, or to act upon a feeling, thus moving us from a position of helplessness toward one of empowerment.

What steps can you take to manage your emotions and feelings more successfully? Are you allowing your brain to be God-educated and Holy Spirit-impressed?

OF LIGHTBULBS AND HEALTH

Hans Diehl

You are the light of the world. A city on a hill cannot be hidden. Neither do people light a lamp and put it under a bowl. Instead they put it on its stand, and it gives light to everyone . . . , let your light shine before men, that they may see your good deeds and praise your Father. Matt. 5:14-16, NIV.

Yesterday I ran into Mr. Ultrahealth. Thirty-one years of age, committed to a daily one-hour workout on his Nautilus machine, he is in fabulous shape. His hobby is rock-climbing and his diet consists of piles of unsprayed fruits and vegetables, mounds of alfalfa sprouts, and barrels of oat bran. He drinks 10 glasses of distilled water a day, sleeps eight hours at night, regards sweets with utter disdain, and never forgets to floss his teeth. In addition, his cholesterol is below 130, he has never been in a hospital, and his physician says he has never seen anybody healthier.

Today, however, I saw him kick the dog, scream obscenities at his wife, and leave the house without saying goodbye to his children. At work he lied to his boss, blaming a colleague for his own mistake. He was unkind, impatient, selfish, immoral, and spiritually bankrupt.

And suddenly a light came on in my mind. Health is more than eating right and exercising daily. Fitness involves more than first meets the eye. Actually, health is more like a lightbulb. The glass may be shiny, clean, and clear on the outside. But if the filament on the inside is broken or disconnected from the core, then there won't be any light. Yet without light the bulb will have missed its purpose.

Lightbulbs aren't ends in themselves. They're only a means to an end, only valuable if they help us get to where we really want to go.

As we look forward to the new year, let us take a closer look at our goal of health. If our lifestyle improvements don't help us to become more loving persons, then we are as worthless as a broken lightbulb. We may look polished on the outside, but without being connected on the inside we are not bringing light to others.

The ultimate purpose of pursuing health remains to become a more efficient lightbulb—to serve others better.

Lord, may my life shine with love to others. Amen.

PROMISES— PROMISES

Watch and pray so that you will not fall into temptation. The spirit is willing, but the body is weak. Matt. 26:41, NIV.

One of the most common New Year's resolutions is in the area of health—either to lose weight, change our diet, or exercise more. Psychologically the new year seems an appropriate time to make a new start, and so we all vow to be better in some way.

Health clubs around the country swell with new memberships every January. You can hardly find a free StairMaster or cycling machine. Aerobics classes are jam-packed. Sporting good stores love the month of January. They sell sweat suits, running shoes, and exercise equipment by the truckload to all the New Year's health converts. January clients besiege weight-loss clinics everywhere. And bookstores brace for a run on health, diet, and fitness books after the new year.

For the first few weeks of the new year we make good on our promise to turn our lives around, for "the spirit" is indeed willing and seems to fuel our determination. But soon reality sets in and "the flesh" begins to rebel. We find that breaking old lifestyle habits is not as easy as a New Year's promise and a brand-new running suit. We begin to invent excuses to neglect our resolution: "It's too cold outside." "It's too late today." "I'm too tired." "My toe hurts." "I'll do it tomorrow." "This isn't fun anymore." And so on. By February we have pretty much returned to our old routines. The health clubs are once again ghost towns, and those brand-new running shoes get lost in the closet.

Jesus summed up the human condition with His memorable quote for today, and He should know, for He shared our frailties while here on earth. But He also showed us that our true source of strength lies not in our own feeble willpower, but in joining forces with divinity.

So, if you have faltered on New Year's resolutions in the past, remember: "I can do all things through Christ who strengthens me" (Phil. 4:13, NKJV) and lace up those walking shoes for a healthy new year.

Make three resolutions for a healthy new year and pray this prayer: "Lord, give me Your strength to keep the resolutions I have made, for my spirit is willing, but my flesh is weak. Amen."

SCRIPTURE INDEX

ACTS

1:8 . . . . June 23
9:36 . . . . Aug. 15
9:36-40 . . . . . Sept. 11

ROMANS

1:20, 21 . . . . . . Oct. 31
3:1, 2 . . . . Mar. 28
8:13, 14 . . . . . Sept. 24
8:28 . . . . Jan. 10
8:28 . . . . Mar. 29
12:2 . . . . Mar. 3
12:2 . . . . Sept. 22
12:12, 13 . . . . . Nov. 1
15:13 . . . . Nov. 6

1 CORINTHIANS

3:16, 17 . . . . . . Apr. 29
6:19, 20 . . . . . . Mar. 21
6:19, 20 . . . . . . Nov. 19
9:24 . . . . Jan. 2
9:24 . . . . July 19
9:25, 26 . . . . . . Aug. 1
10:13 . . . . Mar. 11
10:31 . . . . Apr. 30
12:24-36 . . . . . Aug. 13
12:31 . . . . July 9
13:5 . . . . Sept. 18
13:12 . . . . Mar. 30
13:13 . . . . Jan. 11
13:13 . . . . May 13

2 CORINTHIANS

1:3, 4 . . . . Feb. 2
1:3, 4 . . . . May 21
3:17 . . . . Jan. 3
4:15 . . . . Nov. 21
5:18 . . . . Aug. 22
5:18, 19 . . . . . Sept. 17
9:7 . . . . Oct. 19
12:9 . . . . Nov. 29
12:9 . . . . Dec. 15

GALATIANS

6:4-9 . . . . Mar. 2

6:7, 8 . . . . Aug. 28
6:9 . . . . June 15

EPHESIANS

1:4, 5 . . . . July 12
5:15 . . . . Dec. 11
5:18 . . . . Apr. 20
5:19, 20 . . . . . Dec. 29
6:4 . . . . May 28

PHILIPPIANS

2:3, 4 . . . . Apr. 10
2:5 . . . . June 6
3:7, 8 . . . . Oct. 23
4:4 . . . . Apr. 26
4:8 . . . . Apr. 16
4:8 . . . . Aug. 6
4:13 . . . . Jan. 19
4:19 . . . . Apr. 27
4:19 . . . . May 22

COLOSSIANS

3:11-14 . . . . July 3

1 THESSALONIANS

4:7, 9 . . . . Aug. 3
4:17 . . . . Sept. 7
5:21 . . . . Jan. 7

1 TIMOTHY

6:18, 19 . . . . . . Dec. 1

2 TIMOTHY

1:7 . . . . Sept. 4
1:7 . . . . Nov. 23
4:17 . . . . Apr. 18

TITUS

2:1-7 . . . . May 26
2:4, 5 . . . . May 9

PHILEMON

2:5 . . . . Feb. 20

HEBREWS

3:7, 8 . . . . Sept. 30
4:9, 10 . . . . . . Sept. 13
11:25 . . . . Jan. 17
12:1 . . . . Apr. 4
12:5, 6 . . . . May 2
13:5 . . . . Apr. 15
13:12 . . . . Oct. 22

JAMES

1:13-15 . . . . July 4
1:17 . . . . Jan. 5
1:26 . . . . Nov. 14
2:12, 13 . . . . . Sept. 12
3:17 . . . . Apr. 17
4:17 . . . . Feb. 11
4:8 . . . . Mar. 14
4:8 . . . . Aug. 17
5:14 . . . . Apr. 12
5:14, 15 . . . . . May 30
5:16 . . . . Apr. 13
5:16 . . . . Oct. 3

1 PETER

2:2, 3 . . . . Mar. 18
2:4, 5 . . . . May 27

1 JOHN

1:9 . . . . July 5
4:18 . . . . Dec. 13
5:14, 15 . . . . . . Aug. 8

3 JOHN

2 . . . . Feb. 15
2 . . . . Apr. 8

REVELATION

3:20 . . . . June 10
4:11 . . . . July 14
11:18 . . . . Dec. 10
12:11 . . . . Jan. 12
14:6, 7 . . . . . . Nov. 27
21:4 . . . . Apr. 23
21:5 . . . . July 31